Obsessive–compulsive
and **related disorders in adults**

Written for clinicians, this book presents in detail the diagnosis, clinical picture, and pharmacotherapeutic and psychotherapeutic treatments, both for obsessive–compulsive disorder and for disorders traditionally included in an obsessive–compulsive spectrum. The book draws on the author's extensive experience as well as reviewing the published evidence, including controlled trials, case series and case reports.

This book can improve the clinician's knowledge and skill in treating patients with complicated as well as straightforward clinical presentations. Each chapter ends with treatment planning guidelines summarizing appropriate evaluation and treatment strategies. An extended chapter details the use of all medications that have been reported effective for these disorders and the management of common and uncommon drug interactions and side effects. The book's appendices contain useful symptom rating scales, provide access to mental health organizations and to printed and Internet materials for patient education, and list international proprietary names for the drugs discussed.

This is an essential resource and practical guide to treatment planning for psychiatrists and other mental health professionals, whether they favor pharmacological or cognitive–behavioral approaches. For professionals in training, this book brings together a wealth of information not otherwise available in a single source.

Lorrin M. Koran is Professor of Psychiatry and Director of the Obsessive–Compulsive Disorder Clinic at Stanford University Medical Center, Stanford, California.

Obsessive–compulsive
and **related disorders in adults**

A comprehensive clinical guide

Lorrin M. Koran, M.D.

Department of Psychiatry and Behavioral Sciences
Stanford University Medical Center
Stanford, California

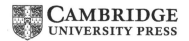
CAMBRIDGE
UNIVERSITY PRESS

PUBLISHED BY THE PRESS SYNDICATE OF THE UNIVERSITY OF CAMBRIDGE
The Pitt Building, Trumpington Street, Cambridge, United Kingdom

CAMBRIDGE UNIVERSITY PRESS
The Edinburgh Building, Cambridge CB2 2RU, UK   http://www.cup.cam.ac.uk
40 West 20th Street, New York, NY 10011-4211, USA   http://www.cup.org
10 Stamford Road, Oakleigh, Melbourne 3166, Australia

First published 1999

Printed in the United Kingdom at the University Press, Cambridge

Typeset in Minion 10.5/14, in QuarkXPress™   [SE]

A catalogue record for this book is available from the British Library

Library of Congress Cataloguing in Publication data

Koran, Lorrin M.
Obsessive–compulsive and related disorders in adults : a
comprehensive clinical guide / Lorrin M. Koran.
     p.   cm.
Includes bibliographical references and index.
ISBN 0 521 55975 8 (pbk.)
1. Obsessive–compulsive disorder – Treatment.   2. Psychiatry.
I. Title.
RC533.K67   1999   98-42347   CIP
616.85′227–dc21

ISBN 0 521 55975 8 paperback

Every effort has been made in preparing this book to provide accurate and up-to-date information which is
in accord with accepted standards and practice at the time of publication. Nevertheless, the author and publisher can make no warranties that the information contained herein is totally free from error, not least
because clinical standards are constantly changing through research and regulation. The authors, editors, and
publisher therefore disclaim all liability for direct or consequential damages resulting from the use of material
contained in this book. Readers are strongly advised to pay careful attention to information provided by the
manufacturer of any drugs or equipment that they plan to use.

This book is dedicated to Stephanie, Joshua and Jessica

Life is short, and the Art long; the occasion fleeting; experience fallacious and judgment difficult.

Hippocrates (460–377 BC), *Aphorisms*

May I never see in the patient anything but a fellow creature in pain.

Attributed to Maimonides (AD 1135–1204)

Contents

Acknowledgments   *page* ix

Part I   The clinical perspective

1   Introduction   3
2   Approach to the patient and treatment of comorbid conditions   7

Part II   Obsessive–compulsive disorder and its treatment

3   Obsessive–compulsive disorder   35
4   Managing the side effects of serotonergic drugs   81
5   Obsessive–compulsive symptoms in schizophrenic disorders   115
6   Medical conditions associated with obsessive and compulsive symptoms 119

Part III   Obsessive–compulsive spectrum disorders

7   Tourette's disorder   135
8   Body dysmorphic disorder   151
9   Hypochondriasis   163
10   Pathological jealousy   178
11   Trichotillomania   185
12   Skin picking   202
13   Nail biting   208
14   Compulsive buying   213
15   Kleptomania   219
16   Pathological gambling   227
17   Nonparaphilic sexual disorders   238
18   Obsessive–compulsive personality disorder   248

Appendixes

1   Accessing patient education materials   256
2   Rating scales for clinical use   275
3   Trademark drug names: an international list   303

   Bibliography   314
   Index   362

Acknowledgments

A book crystallizes a portion of its author's life and captures his or her bonds to others. I am indebted to many who have helped me bring this book into existence.

My patients and their families have been my most valuable teachers. I am deeply grateful to them for the great privilege of sharing in their lives as their physician.

Alan Schatzberg, Chairman of Stanford's Department of Psychiatry and Behavioral Sciences, first suggested that this book be written. His support during its long gestation has been constant.

I wish to express my gratitude to several colleagues (and treasured friends) who kindly offered their time, comments, and criticism: Don W. DeBra, M.D., Floyd R. Sallee, M.D., Ph.D., John Van Natta, M.D., and Sanford R. Weimer, M.D. Their reviews and comments on specific chapters were extremely helpful and resulted in substantial improvements.

Alan Ringold, M.D., my colleague in the Stanford Medical Center OCD Clinic, and Kerry D. Kravitz, M.D., a valued member of the Stanford Clinical Faculty, read the entire manuscript and greatly enriched the material by providing judicious criticism and clinical insights. I acknowledge my very special gratitude to them both. They are hereby absolved of responsibility for my errors of fact and interpretation.

Stefano Pallanti, M.D., Director of the Istituto di Neuroscienze in Florence, Italy, has been a delightful collaborator and cherished friend as we searched together for better treatments for our patients. I learned much from him during my stays in Florence, which were some of my life's happiest days.

I also wish to extend special thanks Kristen Cassic, M.A., Ms. Holly B. Thompson, Ms. Jennifer Ratner, Ms. Sari Kasper, Ms. Karen Lim and Ms. Emi Fukushima for their assistance in obtaining and documenting bibliographic materials. The staff of the Lane Medical Library at Stanford gave generously of their time and expertise to aid my search for relevant materials. I greatly appreciate the assistance of the staff of Cambridge University Press, particularly Ms. Rita A. Owen, who provided fine-tuned editorial assistance, and Richard Barling, M.D., whose comments on early draft chapters helped shape the clincial focus of the book. The assistance of Mehran Farid, M.D. in locating Internet resources for patient education is much appreciated.

I am above all grateful for the unfailing encouragement and understanding of my wife, Stephanie, and my children, Joshua and Jessica, who permitted much time to be taken from our lives together.

Part I

The clinical perspective

Introduction

The Physician that bringeth love and charity to the sick, if he be good and kind and learned and skillful, none can be better than he.

Savonarola

This book is written for clinicians. As a result, it omits a great deal of neuroanatomical, neurochemical and neuropsychological speculation and research regarding the disorders considered. While these hypotheses and investigations will ultimately improve our ability to help patients, the fruits of these labors lie in the future. This book seeks to provide clinicians with information they can use to help patients now.

The disorders considered here, that is, obsessive–compulsive disorder (OCD) and some of the disorders that hypothetically belong to an "obsessive–compulsive spectrum," reflect my experience and interests. Because I am a specialist in adult psychiatry, the perspective centers on adult patients. From among the disorders often considered part of the OCD spectrum (Hollander, 1993), I have selected those with which I have the most experience and for which treatment approaches are reasonably well supported by evidence. For many of these disorders, however, well-controlled treatment trials are scarce or unavailable. Consequently, I have included treatments supported by case reports and case series so that clinicians can explore their utility.

Which diagnoses belong under the umbrella concept of OCD spectrum disorders is a matter of debate. Early advocates of the spectrum concept suggested the following collection (Hollander and Wong, 1995):

(1) Somatoform disorders (body dysmorphic disorder and hypochondriasis).
(2) Dissociative disorders (depersonalization disorder).
(3) Eating disorders (anorexia nervosa and binge-eating disorder).
(4) Schizo-obsessive disorders (OCD with loss of insight, OCD in patients with schizotypal personality disorder, OC symptoms in patients with schizophrenia).
(5) Tic disorders (Tourette's syndrome).
(6) Neurological conditions (Tourette's syndrome, Huntington's disease, autism, epilepsy, Sydenham's chorea).
(7) Impulse control disorders (compulsive buying, kleptomania, self-injurious

behaviors, sexual compulsions [nonparaphilic sexual disorders], trichotillomania and pathological gambling).

(8) Impulsive personality disorders (borderline and antisocial).

Others have suggested including certain habit disorders (skin picking and nail biting), phobias, post-traumatic stress disorder, intermittent explosive disorder, obsessive–compulsive personality disorder and tic disorders other than Tourette's syndrome (McElroy, Phillips and Keck, 1994b).

The clearest case for a relationship among these disorders lies in their phenomenology – each disorder is characterized by "obsessional" thoughts (repetitive, often senseless, preoccupying, unwanted ideation) and "compulsive" behaviors (repetitive behaviors performed in response to a strong urge that is often felt to be "irresistible," followed by tension or anxiety relief). Shared phenomenology is, however, an untrustworthy guide to shared pathophysiology or etiology. The history of psychiatric diagnostic systems from the eighteenth century through the twentieth is littered with the discarded remains of classifications built on phenomenology alone. Phenomenological comparisons generate hypotheses about pathophysiology or etiology; the tests that weed out error take place in biological terrain, albeit taking cognizance of how psychosocial characteristics of the individual, the family and the community modify disease.

Even within the realm of phenomenology, OCD and the spectrum disorders have been noted to differ (McElroy et al., 1993, 1994b; Black et al., 1994). The signs and symptoms of OCD usually express harm avoidance, whereas those of many spectrum disorders more often express stimulation or pleasure seeking and have harmful consequences. OCD patients usually retain insight, resist their symptoms and experience only tension relief while performing or completing compulsions. Patients with impulse control disorders often lack insight into the irrationality of their behaviors, do not resist urges and experience pleasure or excitement while performing impulsive behaviors (despite later painful consequences, sadness and remorse). Whether arraying OCD and the OCD spectrum disorders along a continuum from compulsivity (risk or harm avoidance) to impulsivity (excitement or pleasure seeking) (Hollander and Wong, 1995) will help clinicians choose among pharmacotherapies and psychotherapeutic approaches remains to be seen.

Hollander and Wong (1995) believe that the spectrum disorders and OCD share many features other than phenomenology, i.e., symptom profile; patterns of demography, family history, comorbidity, and clinical course; neurobiology; and, response to behavioral and pharmacological therapies. Others caution that the spectrum concept may be overly inclusive (Rasmussen, 1994), a caution its proponents acknowledge. Skeptics note that the spectrum disorders vary widely in how closely they resemble OCD, that the data needed to judge the degrees of resemblance are mostly missing, and, that OCD and each spectrum disorder may all turn out to be collections of diseases, so that a shared pathophysiology may not span all of the entities inhabiting each current diagnostic label. In addition, differences exist among the spectrum conditions with regard to gender distribution, neurobiology, patterns of comorbidity and treatment response (McElroy et al., 1994b).

In my view, the spectrum concept is valuable primarily as a stimulus to basic and clinical research. Investigators and funding sources may become more interested in disorders that have attracted less attention than the mood disorders and schizophrenia. In addition, since some treatments, such as serotonin reuptake inhibitors and behavioral therapies, have application to many spectrum disorders, clinicians who become skilled in treating one disorder may become more interested in treating others. A shared therapeutic response to serotonin reuptake inhibitors is not, however, a strong indicator of pathophysiological relationships. Aspirin, for example, is useful in rheumatoid arthritis, headache and the prevention of myocardial infarction, but no one would argue on this basis for a shared etiology.

Clinicians applying a diagnostic system to the human problems brought for their care can increase the clarity of analysis by keeping in mind the distinctions between a disease, a disorder, an illness and a diagnosis. A disease is a pathological anatomical or physiological condition of known cause or causes. A disorder is a collection of pathological signs and symptoms (mental or physical) believed by physicians to cohere fairly well in onset, course, prognosis and treatment response, but whose etiology is unknown. Disorders are carved from a body of repeated observations of patients whose conditions seem similar. An illness is a disease or disorder as experienced by the patient, physically, psychologically and socially. A diagnosis, Scadding reminds us, is simply a label applied by the clinician to a disease, disorder or illness in order to bring medical knowledge to bear on altering its course or consequences (Mindham, Scadding and Cawley, 1992). None of the pathological conditions discussed in this book have attained the conceptual level of disease; all are disorders whose biological causes remain unknown.

Each chapter presents for the disorder it discusses the diagnostic criteria given in the *Diagnostic and Statistical Manual of Mental Disorders,* Fourth Edition (American Psychiatric Association, 1994) and notes any important differences between these criteria and the diagnostic guidelines set out in the *ICD-10 Classification of Mental and Behavioural Disorders* (World Health Organization, 1992). The comparisons remind us that these two diagnostic classification systems are simply tools, not truths. The chapters next describe the differential diagnosis for each disorder, summarize the available epidemiological data and describe the clinical picture, including common comorbid conditions. In discussing treatments, the results of controlled trials, case series and cases are presented. Pharmacological and psychotherapeutic approaches are described in sufficient detail that the clinician can apply these treatments with an informed expectation of the results. Some treatment recommendations identified are derived from my clinical experience. At times, clinical research that may widen the range of effective treatments is suggested to encourage clinicians to publish novel observations. Physicians (and scientists) concerned about the care of individual patients have often made observations that ultimately have led to previously unimagined treatments.

Fortunately, medical science is continually progressing. As a consequence, however, some ideas and recommendations contained in this text will be outdated by the time they are read. For this I am both grateful and chagrined.

I could find no smooth phrasing to encompass both genders when writing of clinicians and patients. As a result, I have settled on the male gender in referring to clinicians and have utilized the male or female gender, as reflected in the studies cited, to refer to patients. I happily acknowledge that wisdom, caring and clinical skill are independent of the clinician's gender and hope that my phrasing engenders no offense.

2

Approach to the patient and treatment of comorbid conditions

What a piece of work is a man! How noble in reason! how infinite in faculty! in form, in moving, how express and admirable! in action how like an angel! in apprehension how like a god! the beauty of the world! the paragon of animals!

Shakespeare, *Hamlet*

Patients come to us driven by distress and dysfunction, hopeful of relief, fearful of our pronouncements. They often know little of the nature, biology, clinical course or treatment of their conditions, and may mistake symptoms for aspects of their innate selves. They struggle against the implied weakness and social stigma that come with seeking mental health care. Despite our caring and our desire to relieve their suffering, they may resist taking the actions we recommend. Our responsibilities as physicians have remained constant for several thousand years – to express genuine caring, to relieve suffering and restore functioning as best we can, to find the most recent knowledge and use it to benefit the patient, to educate, to maintain hope and to share our discoveries with our colleagues.

A comprehensive clinical assessment precedes good treatment. Experienced clincians routinely pursue the elements of a case history:
* Chief complaint (in the patient's own words).
* History of the present illness.
* Concurrent diseases and disorders.
* Current conflicts, stressors and social environment.
* Past psychiatric history.
* Medical history.
* Review of systems.
* Family history.
* Social history.
* Current medications.
* Indicated mental status examination.
  Complementing this rather dry compilation are certain questions that can help clinicians fulfill the full range of their responsibilities. The answers to these questions may not be immediately evident.
* Why has the patient come to you, and why now? What does the patient want or

expect, and how does this relate to what you perceive the patient needs, should want or can expect?

- Could patients' symptoms be the result of an occult medical disease or disorder? Although this is less likely in patients with obsessive–compulsive disorder (OCD) and OCD spectrum symptoms than in patients with affective symptoms, this question should always be addressed.
- How do patients' beliefs about their condition, their view of past treatments, their experiences with the illnesses of family members and their cultural background affect what they want or expect?
- Who else is affected by the patient's disorder, and what is this person's role in initiating, maintaining, exacerbating or relieving the patient's condition?
- What comorbid psychiatric *and medical* conditions are present, and how should their treatment be integrated with treatment of the presenting disorder?
- How will you measure the outcome of your treatment? Will you evaluate specific symptoms, the patient's ability to perform various social role functions, the opinions of concerned others? To help in measuring change, I have included well-validated assessment instruments in Appendix 2.
- Has any new treatment been proven effective or been suggested for treatment-resistant cases since you last encountered this disorder?

Bearing in mind other considerations that influence treatment is also helpful:

What physical and social atmospheres pervade your office? What physical atmosphere is created by the building in which your office is located? Is the social atmosphere in your office professional and educative? If you have support staff such as a receptionist, nurse or billing service, are these staff members contributing to the patient's confidence in your treatment plan and his belief that you are devoted to his welfare?

Too much has been written about patient compliance, transference, countertransference, secondary gain and the elements of a therapeutic relationship to summarize this literature here. Because the success or failure of treatment, however, usually hinges on keeping these concepts in mind, a few comments seem in order.

What must the patient do in order to cooperate with the treatment you prescribe, and how does this required action match his methods of coping with past adversities and trials? What must you do to minimize lapses in the patient's cooperation?

How do you feel about this patient? Do you feel like rescuing or overindulging the patient? Or, on the contrary, do you find yourself wishing you did not have to be responsible for his care?

What are your requirements for a continuing relationship? What can you tolerate and what can you not? Do not forget that the patient is responsible for working with you; you are only one member of the therapeutic team. In Hippocrates' eloquent formulation: "The art has three factors, the disease, the patient, the physician. The physician is the servant of the art. The patient must co-operate with the physician in combating the disease." (*Epidemics*, I.XI).

Finally, who is paying for the treatment, and has this payment source influenced the nature and amount of treatment?

Therapeutic activities that fall under the rubric of "supportive psychotherapy" are part of the care of every patient. Some, such as uncovering and evaluating all of the disorders affecting patients, their relationships and their functioning, have already been mentioned. Others include establishing and maintaining a therapeutic alliance; communicating that one accepts and respects the patient despite his problems or disorders; expressing genuine caring; educating the patient and his concerned others about the disorders and their treatment; providing appropriate reassurance, guidance and hope; and, enlisting, as indicated, the help of other professionals and of the patient's concerned others. The artful clinician weaves these therapeutic activities into the care of all patients.

Treating comorbid conditions

Patients presenting for treatment of OCD or an OCD spectrum disorder will frequently be suffering from one or more comorbid disorders. Common comorbid Axis I disorders are major depression, social phobia and panic disorder (Rasmussen and Eisen, 1992b), while common Axis II disorders include avoidant and dependent personality disorders or traits (Oldham et al., 1995; Torres and Del Porto, 1995). Although complete discussions of the treatment of these and other comorbid disorders is beyond the scope of this book, I would like to offer some guidance for commonly encountered clinical situations. My recommendations for additive pharmacotherapies are meant to apply to situations in which OCD or an OCD spectrum disorder is associated with only one comorbid condition. The management of more complex combinations of disorders has not been subjected to study and depends on clinical judgment applied to the individual case. More complete discussions of the isolated treatment of the comorbid conditions considered here can be found in standard texts, such as, *Treatments of Psychiatric Disorders* (Gabbard, 1995) or *Current Psychiatric Therapy* (Dunner, 1997), in specialized monographs, such as, *Drug Use in the Medically Ill* (Silver, 1994), or in the review and update articles that are staples of the scientific literature.

Treating comorbid major depression

The DSM-IV (*Diagnostic and Statistical Manual*, Fourth Edition) criteria for major depression are shown, for purposes of review, in Table 2.1. Faced with comorbid major depression of mild to moderate severity, the clinician has available many

Table 2.1. DSM-IV diagnostic criteria for major depressive episode

A. Five (or more) of the following symptoms have been present during the same two-week period and represent a change from previous function; at least one of the symptoms is either (1) depressed mood or (2) loss of interest or pleasure.
Note: Do not include symptoms that are clearly due to a general medical condition, or mood-incongruent delusions or hallucinations.
   (1) depressed mood most of the day, nearly every day, as indicated by either subjective report (e.g., feels sad or empty) or observation made by others (e.g., appears tearful).
   (2) markedly diminished interest or pleasure in all, or almost all, activities most of the day, nearly every day (as indicated by either subjective account or observation made by others).
   (3) significant weight loss when not dieting or weight gain (e.g., a change of more than 5% of body weight in a month), or decrease or increase in appetite nearly every day.
   (4) insomnia or hypersomnia nearly every day.
   (5) psychomotor agitation or retardation nearly every day (observable by others, not merely subjective feelings of restlessness or being slowed down).
   (6) fatigue or loss of energy nearly every day.
   (7) feelings of worthlessness or excessive or inappropriate guilt (which may be delusional) nearly every day (not merely self-reproach or guilt about being sick).
   (8) diminished ability to think or concentrate, or indecisiveness, nearly every day (either by subjective account or as observed by others).
   (9) recurrent thoughts of death (not just fear of dying), recurrent suicidal ideation without a specific plan, or a suicide attempt or a specific plan for committing suicide.
B. The symptoms do not meet criteria for a Mixed Episode [mixed mania and depression].
C. The symptoms cause clinically significant distress or impairment in social, occupational, or other important areas of functioning.
D. The symptoms are not due to the direct physiological effects of a substance (e.g., a drug of abuse, a medication) or a general medical condition (e.g., hypothyroidism).
E. The symptoms are not better accounted for by Bereavement, i.e., after the loss of a loved one, the symptoms persist for longer than two months or are characterized by marked functional impairment, morbid preoccupation with worthlessness, suicidal ideation, psychotic symptoms, or psychomotor retardation.

Source: Reprinted with permission from the *Diagnostic and Statistical Manual of Mental Disorders,* Fourth Edition. Copyright 1994 American Psychiatric Association, p. 327.

medications and several forms of psychotherapy known to be effective, but not well studied in the comorbid circumstance. In light of this uncertainty, the clinician must decide whether to utilize a specific form of psychotherapy alone or to combine it with an added medication. The factors influencing this judgment include the nature and extent of significant intrapsychic conflicts, social supports and stressors, and the patient's willingness and capacity to undergo different forms of treatment (American Psychiatric Association, 1993).

Certain general principles applicable to treating uncomplicated major depression can be extended to treating comorbid depressions:

- Look for an organic cause. Take a careful medical history and order any indicated laboratory tests, including a thyroid stimulating hormone assay. Consider both general medical conditions, such as hypothyroidism, nutritional deficiencies, renal failure and neurosyphilis, and drugs, such as methyldopa, corticosteroids and drugs of abuse, including alcohol (Koran et al., 1989).
- Evaluate suicide risk and intervene. Selective serotonin reuptake inhibitors (SSRIs) are safer than tricyclic antidepressants (an overdose of 1.5 g of a tricyclic can be fatal). Electroconvulsive therapy (ECT) can be life-saving.
- Evaluate the patient's living situation and the help that can be expected from his environmental support system.
- Ask about personal and family histories of hypomania, mania and substance abuse.
- Educate the patient and, with his permission, his concerned others, about the nature and treatment of depression. The myths that depression is a sign of character weakness, is the patient's fault or can be overcome by an effort of the will, must still be dispelled (See Appendix 1).
- Although SSRIs have a flat dose-response curve, individual patients may benefit from an increased dose (Fava et al., 1994). For drugs with an ascending dose-response curve (e.g., tricyclics, venlafaxine), titrate the dose steadily upward based on response and side effects.
- Inform the patient that it may take two to four weeks for medication to produce a substantial therapeutic effect, and six to eight weeks at the therapeutic dose for the drug's full effect to be evident (American Psychiatric Association, 1993; Phillips and Nierenberg, 1994). In chronic major depression (an episode lasting two years or more), full remission may take 12 weeks (Keller et al., 1998) or longer (Koran et al., 1999, unpublished data).
- The aim of treatment is full remission of all symptoms.
- Treat an initial episode for at least four to five months after remission has occurred in order to prevent relapse (Kupfer, 1991). Even longer continuation treatment may be in order. Patients in remission after 12 weeks of fluoxetine who continued the drug for nine months had significantly lower relapse rates than those randomly assigned to double-blind placebo (Reimherr et al., 1998).
- Maintain drug treatment in cases of recurrent depression (patients with three or more episodes) at full therapeutic dose for three years or more to prevent recurrence (Kupfer et al., 1992). Long-term treatment is also advisable when the initial episode occurs after age 50, has been chronic or is marked by high suicide risk, disability or other indications of considerable severity.

- Treat atypical depression (characterized by hypersomnia, increased appetite or weight gain, mood reactivity, rejection sensitivity and leaden heaviness of the limbs) with a monoamine oxidase inhibitor (MAOI) or a selective serotonine reuptake inhibitor (SSRI) (Phillips and Nierenberg, 1994).
- Treat psychotic depression with ECT or a combination of an antidepressant and a neuroleptic (Phillips and Nierenberg, 1994). ECT is also useful in acutely suicidal and in elderly patients.
- When stopping treatment, taper the medication slowly, i.e., over eight weeks or more (Kupfer, 1991). Fluoxetine's long half-life allows a somewhat more rapid taper schedule.

Pharmacotherapy

Table 2.2 displays pharmacotherapies to consider, taking into account the medication producing a good response or remission of the primary psychiatric condition.

When a comorbid depression appears or fails to respond despite treatment of the primary psychiatric condition with an SSRI, the situation can be considered analogous to a treatment-resistant depression (although treatment resistance is variously defined as failure to respond to two, three or four adequate antidepressant trials). In this circumstance, the clinician can obtain some help from the literature concerning treatment-resistant depression.

The treatment of depressive episodes is divided into an acute phase 6–12 weeks long and aimed at symptom resolution, a continuation phase four to nine months long and aimed at preventing relapse and a maintenance phase of one year or longer aimed at preventing recurrence (Kupfer, 1991). Although acute phase studies of treatment-resistant depression abound, little is known about continuation and maintenance phase treatment.

Controlled trials in patients with treatment-resistant depression suggest that a comorbid depression may respond to increasing fluoxetine from 20 mg/day to a higher dose; improvement is more likely to occur in patients with a partial than with no initial response (Fava et al., 1994). Whether increasing the doses of other SSRIs raises response rates has not been established. After an unsuccessful initial trial of an SSRI, open-label studies suggest that treatment with a second SSRI is effective in about half of cases (Thase and Rush, 1997). A substitution strategy runs the risk, however, that the second SSRI will not be effective for the primary psychiatric condition. Adding lithium carbonate to fluoxetine in doses producing serum levels of 0.4–1.0 mEq/L (or, mmol/L) is effective in perhaps half of cases after periods ranging up to six weeks (Fava et al., 1994; Katona et al., 1995; Bauer et al., 1996b). Severely depressed patients are less likely to respond. The combination is generally well tolerated, with no significant increase in the side effect rate. A small case series supports the addition of lithium to sertraline (Dinan, 1993).

Table 2.2. Pharmacotherapies to consider for comorbid major depression

Medication prescribed for the primary psychiatric condition	Added medication to consider for comorbid major depression
An SSRI	The same SSRI, ↑ dose
	Lithium[a]
	Desipramine or nortriptyline[b]
	Buspirone
	Pindolol
	Bupropion
	An alternative SSRI for both conditions[c]
A tricyclic antidepressant	Lithium[a]
	Triiodothyronine
	An SSRI[b]
A benzodiazepine	An SSRI or a tricyclic are first-line choices, but
Buspirone	other classes may be used. Check for drug
A neuroleptic[d]	interactions
Valproate	

Notes:
SSRI: selective serotonin reuptake inhibitor.
[a] Rare instances of confusional states, lithium toxicity and serotonin syndrome (with SSRIs or clomipramine) have been reported, but the combination is generally regarded as safe (Ciraulo et al., 1995).
[b] Because SSRIs impair tricyclic antidepressant metabolism, one should start with low doses and consider monitoring plasma levels.
[c] The alternate SSRI may not be effective in this individual for the primary psychiatric condition.
[d] e.g., Fluoxetine and paroxetine may increase plasma levels of neuroleptics (Chapter 4. See also: Ciraulo et al., 1995; Nemeroff, DeVane and Pollock, 1996). Watch for additive adverse effects on alertness and cognitive functions, anticholinergic effects and postural hypotension.

Case reports and open-label studies in treatment-resistant depression suggest that adding a tricyclic antidepressant such as desipramine or nortriptyline may be effective within one to four weeks (Weilburg et al., 1991). Reported response rates vary from 35% (Zajecka, Jeffriess and Fawcett, 1995) to 87% (Weilburg et al., 1989b). Because SSRIs raise tricyclic plasma levels, the initial dose should be small (e.g., 10–25 mg/day) and monitoring plasma levels to avoid central nervous system (CNS) and cardiac toxicity should be considered.

Tricyclic antidepressants can cause confusion, delirium and seizures. Their blockade of fast sodium channels can induce delayed intracardiac conduction, arrhythmias (at high concentrations) and seizures. Their anticholinergic effects lead to sinus tachycardia and memory impairment, while their blockade of α_1-adrenergic receptors produces postural hypotension (Preskorn, 1989).

Nortriptyline, which has a therapeutic plasma level range of 50–150 ng/ml, delays intraventricular conduction at levels of ≥ 200 ng/ml, while imipramine often does so at ordinary therapeutic levels (Glassman and Bigger, 1981). Low tricyclic plasma levels, however, are not absolute guides to safety nor are high levels absolute contraindications to continued treatment. For example, one healthy young adult exhibited a prolonged QRS interval at desipramine plasma levels of 40–69 ng/ml while another had a plasma level of 453 ng/ml without electrocardiogram (ECG) changes (Veith et al., 1980).

High plasma levels of clomipramine have been tolerated without incident. Twelve of 22 depressed patients tolerated combined plasma levels of clomipramine and desmethylclomipramine of 516–1484 ng/ml without ECG changes, while four exhibited changes at levels of 185, 602, 956 and 1360 ng/ml, but without clinically significant adverse effects (Szegedi et al., 1996). This patient series, however, is small, and caution is in order when combined plasma levels approach 450 ng/ml.

In healthy adults, the ECG changes associated with tricyclic antidepressants at normal therapeutic levels are rarely significant. Patients older than 50 years or those suspected of having cardiac disease should have a pretreatment ECG (Glassman and Bigger, 1981).

For tertiary tricyclic antidepressants (e.g., amitriptyline and imipramine), plasma levels above 300 ng/ml and 450 ng/ml increase the risk for delirium by 14.7- and 37-fold respectively, to 33% and 67% of patients (Preskorn, 1989, 1993). Because they are less anticholinergic, nortriptyline and desipramine are safer in this regard.

Prescribing tricyclic dose increases every 6th to 8th day will allow steady-state plasma levels to be attained between increments and permit associated side effects to become apparent. Tremor and mild ataxia are warning signs of CNS toxicity (Preskorn, 1989). Sertraline 50 mg/day may decrease tricyclic metabolism less than comparable doses of other SSRIs (Preskorn, 1996a), but most patients treated with sertraline and having little response will be receiving higher doses.

An open-label study of buspirone augmentation with 20–50 mg/day in 25 patients unresponsive to fluoxetine or fluvoxamine reported that one-third experienced a marked and one-third a complete response after three weeks (Joffe and Schuller, 1993).

Another well-tolerated augmentation strategy, supported by two small open-label trials, is a 1- to 3-week trial of adding pindolol 2.5 mg three times daily (Artigas, Perez and Alvarez, 1994; Blier and Bergeron, 1995a). Although pindolol is marketed as a beta-blocker, it blocks the presynaptic $5HT_{1A}$ autoreceptor as well, presumably facilitating increased release of serotonin. Irritability and sweating are occasionally troubling side effects, but clinically significant pulse or blood pressure changes have not been reported. If the patient responds, pindolol should be continued throughout the acute and continuation phases of treatment (4–6 months) (Zanardi et al., 1997). Whether pindolol hastens the antidepressant response to SSRIs is a matter of controversy (Berman, et al., 1997).

I have had successes and failures with each of these strategies. Adding bupropion to an SSRI has also brought about response or remission, although this approach has not been evaluated in controlled trials. I start with 75 mg/day of the immediate-release formulation and increase the dose by 75 mg/day every five to seven days to 300 mg/day, as tolerated. Dose limiting side effects have included insomnia, jitteriness and feeling overstimulated. Bupropion carries a seizure risk of 0.4% in doses of 300–450 mg/day (Medical Economics Company, 1998), and should not be used in patients with an increased seizure risk (e.g., patients with a history of head trauma, seizures or eating disorders). To avoid increasing the seizure risk, doses of the immediate-release formulation should be taken at least six hours apart, and doses of the sustained-release formulation at least eight hours apart. A side benefit of adding bupropion is that it may counteract SSRI-induced sexual dysfunction if this is present (see Chapter 4). Fluoxetine can raise the plasma levels of the active metabolites of bupropion, but the clinical significance of this effect is unclear (Preskorn, 1996b).

When patients exhibit or develop a comorbid depression unresponsive to an SSRI, I usually start with trials of adding a tricyclic or bupropion, because of their ease of administration and established antidepressant efficacy. If additional trials are needed, the weight of evidence favors trials of lithium, followed by pindolol and buspirone.

The literature on depressions unresponsive to an SSRI provides little guidance on how long to continue the added drug. Until data are available, it is clinically appropriate to continue the combination for the length of an adequate period of antidepressant treatment, i.e., four to nine months after remission occurs (Reimherr et al., 1998). The added agent can then be tapered over a two-month period, while the patient is observed for recurrence of symptoms.

When a tricyclic antidepressant has been successfully prescribed for the primary psychiatric condition, the literature on treatment-resistant depression suggests several approaches. Double-blind, placebo-controlled trials indicate that adding lithium in doses producing serum levels of 0.5–1.2 mEq/L (or, mmol/L) is effective in 30% to 65% of patients after four to six weeks (Phillips and Nierenberg, 1994; Schweitzer, Tuckwell and Johnson, 1997). Troublesome side effects can include feeling mentally slowed, memory impairment, tremor and weight gain. The literature provides no firm guidance regarding the indicated length of combined treatment; judging from the length of an adequate treatment period for acute depressive episodes, tapering the lithium dose should begin four months or more after a positive response has been established. Hypothyroidism may be seen in a small minority of patients after a year of lithium treatment.

The strategy of adding triiodothyronine (T_3) in doses of 25–50 µg/day for a two- to three-week trial has been less well studied than lithium augmentation, but appears to be about as effective (Schweitzer et al., 1997). Side effects are usually absent or mild, but may include anxiety, tachycardia, sweating or insomnia. Elderly patients should be monitored for iatrogenic thyrotoxicosis manifesting as atrial fibrillation. No studies have established the necessary duration of treatment, but Schatzberg, Cole and DeBattista (1997) recommend tapering by 12.5 µg every three days, beginning about two months after a positive response has occurred. The risk of inducing hypothyroidism must be considered in deciding how long to treat.

As noted earlier, combining a tricyclic antidepressant with an SSRI appears to be effective for many patients. Again, it may be necessary to monitor tricyclic plasma levels in order to guard against CNS or cardiac toxicity.

When the primary psychiatric condition is responding well to a benzodiazepine, a neuroleptic or buspirone, comorbid or emergent major depression is not analogous to treatment-resistant major depression. If the emergent depression is not a benzodiazepine or neuroleptic drug side effect, the choice of an antidepressant depends on the same factors that operate when major depression is the primary focus:
• safety;
• side effects;
• evidence of efficacy beyond the acute phase of treatment;
• ease of administration (affecting likely compliance);
• patient preference;
• possible interactions with the patient's other medications.
(See Chapter 4; Ciraulo et al., 1995; Preskorn, 1995; Nemeroff, DeVane and Pollack, 1996.)
Taking into account these factors and the extent of published experience with different antidepressants, an SSRI is the first-line choice. Although the tricyclic antidepressants, nortriptyline and desipramine, are equally effective and are well-tolerated, their narrower therapeutic index is a disadvantage. Since less is known, in cases of comorbidity, about the newer antidepressants, bupropion, mirtazapine, nefazodone and venlafaxine, they remain second or third choice drugs in these situations. A few drug interactions are known. Venlafaxine raises haloperidol serum levels; and, nefazodone raises serum levels of drugs metabolized by cytochrome P450 isoenzyme 3A4, e.g., alprazolam and triazolam (Medical Economics Company, 1998).

Psychotherapy

Most readers will be amply experienced in psychotherapeutic management of depression, and a complete account of such treatment is beyond the scope of this book. Nonetheless, a few comments are in order. Controlled trials have shown that interpersonal psychotherapy, behavior therapy and cognitive–behavioral therapy are effective in treating nonmelancholic depressions of mild to moderate severity (American Psychiatric Association, 1993). When combined with medication, interpersonal psychotherapy appears to have some value in maintenance phase treatment, but the utility of longer-term behavioral and cognitive-behavioral therapy and their prophylactic effects remain uncertain, despite some suggestions of benefit (Clarkin, Pilkonis and Magruder, 1996). Psychodynamic psychotherapy, despite its wide usage, and psychoanalysis, despite its long history, await evaluation in controlled trials.

When a patient with OCD or a spectrum disorder suffers from a comorbid depression, the complexities of the clinical situation usually require psychotherapeutic intervention in addition to any pharmacotherapy selected. My practice is to intervene with a mixture of approaches influenced by the individual patient's needs, areas of resourcefulness and desires. Treatment entails some combination of attending to social stressors, relationship issues and social skill deficits; eliciting and teaching the patient to combat automatic negative thoughts; problem solving and teaching problem-solving skills; and, seeking to identify and change maladaptive patterns of thought and behavior that originated in early life experiences. In other words, treatment draws on elements from all of the therapeutic schools mentioned earlier. At times, marital or family therapy is indicated. In these cases, I arrange for an independent therapist so that I can remain the patient's agent. Eclectic approaches such as this one are consistent with professional practice guidelines (American Psychiatric Association, 1993) and the present state of knowledge.

Clinicians wishing more information regarding the effectiveness of psychotherapies for major depression or about how to implement them are referred to recent reviews (American Psychiatric Association, 1993; Clarkin et al., 1996) and to the more detailed literature reviews and treatment manuals these references cite.

Treating comorbid social phobia

The generalized type of social phobia is characterized by intense fear in social situations in which the individual may be scrutinized (Table 2.3). This type of social phobia is probably related to avoidant personality disorder (Table 2.8), and the two conditions are highly comorbid (Schneier et al., 1991). Current diagnostic conventions, as codified in DSM-IV, define social phobia more in terms of phobic anxiety, and avoidant personality disorder more in terms of social dysfunction. Excessive fear of public speaking is the most common symptom of social phobia, but the

Table 2.3. DSM-IV criteria for social phobia (300.23)

A. A marked and persistent fear of one or more social or performance situations in which the person is exposed to unfamiliar people or to possible scrutiny by others. The individual fears that he or she will act in a way (or show anxiety symptoms) that will be humiliating or embarrassing.

B. Exposure to the feared social situation almost invariably provokes anxiety, which may take the form of a situationally bound or situationally predisposed panic attack.

C. The person recognizes that the fear is excessive or unreasonable.

D. The feared social or performance situations are avoided or else are endured with intense anxiety or distress.

E. The avoidance, anxious anticipation, or distress in the feared social or performance situation(s) interferes significantly with the person's normal routine, occupational (academic) functioning, or social activities or relationships, or there is marked distress about having the phobia.

F. In individuals under age 18 years, the duration is at least six months.

G. The fear or avoidance is not due to the direct physiological effects of a substance (e.g., a drug of abuse, a medication) or a general medical condition and is not better accounted for by another mental disorder (e.g., Panic Disorder With or Without Agoraphobia, Separation Anxiety Disorder, Body Dysmorphic Disorder, A Pervasive Development Disorder, or Schizoid Personality Disorder).

H. If a general medical condition or another mental disorder is present, the fear in criterion A is unrelated to it, e.g., the fear is not of stuttering, trembling in Parkinson's disease or exhibiting abnormal eating behavior in Anorexia Nervosa or Bulimia Nervosa.

Specify if:

Generalized: if the fears include most social situations also consider the additional diagnosis of Avoidant Personality Disorder.

Source: Reprinted with permission from the *Diagnostic and Statistical Manual of Mental Disorders,* Fourth Edition. Copyright 1994 American Psychiatric Association, pp. 416–7.

material that follows pertains to patients who are troubled in multiple social situations.

In judging the effectiveness of any treatment program for social phobia, the clinician should evaluate change in several domains: anxiety or distress; avoidance behavior; social interaction; occupational functioning; and ability to engage in rational internal dialogue regarding stressful situations. Two brief self-rating scales, the Liebowitz Social Anxiety Scale (Liebowitz, 1987) (Appendix 2) and the Sheehan Disability Scale (Sheehan, Harnett-Sheehan and Raj, 1996) (Appendix 2), are useful in measuring and documenting these dimensions of treatment outcome. Symptoms and disability may improve at different rates and to different degrees (Sheehan et al., 1996).

Pharmacotherapy

Double-blind studies indicate that phenelzine (Liebowitz et al., 1992), reversible MAOIs available in Europe (meclobemide and brofaromine), clonazepam (Davidson, Tupler and Potts, 1994), and the SSRIs fluvoxamine (Van Vliet, den Boer and Westenberg, 1994) and sertraline (Jefferson, 1995) are effective. Open-label trials, usually involving fewer than 20 patients, suggest efficacy for fluoxetine, paroxetine and alprazolam (Jefferson, 1995) and citalopram (Lepold, Koponow and Leinonen, 1994). Table 2.4 displays medication approaches to consider, taking into account the medication producing a good response or remission for the primary condition.

About two-thirds to three-quarters of patients respond to phenelzine (60–90 mg/day) after eight weeks of treatment, but its disadvantages are serious: dietary limitations; troubling side effects; and the inability to co-prescribe certain drugs that may be needed for the primary psychiatric condition, e.g., an SSRI or buspirone (Liebowitz et al., 1992; Jefferson, 1995).

Fluvoxamine 50 mg three times daily (Van Vliet et al., 1994) and sertraline 50–200 mg/day (Katzelnick et al., 1995) bring substantial relief to half, or more, of patients within 8–12 weeks. Similar results have been reported from open-label trials of fluoxetine and sertraline. The dosing procedures are the same as in the treatment of major depression.

Clonazepam 1–6 mg/day benefits three-quarters or more of patients, with symptomatic improvement often occurring within the first two weeks (Davidson et al., 1994). One can start with a dose of 0.5 mg/day and increase the dose by 0.5 to 1.0 mg every five to seven days as tolerated and needed. Somnolence is a common side effect, but tends to diminish after one to two weeks at a given dose. Patients prescribed higher doses should be warned about possible incoordination, ataxia and impairment of recent memory. All patients should be warned about possible diminished alertness, e.g., while driving. Preliminary evidence suggests that continuing clonazepam for a year produces a better outcome than tapering medication off after six months (Connor et al., 1998).

Somewhat less than half of patients treated with buspirone 50–60 mg/day seem to benefit (Schneier et al., 1993). Maximal benefit is seen after about four weeks of treatment. Patients rated severely ill appear to be less likely to respond than those rated moderately ill. Dizziness (distinct from true vertigo) may be troubling; mild nausea, headache and fatigue also occur.

Psychotherapy

Although neither the essential nor the optimal elements of psychotherapy for social phobia have been identified, controlled studies suggest that cognitive and behavioral approaches are effective for many patients (Heimberg, 1993). The data are too few

Table 2.4. Pharmacotherapies to consider for comorbid social phobia

Medication prescribed for the primary psychiatric condition	Added medication to consider for comorbid social phobia
An SSRI	The same SSRI
	Clonazepam[a]
	Buspirone
	An alternative SSRI for both conditions[b]
A tricyclic antidepressant	An SSRI[c]
	Clonazepam
	Buspirone
A benzodiazepine	Switch to clonazepam
	An SSRI[c]
	Phenelzine
Buspirone	An increased buspirone dose
	An SSRI[c]
A neuroleptic	An SSRI[d]
	Clonazepam[e]
	Phenelzine[f]
Lithium	Clonazepam
	An SSRI[g]
	Phenelzine
Valproate	An SSRI[c]
	Clonazepam

Notes:
SSRI: selective serotonin reuptake inhibitor.
[a] Fluvoxamine and fluoxetine inhibit the metabolism of alprazolam but not clonazepam.
[b] The alternative SSRI may not be effective in this individual for the primary psychiatric condition.
[c] Fluvoxamine and sertraline are the best studied SSRIs in social phobia. Since SSRIs increase tricyclic plasma levels to varying degrees, monitoring these levels may be advisable.
[d] Fluoxetine and paroxetine may increase plasma levels of neuroleptics.
[e] Watch for additive adverse effects on alertness and cognitive functions.
[f] Watch for additive anticholinergic effects and postural hypotension.
[g] Rare instances of confusional states, lithium toxicity, and serotonin syndrome have been reported, but the combination is generally regarded as safe (Ciraulo et al., 1995).

and the methodological problems too many to permit firm conclusions about the comparative efficacy of cognitive–behavioral therapies and medications, the role of combined therapy or the proper way to match patients to treatments. Nonetheless, when social phobia complicates the presentation of OCD or a spectrum disorder, implementing a cognitive–behavioral or behavioral approach instead of or in addition to prescribing an additional medication is clinically appropriate.

Cognitive–behavioral techniques utilized successfully with patients suffering from social phobia include: education regarding the cognitive–behavioral model for the disorder; social skills training; cognitive restructuring; graded exposure; and, anxiety management training (Heimberg, 1993). Cognitive restructuring involves teaching the patient to identify, analyze logically and refute negative thoughts evoked in feared situations. In graded exposure therapy, the clinician asks the patient to construct a list of feared situations ranked in order of increasing anxiety. Then the clinician systematically encourages sequential exposure to these situations, first in imagination or in the therapy situation (e.g., in role-playing), and subsequently, in vivo. Anxiety management training is a combination of training in relaxation and distraction techniques and in replacing irrational with rational internal dialogues.

Heimberg and his colleagues have created and evaluated a program of 12, weekly 2½-hour group psychotherapy sessions that seems to have long-term effectiveness (Heimberg and Juster, 1994). Descriptions of this and other therapeutic techniques offer the clinician a variety of reasonable approaches (Butler et al., 1984; Stravynski et al., 1994).

Treating Comorbid Panic Disorder

The DSM-IV diagnostic criteria for panic disorder without agoraphobia are shown in Table 2.5. Panic attacks are periods, usually lasting 10 minutes or so (but occasionally hours), in which the individual suddenly experiences intense fear and at least 4 of 13 specified somatic or cognitive symptoms (Table 2.6). Panic disorder may be accompanied by agoraphobia, which DSM-IV describes as:

Anxiety about being in places or situations from which escape might be difficult (or embarrassing) or in which help may not be available in the event of having an unexpected or situationally predisposed Panic Attack or panic-like symptoms. (American Psychiatric Association, 1994, p. 396.)

Before deciding on a treatment plan, the clinician should carefully explore the possibility that the panic symptoms reflect a medical cause (Ballenger, 1997). The more likely masqueraders are excessive caffeine intake, stimulant abuse, hyperthyroidism, a cardiac arrhythmia and chronic obstructive pulmonary disease. Less likely causes are hypoparathyroidism, vestibular disturbances, temporal lobe

Table 2.5. DSM-IV diagnostic criteria for panic disorder without agoraphobia (300.01)

A. Both (1) and (2):
   (1) Recurrent unexpected panic attacks.
   (2) At least one of the attacks has been followed by one month (or more) of one (or more) of the following:
      a. persistent concern about having additional attacks;
      b. worry about the implications of the attack or its consequences (e.g., losing control, having a heart attack, "going crazy");
      c. a significant change in behavior related to the attacks.
B. Absence of agoraphobia.
C. The panic attacks are not due to the direct physiological effects of a substance (e.g., a drug of abuse, a medication) or a general medical condition (e.g., hyperthyroidism).
D. The panic attacks are not better accounted for by another mental disorder, such as social phobia (e.g., occurring on exposure to feared social situations), specific phobia (e.g., on exposure to a specific phobic situation), obsessive–compulsive disorder (e.g., on exposure to dirt in someone with an obsession about contamination), post-traumatic stress disorder (e.g., in response to stimuli associated with a severe stressor), or separation anxiety disorder (e.g., in response to being away from home or close relative).

Source: Reprinted with permission from the *Diagnostic and Statistical Manual of Mental Disorders,* Fourth Edition. Copyright 1994 American Psychiatric Association, p. 402.

Table 2.6. DSM-IV criteria for panic attack

A discrete period of intense fear or discomfort, in which four (or more) of the following symptoms developed abruptly and reached a peak within 10 minutes:
  (1) palpitations, pounding heart, or accelerated heart rate;
  (2) sweating;
  (3) trembling or shaking;
  (4) sensations of shortness of breath or smothering;
  (5) feeling of choking;
  (6) chest pain or discomfort;
  (7) nausea or abdominal distress;
  (8) feeling dizzy, unsteady, lightheaded, or faint;
  (9) derealization (feelings of unreality) or depersonalization (being detached from oneself);
 (10) fear of losing control or going crazy;
 (11) fear of dying;
 (12) paresthesias (numbness or tingling sensations);
 (13) chills or hot flushes.

Source: Reprinted with permission from the *Diagnostic and Statistical Manual of Mental Disorders,* Fourth Edition. Copyright 1994 American Psychiatric Association, p. 395.

epilepsy, the use of steroids or stimulating bronchodilators such as theophylline, and alcohol withdrawal. Pheochromocytoma and hypoglycemia are quite rare.

The clinician should evaluate not only changes in the patient's panic symptoms, but also his degree of avoidance behavior and his occupational functioning. The Sheehan Disability Scale (Appendix 2) is a useful measure, providing disability scores reflecting the effects of symptoms on work, social function and family life. In one study, these scores decreased about 30%, 36% and 44% respectively after eight weeks of treatment with alprazolam (Sheehan et al., 1993). As with social phobia, symptoms and disability may improve at different rates and to different degrees (Sheehan et al., 1996).

Pharmacotherapy

Therapy should aim at abolishing panic attacks, not simply ameliorating them. Panic disorder responds well to tricyclic antidepressants, SSRIs, high potency benzodiazepines and MAOIs. Table 2.7 displays medication approaches to consider, taking into account the medication that is producing a good response or remission of the primary psychiatric condition. Since panic disorder tends to be a chronic condition, pharmacotherapy is likely to be prolonged (Pollack and Otto, 1997). For example, relapse rates following discontinuation of imipramine are lower after 18 months than after six months of treatment (Mavissakalian and Perel, 1992). My practice has been to continue pharmacotherapy for at least a year while trying to modify the patient's panic-related cognitions and behaviors.

When alcoholism complicates apparent panic disorder, some authorities suggest withholding this diagnosis and anti-panic medications to see whether six weeks of abstinence will resolve the symptoms. Others prefer to start an SSRI while attending to the alcohol problem, feeling that the SSRI may benefit both conditions. No consensus exists (Marshall, 1997, and Discussion).

The SSRIs, fluvoxamine (150–250 mg/day), sertraline (50–200 mg/day), citalopram (20–60 mg/day), and paroxetine (40 mg/day) have been found effective for panic disorder in large, double-blind, placebo-controlled trials (Jefferson, 1997; Wade et al., 1997; Lepola et al., 1998; Pollack et al., 1998). Small trials support the efficacy of fluoxetine (Jefferson, 1997). Again, initial doses should be low and upward titration gradual to avoid side effects and noncompliance. Because fluoxetine may be more activating than other SSRIs, a starting dose of 5 mg/day or less is recommended. The comparative tolerability and efficacy of the SSRIs has not been established. Whether nonresponders to one SSRI will respond to another is also unknown. When prescribing either a tricyclic or an SSRI, the clinician can consider providing the patient with immediate symptom relief and protection against exacerbation by also prescribing a high potency benzodiazepine for four to six weeks, followed by a slow taper to zero.

Table 2.7. Pharmacotherapies to consider for comorbid panic disorder

Medication prescribed for the primary psychiatric condition	Added medication to consider for comorbid panic disorder
An SSRI	The same SSRI Clonazepam, lorazepam or alprazolam[a] Imipramine[b] Clomipramine[b] An alternative SSRI for both conditions[c]
A tricyclic antidepressant	Clonazepam, lorazepam or alprazolam An SSRI[b]
A benzodiazepine	Switch to clonazepam, lorazepam or alprazolam An SSRI[a] Imipramine or clomipramine
Buspirone	Clonazepam, lorazepam or alprazolam An SSRI Clomipramine or imipramine
A neuroleptic	An SSRI[d] Clonazepam, lorazepam or alprazolam[e] Imipramine or clomipramine[f]
Lithium	Clonazepam, lorazepam or alprazolam An SSRI[g] Clomipramine or imipramine[g]
Valproate	An SSRI Imipramine or clomipramine Clonazepam[h], lorazepam or alprazolam

Notes:
SSRI: selective serotonin reuptake inhibitor.
[a] Fluvoxamine and fluoxetine inhibit the metabolism of alprazolam, but not of clonazepam or lorazepam.
[b] Because SSRIs impair tricyclic antidepressant metabolism, one should start with low doses and consider monitoring plasma levels.
[c] The alternate SSRI may not be effective in this individual for the primary psychiatric condition.
[d] Fluoxetine and paroxetine may increase plasma levels of neuroleptics (Chapter 4).
[e] Watch for additive adverse effects on alertness and cognitive functions.
[f] Watch for additive anticholinergic effects and postural hypotension.
[g] Rare instances of confusional states, lithium toxicity and serotonin syndrome have been reported, but the combination is generally regarded as safe (Ciraulo et al., 1995).
[h] Watch for added central nervous system depression. Combined use has resulted in absence status in patients with temporal lobe epilepsy.

Among the tricyclics, the best studied are imipramine and clomipramine, both of which are clearly effective (Jefferson, 1997). Dosing should begin at the lowest practical dose and be increased in small weekly steps in order to avoid exacerbating the panic disorder or causing noncompliance because of side effects that may frighten the patient. Imipramine can be started at 10 mg or 25 mg/day and clomipramine at 25 mg daily or every other day. The therapeutic effect may not be apparent until six to eight weeks after achieving the target dose of 200 mg/day for imipramine (Mavissakalian and Perel, 1989) or 75–250 mg/day for clomipramine (Papp et al., 1997). The disadvantages of these medications are their side effects, particularly postural hypotension, increased heart rate, anticholinergic side effects and weight gain. These are associated with a high rate of intolerance (Papp et al., 1997). In addition, if an SSRI is the primary prescribed drug, plasma tricyclic levels require attention to avoid side effects or toxicity.

The efficacy of the high potency benzodiazepines, clonazepam (1–8 mg/day), lorazepam (1.5 to 8 mg/day) and alprazolam (1–10 mg/day) in panic disorder is well established (Schweizer et al., 1990; Davidson, 1997). Their advantages include rapid onset (within the first week), effect on the characteristic anticipatory anxiety, and their high rate of patient acceptance. Patients without a substance abuse history do not escalate their doses over time (Pollack et al., 1993). Clonazepam has advantages over the shorter acting agents; its long duration of action is associated with less interdose anxiety, less "clock-watching," and perhaps with fewer and less intense withdrawal symptoms during tapering (see Table 4.4 in Chapter 4). However, treatment-emergent depression has been reported in a small proportion of patients treated with clonazepam and may require dose reduction, adding an antidepressant drug or discontinuing clonazepam. The disadvantages of the high potency benzodiazepines include sedation, which usually clears within one to two weeks of dose change, impaired psychomotor function, impaired recent memory and the possibility of a withdrawal syndrome. Since alprazolam plasma levels are increased by fluoxetine, fluvoxamine and nefazodone (Nemeroff et al., 1996), clonazepam or lorazepam is preferred when patients are taking these drugs.

The MAOI phenelzine has been found effective for panic disorder in placebo-controlled and open label trials (Jefferson, 1997), but the dietary restrictions on foods containing tyramine, potentially serious consequences of dietary indiscretion, inability to combine phenelzine with an SSRI or buspirone, and often troubling side effects make it a less attractive choice in patients with comorbid panic disorder.

Psychotherapy

A growing body of evidence strongly suggests the efficacy of cognitive–behavioral and some behavioral psychotherapeutic techniques in the treatment of panic disorder, although the relative value of various treatment elements is uncertain (Barlow, 1997). The comparative efficacy of pharmacotherapy, specific psychotherapies and combined treatments has not been established. Nonetheless, when panic disorder complicates the presentation of OCD or a spectrum disorder, implementing a cognitive–behavioral or behavioral approach instead of or in addition to prescribing an anti-panic medication is clinically appropriate.

Barlow (1997) recommends a cognitive–behavioral intervention he terms "panic control treatment." It consists of a combination of cognitive restructuring, breathing retraining and structured exposure to bodily sensations associated with panic attacks. Cognitive restructuring aims at correcting the patient's beliefs that the bodily sensations associated with panic attacks portend dangerous loss of control or perhaps death. Breathing retraining teaches the patient to feel comfortable with diaphragmatic breathing, 8–10 breathes per minute, and to use this breathing technique in stressful situations. To expose the patient to feared bodily sensations, the therapist asks him to engage under observation in activities that will elicit them, e.g., running in place or breathing through a narrow straw to induce respiratory distress, or spinning in a swivel chair to induce dizziness. As the patient learns that these sensations are not dangerous, he is asked to perform symptom-provoking activities in naturalistic situations.

Agoraphobic avoidance requires specific treatment, e.g., graded exposure, since it does not remit spontaneously when panic attacks are brought under control. In my experience, patients with panic-related avoidance behaviors comorbid with OCD can be extremely reluctant to confront their fears. For example, in one case, after many months spent in providing cognitive therapy, relaxation training, exposure in imagination and prescribing visits to the airport to an OCD patient whose panic symptoms were in remission in response to clonazepam, I had to accompany him to the airport before he would agree to board a plane for a short flight to expose himself to a feared panic attack. Short of this intervention, the patient was unable to confront his fear in vivo even though his professional work required travel by air and he was in danger of losing his job.

Shear and Weiner (1997) recommend psychotherapeutic attention to the agoraphobic patient's concerns about abandonment, feeling trapped in relationships and tendency to avoid dealing with negative emotions. Whether panic disorder with agoraphobia is as responsive as uncomplicated panic disorder to cognitive–behavioral treatments is unknown.

Barlow (1997) reports that nearly half of 63 patients evaluated two years after completing 12–sessions of panic control treatment were doing well without further treatment; however, many had had panic attacks in the previous year. In addition, he cites studies (e.g., Shear et al., 1994) that found no difference in short-term outcome between reflective listening or instruction in relaxation techniques and

Table 2.8. DSM-IV criteria for avoidant personality disorder (301.82)

A pervasive pattern of social inhibition, feelings of inadequacy and hypersensitivity to negative evaluation, beginning by early adulthood and present in a variety of contexts, as indicated by four (or more) of the following:

(1) avoids occupational activities that involve significant interpersonal contact, because of fears of criticism, disapproval, or rejection;

(2) is unwilling to get involved with people unless certain of being liked;

(3) shows restraint within intimate relationships because of the fear of being shamed or ridiculed;

(4) is preoccupied with being criticized or rejected in social situations;

(5) is inhibited in new interpersonal situations because of feelings of inadequacy;

(6) views self as socially inept, personally unappealing, or inferior to others;

(7) is unusually reluctant to take personal risks or to engage in any new activities because they may prove embarrassing.

Source: Reprinted with permission from the *Diagnostic and Statistical Manual of Mental Disorders*, Fourth Edition. Copyright 1994 American Psychiatric Association, pp. 664–5.

more complex cognitive–behavioral interventions. Thus, the therapeutic power of the elements of cognitive–behavioral therapy for panic disorder remain to be incontrovertibly established.

Treating comorbid avoidant personality disorder

The validity of the DSM-IV personality disorder categories is much less well established than the categories defining most Axis I disorders (Perry, 1992). In addition, the necessity of making judgments about symptoms and functioning over long periods of time and the limitations inherent in available assessment instruments (Stone, 1993) severely compromise the reliability of personality disorder diagnoses. As a result, descriptive and intervention studies are difficult to evaluate. In the face of this uncertainty, the clinician is nonetheless required to act. Valuable suggestions from the sparse literature concerning pharmacotherapy and psychotherapeutic interventions are summarized below.

The defining characteristics of avoidant personality disorder are feelings of inadequacy, fear of criticism and resultant social inhibition. The DSM-IV diagnostic criteria are shown in Table 2.8.

Pharmacotherapy

When avoidant personality disorder is comorbid with social phobia, both disorders may respond in parallel to pharmacological treatment (Gitlin, 1993). Given the great resemblance between the two disorders, patients with avoidant personality disorder deserve trials of the medications known to be effective for social phobia. The MAOIs phenelzine and tranylcypromine, for example, were helpful in isolated case reports, producing marked improvement after four to six weeks in the patients' ability to socialize (Deltito and Stam, 1989). Two small medication studies of OCD patients suggest that comorbid avoidant personality disorder and traits are sometimes epiphenomena (Mavissakalian, Hamann and Jones, 1990b; Ricciardi et al., 1992). Avoidant personality disorder or traits improved or disappeared in patients whose OCD markedly improved. In my experience, avoidant personality traits in patients with severe OCD and OCD spectrum disorders are less likely to dramatically diminish.

Psychotherapy

A small number of well-designed studies have documented that 10–14 weekly sessions of social skills training and graded exposure to feared situations can produce clinically worthwhile improvement in avoidant personality disorder (Alden, 1989; Stravynski et al., 1994). Whether psychodynamic, interpersonal, cognitive–behavioral or other forms of psychotherapy are effective is unknown. In light of this uncertainty, I usually attempt an eclectic mixture of treatment elements that includes social skills training, cognitive therapy and graded exposure. Pharmacotherapy to treat concomitant mood or anxiety disorders may be necessary (Oldham et al., 1995). Couple or family therapy may be needed to change the behaviors of others who are eliciting or reinforcing the patient's maladaptive thoughts, feelings and behaviors.

Beck and Padefsky (1990), drawing on the cognitive–behavioral models of Aaron Beck (1976), have put forward plausible therapeutic interventions for avoidant personality disorder. They note that these patients expect disapproval, criticism and rejection in the therapeutic encounter, have difficulty trusting the clinician's caring and believe that they can know the clinician's (negative) attitudes without asking. They habitually use judgmental, all-or-none thinking.

To begin correcting habitual negative expectations, the clinician examines with the patient a situation in which these occurred. The clinician exposes the ways in which negative expectations elicited dysphoric feelings. He connects the feelings to the patient's avoidant behavior, illustrating how the behavior led away from desired outcomes. The clinician guides the patient into exploring the childhood sources of his negative expectations. As in psychodynamic therapy, attaining insight and distinguishing the past from the present may facilitate emotional and behavioral change. The patient is asked to bring a log of negative thoughts and feelings to the therapy sessions for mutual analysis.

Avoidant patients hide painful topics. The clinician should help the patient make a hierarchical list of such topics. As these are gradually explored, the patient is asked to test his expectation that discussing them would lead to rejection, loss of control or other feared consequences. Once rapport seems well established, the clinician inquires periodically about other thoughts or experiences that the patient is afraid to reveal because of feared rejection.

Because interpersonal trust is a central issue in this disorder, the clinician should periodically ask the patient to indicate the degree to which he trusts the clinician's feedback. Beck and Padefsky (1990) suggest using a 0–100% scale.

To combat judgmental thinking applied to the self and expected from others, the patient can be asked to explore his views about a friend's behaviors in a hypothetical situation like one that produced a particular instance of self-criticism. As the patient arrives at less judgmental attitudes and conclusions regarding the friend's behaviors, he is encouraged to recognize that others are more likely to share these conclusions than the judgments he reflexively applies to himself.

Beck and Padefsky (1990) also suggest role-playing new behaviors in the therapy session, having the patient keep a record of successes to counteract his habitual negative expectations, and conducting or arranging for social skills training. As with any personality disorder, change is expected to be slow.

Recommended strategies and understandings embedded in psychodynamic psychotherapeutic approaches to avoidant personality disorder are summarized elsewhere (Quality Assurance Project, 1991; Gabbard, 1994).

Treating comorbid dependent personality disorder

Like avoidant personality disorder, dependent personality disorder is characterized by feelings of inadequacy. The feelings pertain, however, to making the simple decisions of everyday life rather than to the likelihood of encountering social criticism. The DSM-IV diagnostic criteria are shown in Table 2.9. Dependent traits, especially difficulty accepting responsibility and reluctance to undertake projects independently, are much more common than the full syndrome.

The effectiveness of various forms of psychotherapy is untested and I know of no controlled pharmacotherapy trials. In my experience, eclectic individual therapy can be moderately helpful, especially if combined with couple or family therapy. As in avoidant personality disorder, concerned others may be inadvertently reinforcing the patient's maladaptive thoughts, feelings and behaviors. If the patient is receiving disability income based on the presence of a comorbid mental disorder, motivating him to take on independent functioning and self support is exceptionally difficult and requires great energy and patience. As in avoidant personality disorder, medication for a concomitant mood or anxiety disorder may be indicated (Oldham et al., 1995). Clinical consensus suggests caution in prescribing anxiolytics because of an increased risk of drug dependency (Quality Assurance Project, 1991). A tricyclic antidepressant or an SSRI may alleviate anxiety symp-

Table 2.9. DSM-IV diagnostic criteria for dependent personality disorder (301.6)

*A pervasive and excessive need to be taken care of that leads to submissive and clinging behavior
and fears of separation, beginning by early adulthood and present in a variety of contexts, as
indicated by five (or more) of the following:*

(1) has difficulty making everyday decisions without an excessive amount of advice and
    reassurance from others;
(2) needs others to assume responsibility for most major areas of his or her life;
(3) has difficulty expressing disagreement with others because of fear of loss of support or
    approval. *Note:* Do not include realistic fears of retribution;
(4) has difficulty initiating projects or doing things on his or her own (because of a lack of
    self-confidence in judgment or abilities rather than a lack of motivation or energy);
(5) goes to excessive lengths to obtain nurturance and support from others, to the point of
    volunteering to do things that are unpleasant;
(6) feels uncomfortable or helpless when alone because of exaggerated fears of being unable to
    care for himself or herself;
(7) urgently seeks another relationship as a source of care and support when a close
    relationship ends;
(8) is unrealistically preoccupied with fears of being left to take care of himself or herself.

Source: Reprinted with permission from the *Diagnostic and Statistical Manual of Mental
Disorders,* Fourth Edition. Copyright 1994 American Psychiatric Association, pp. 668–9.

toms; whether diminished anxiety increases the patient's willingness to make decisions, accept responsibility and seek less care and support is unknown, but deserves
study.

Fleming (1990) describes a cognitive–behavioral approach to dependent personality disorder. I meld some of these techniques with behavioral and interpretive
interventions, but have not engaged patients with comorbid dependent personality disorder or traits in intensive psychotherapy. Perhaps as a result, I have observed
only modest improvements.

Fleming (1990) warns that the patient will seek to place the clinician in the role
of the expert who will provide the guidance, advice and decisions that the patient
feels so incapable of providing himself. In the early stages of treatment, some practical advice and a more active role in structuring decision analyses may be necessary to manage the patient's anxiety; but, as treatment progresses, the emphasis
should shift to teaching the patient decision-making skills. The clinician should
progressively shift responsibility to the patient for choosing subjects to talk about
during the session and should explore the patient's fear that his choices will be
wrong. The therapist must resist the temptation to play the admired expert if the
patient's dependency is to be reversed.

The patient is instructed to keep a daily log of automatic negative or self-denigrating thoughts. The log should record the situation in which these occur, the evoked emotional responses, their intensities and the situation's outcome. The clinician and patient analyze these vignettes together, and the patient is taught how to use rational analysis to combat the negative thoughts. A need for assertiveness or social skills training may become evident.

When little progress is being made, I find it helpful to invite the patient to make a list of the advantages and disadvantages of remaining "dependent" or "helpless" or "ill." The invitation must be offered in a spirit of genuine inquiry and without suggestion of criticism. Often the patient is surprised to discover that powerful motivating advantages exist. Once these have been acknowledged, I explore with the patient whether and to what degree he is willing to give up these advantages in hopes of achieving a more satisfying life.

Fleming (1990) cautions that a strong erotic transference may develop, and that the patient may fall in love with the clinician. She suggests that the clinician strive to keep the relationship professional at all times, avoid physical contact and if a patient's romantic feelings become a problem, make clear that a personal relationship is not desired and is not possible.

Recommended strategies and understandings embedded in psychodynamic psychotherapeutic approaches to dependent personality disorder are summarized elsewhere (Quality Assurance Project, 1991; Perry, 1995).

Part II

Obsessive–compulsive disorder and its treatment

3

Obsessive–compulsive disorder

[The patient] is chained to actions that neither his reason or emotion have originated, that his conscience rejects and his will cannot suppress.

Esquirol, *Des Maladies Mentales Considerées Sur les Rapports Médical, Hygienique et Médico-Legal,* 1838

Time changes all concepts. "Obsessive–compulsive disorder" is no exception. In the seventeenth century, obsessions and compulsions were often described as symptoms of religious melancholy. The Oxford Don, Robert Burton, reported a case in his compendium, *The Anatomy of Melancholy* (1621): "If he be in a silent auditory, as at a sermon, he is afraid he shall speak aloud and unaware, something indecent, unfit to be said." (Goshen, 1967). In 1660, Jeremy Taylor, Bishop of Down and Connor, Ireland, was referring to obsessional doubting when he wrote of "scruples" (religious preoccupations): "[A scruple] is a trouble where the trouble is over, a doubt when doubts are resolved." (*Ductor dubitantium, or the Rule of Conscience*) (Hunter and Macalpine, 1963). In his 1691 sermon on religious melancholy, John Moore, Bishop of Norwich, England, referred to individuals obsessed by "naughty, and sometimes Blasphemous Thoughts [which] start in their Minds, while they are exercised in the Worship of God [despite] all their endeavours to stifle and suppress them . . . the more they struggle with them, the more they encrease" (Hunter and Macalpine, 1963).

Modern concepts of OCD began to evolve in the nineteenth century, when Faculty Psychology, phrenology and Mesmerism were popular theories and when "neurosis" implied a neuropathological condition. Like ourselves, psychiatrists then struggling to understand the mentally ill were influenced by intellectual currents coursing through philosophy, physiology, physics, chemistry and political thought (Zilboorg, 1967). Obsessions, in which insight was preserved, were gradually distinguished from delusions, in which it was not. Compulsions were distinguished from "impulsions," which included various forms of paroxysmal, stereotyped and irresistible behavior (Berrios, 1996). Influential psychiatrists disagreed about whether the source of OCD lay in disorders of the will, the emotions or the intellect. Berrios (1996) details this history, of which a brief summary is as follows:

In his 1838 psychiatric textbook, Esquirol (1772–1840) described OCD as a form of monomania, or partial insanity. He fluctuated between attributing OCD to disordered intellect and disordered will. After French psychiatrists abandoned the concept of monomania in the 1850s, they attempted to understand obsessions and compulsions within various broad nosological categories. These often included the conditions we now identify as phobias, panic disorder, agoraphobia and hypochondriasis; certain classification schemes also included sexual perversions, manic behavior and even some forms of epilepsy. Dagonet (1823–1902), for example, considered compulsions to be a kind of impulsion and OCD a form of *folie impulsive* (impulsive insanity). In this illness, *impulsions violentes, irresistibles* overcame the will and became manifest in obsessions or compulsions. Morel (1809–1873) placed OCD within the category, "*délire emotif*" (diseases of the emotions), which he believed originated from pathology affecting the autonomic nervous system. He felt that attempts to explain obsessions and compulsions as arising from a disorder of intellect did not account for the accompanying anxiety. Magnan (1835–1916) considered OCD a "*folie des dégénérés*" (psychosis of degeneration), indicating cerebral pathology due to defective heredity.

While the emotive and volitional views held sway in France, German psychiatry regarded OCD, along with paranoia, as a disorder of intellect (Berrios, 1996). In 1868, Griesenger published three cases of OCD, which he termed "*Grübelnsucht*," a ruminatory or questioning illness (from the Old German, *Grübeln*, racking one's brains). In 1877, Westphal ascribed obsessions to disordered intellectual function. Westphal's use of the term *Zwangsvorstellung* (compelled presentation or idea) gave rise to our current terminology, since the concept of "presentation" encompassed both mental experiences and actions. In Great Britain *Zwangsvorstellung* was translated as "obsession," while in the United States it became "compulsion." The term "obsessive–compulsive disorder" emerged as a compromise.

In the last quarter of the nineteenth century, the diagnostic category, neurasthenia (inadequate "tonus" of the nervous system), engulfed OCD along with numerous other disorders. As the twentieth century opened, both Pierre Janet (1859–1947) and Sigmund Freud (1856–1939) isolated OCD from neurasthenia. In his highly regarded work, *Les Obsessions et la Psychasthénie* (*Obsessions and Psychasthenia*), Janet proposed that obsessions and compulsions arise in the third (deepest) stage of psychasthenic illness. Because the individual lacks sufficient psychological tension (a form of nervous energy) to complete higher level mental activities (those of will and directed attention), nervous energy is diverted into and activates more primitive psychological operations that include obsessions and compulsions (Pitman, 1987).

Freud gradually evolved a conceptualization of OCD that influenced and then drew upon his ideas of mental structure, mental energies, and defense mechanisms (Freud, 1909, 1913, 1926). In Freud's view, the patient's mind responded maladaptively to conflicts between unacceptable, unconscious sexual or aggressive id impulses and the demands of conscience and reality. It regressed to concerns with control and to modes of thinking characteristic of the anal–sadistic stage of psycho-sexual development: ambivalence, which produced doubting, and magical think-ing, which produced superstitious compulsive acts. The ego marshalled certain defenses: intellectualization and isolation (warding off the affects associated with the unacceptable ideas and impulses), undoing (carrying out compulsions to neutralize the offending ideas and impulses) and reaction formation (adopting character traits exactly opposite of the feared impulses). The imperfect success of these defenses gave rise to OCD symptoms: anxiety; preoccupation with dirt or germs or moral questions; and, fears of acting on unacceptable impulses.

As the twentieth century closes, advances in pharmacology, neuroanatomy, neurophysiology and learning theory have allowed us to reach a more therapeuti-cally useful conceptualization of OCD. Although the causes of the disorder still elude us, the recent identification of children with OCD caused by an autoimmune response to group A β-hemolytic streptococcal infection promises to bring increased understanding of the disorder's pathogenesis (Swedo et al., 1998; see dis-cussion of OCD related to Sydenham's chorea in Chapter 6).

Diagnosis and differential diagnosis

DSM-IV diagnostic criteria (300.3)

DSM-IV reexamined the mid-nineteenth century controversy about whether insight is required for a diagnosis of OCD and abandoned the DSM-III-R criterion mandating its presence (American Psychiatric Association, 1994) (Table 3.1). Because a field trial of the DSM-IV criteria found that 8% of patients currently lacked insight and 5% had never had insight into the senselessness of their symp-toms, the DSM-IV work group proposed the subtype, "with poor insight" (Foa and Kozak, 1995). The workgroup hoped that this inclusion would prevent less experi-enced clinicians from treating delusional OCD patients with antipsychotic drugs, instead of appropriate antiobsessional drugs or behavior therapy. When obsessions are of delusional intensity, DSM-IV allows an additional diagnosis of Delusional Disorder (297.1) or Psychotic Disorder Not Otherwise Specified (298.9).

The DSM-IV field trial revealed that nearly 80% of patients had mental as well as behavioral compulsions, and that mental compulsions, like behavioral compul-sions, usually served to reduce distress or prevent feared events (Foa and Kozak, 1995). As a result, DSM-IV made explicit that the "neutralizing thoughts" of DSM-III-R included mental compulsions.

The field trial also investigated the clinical applicability of the ICD-10 sub-categories of OCD: Predominantly obsessional thoughts or ruminations (F42.0), Predominantly Compulsive Acts [obsessional rituals] (F42.1), and Mixed Obses-sional Thoughts and Acts (F42.2). Yale–Brown Obsessive–Compulsive Scale

Table 3.1. DSM-IV diagnostic criteria for obsessive-compulsive disorder (300.3)

A. Either obsessions or compulsions:

Obsessions as defined by (1), (2), (3), and (4):

(1) recurrent and persistent thoughts, impulses, or images that are experienced, at some time during the disturbance, as intrusive and inappropriate and that cause marked anxiety or distress;

(2) the thought, impulses or images are not simply excessive worries about real-life problems;

(3) the person attempts to ignore or suppress such thoughts, impulses or images, or to neutralize them with some other thought or action;

(4) the person recognizes that the obsessional thoughts, impulses or images are a product of his or her own mind (not imposed from without as in thought insertion).

Compulsions as defined by (1) and (2):

(1) repetitive behaviors (e.g., hand washing, ordering, checking) or mental acts (e.g., praying, counting, repeating words silently) that the person feels driven to perform in response to an obsession, or according to rules that must be applied rigidly;

(2) the behaviors or mental acts are aimed at preventing or reducing distress or preventing some dreaded event or situation; however, these behaviors or mental acts either are not connected in a realistic way with what they are designed to neutralize or prevent or are clearly excessive.

B. At some point during the course of the disorder, the person has recognized that the obsessions or compulsion are excessive or unreasonable. *Note:* This does not apply to children.

C. The obsessions or compulsions cause marked distress, are time consuming (take more than 1 hour a day), or significantly interfere with the person's normal routine, occupation (or academic) function, or usual social activities or relationships.

D. If another Axis I disorder is present, the content of the obsession or compulsion is not restricted to it (e.g., preoccupation with food in the presence of an Eating Disorder; hair pulling in the presence of Trichotillomania; concern with appearance in the presence of Body Dysmorphic Disorder; preoccupation with drugs in the presence of a Substance Use Disorder; preoccupation with having a serious illness in the presence of Hypochondriasis; preoccupation with sexual urges or fantasies in the presence of a Paraphilia; or guilty rumination in the presence of Major Depressive Disorder).

E. The disturbance is not due to the direct physiological effects of a substance (e.g., a drug of abuse, a medication) or a general medical condition.

Specify if:

With poor Insight: if, for most of the time during the current episode, the person does not recognize that the obsessions and compulsions are excessive or unreasonable.

Source: Reprinted with permission from the *Diagnostic and Statistical Manual of Mental Disorders,* Fourth Edition. Copyright 1994 American Psychiatric Association, pp. 422–3.

(Y–BOCS) severity scores for obsessions and compulsions indicated that the vast majority of patients (91%) fell into the mixed category, while few had predominantly obsessions (8.5%) and very few had predominantly compulsions (0.5%) (Foa and Kozak, 1995). Clinicians' ratings presented a different picture: clinicians rated nearly 30% of patients as bothered predominantly by obsessions, about 21% by compulsions, and about 49% as bothered equally by both. In view of these mixed data, the Task Force omitted these subtypes from DSM-IV.

ICD-10 diagnostic criteria (F42)

The ICD-10 diagnostic guidelines (World Health Organization, 1992) are consistent with the DSM-IV criteria, but omit certain details and include the subcategories just described. ICD-10 does not expressly exclude worries about real-life problems or mention that time consumed is one indicator of clinically significant obsessions. Obsessions occurring in the presence of schizophrenia, Tourette's syndrome and organic mental disorder are distinguished from OCD, but ICD-10 does not list various DSM-IV exclusions, such as eating disorders, body dysmorphic disorder or hypochondriasis. Even so, ICD-10 does not intend that "obsessional" symptoms in these disorders should trigger the diagnosis of comorbid OCD. Unlike DSM-IV, ICD-10 does not distinguish mental compulsions from obsessions, a distinction which is useful for purposes of cognitive-behavioral treatment. ICD-10 requires symptoms to have been present on most days for two weeks or more, whereas DSM-IV does not specify a minimum duration except in individuals younger than 18 years of age (Table 3.1). Finally, ICD-10 specifies that insight must be present with regard to "at least one thought or act," whereas DSM-IV requires only that insight has been present "at some point during the course of the disorder."

Differential diagnosis

Depressive ruminations are not ego-dystonic and usually focus on past events, self-castigation, or matters about which the patient feels guilty or regretful. The somatic or paranoid delusions of *psychotic depression* may have a ruminative quality, but the clinical picture of depression is clear. The worries of *generalized anxiety disorder* concern real-life problems, such as job loss, potential financial difficulties or plausible, if improbable, harm to a loved one. No rituals are performed to resolve these anxieties and again, they are not ego-dystonic. In OCD, fears about harm to a loved one are either implausible or extremely unlikely, are rarely if ever the only obsessional content, and elicit compulsions. The intrusive thoughts and images of *post-traumatic stress disorder* are the aftermath of actual traumatic experiences, in contrast to the feared future events of OCD. The delusional ruminations and odd stereotyped behaviors of *schizophrenia* are ego-syntonic and insulated from reality testing (See Chapter 5).

Medical disorders giving rise to obsessive and compulsive symptoms are discussed in Chapter 6. In the early stages of dementia, the individual may engage in excessive list-making, hoarding or repeating rituals, but the motive is compensation for declining intellectual function.

Complex motor or vocal tics can be difficult to distinguish from compulsions, particularly in individuals with comorbid Tourette's Syndrome. Unlike compulsions, tics are purposeless; they are not aimed at warding off or undoing a negative event. Moreover, tics are frequently preceded by premonitory sensory experiences such as muscular tension, whereas compulsions are usually preceded by obsessions or by autonomic or psychic anxiety symptoms (See Chapter 7).

The recurrent and intrusive preoccupations in *body dysmorphic disorder* are limited to fears or beliefs that the individual is ugly or has troubling defects in appearance. These ideas are ego-syntonic, though painful, and are less likely to be resisted (see Chapter 8).

In *hypochondriasis*, inviduals' fear or belief that they have a serious disease arises out of misinterpretations of bodily signs or symptoms. In addition, hypochondriacal patients do not resist their frightening thoughts or their urges to seek medical consultation and care. Whereas hypochondriacal fears of diseases like cancer or AIDS are triggered by somatic signals, the OCD patient usually, though not always, obsesses spontaneously or because of exposure to objects, activities or events that bear no medically recognized causal connection to the feared disease (see Chapter 9). When a patient has hypochondriacal fears and rituals and unrelated obsessions and compulsions, both diagnoses may be given.

A number of other behaviors are referred to as "compulsive," e.g., *buying* (Chapter 14), *kleptomania* (Chapter 15), *gambling* (Chapter 16), certain *sexual behaviors* (Chapter 17) and *alcohol and illicit drug use*. These behaviors are associated with pleasure or tension relief during the consummatory act, in contrast to the post hoc anxiety relief brought about by OCD compulsions.

The obsessive concern with body weight, calories and diet, excessive fear of obesity, and compulsive exercising seen in *anorexia nervosa* and *bulimia nervosa* are not considered forms of OCD. The intrusive ideation and irrational behavior center on weight and appearance as the keys to happiness and self-esteem, whereas OCD symptoms center on issues such as harm avoidance, cleanliness, order and hoarding as means of anxiety reduction.

Obsessive–compulsive personality disorder (OCPD) is not associated with obsessions or compulsions, although hoarding behaviors are symptomatic of OCPD as well as OCD. The stubbornness, preoccupation with details and rules, perfectionism, moral inflexibility and need for control characteristic of OCPD are ego-syntonic (Chapter 18).

Table 3.2. Frequency of obsessional themes

	Percent of patients	
Theme	Study A[a]	Study B[b]
Contamination	50	38
Pathologic doubt[c]	42	–
Somatic	33	7
Symmetry	32	10
Aggressive	31	24
Sexual	24	6
Multiple obsessions	72	–
Religious	–	6
Hoarding	–	5
Unacceptable urges	–	4

Notes:

[a] Rasmussen and Eisen (1992a). $N = 560$ patients meeting DSM-III or DSM-III-R criteria. Symptoms determined by structured interview. The frequency of somatic, symmetry-related and sexual obsessions derives from tabulating all symptoms, rather than patients' three primary symptoms.

[b] Foa and Kozak (1995). $N = 425$ patients meeting DSM-IV criteria. Symptoms tabulated from the patients' "three primary obsessions" from the Y–BOCS symptom checklist.

[c] Fear or doubt regarding responsibility for a terrible event.

Clinical picture

Obsessions and compulsions present as infinitely personalized variations on a small number of morbid themes: aggression, harm avoidance, contamination, distasteful or excessive sexual ideation, religious concerns, collecting, need for symmetry or order, need to know, and fear of illness (Tables 3.2 and 3.3., and Y–BOCS Symptom Checklist, Appendix 2). The patient's inner experience is disturbed by persistent, intrusive fears, dread of being guilty, pathological doubt, repugnant images or urges, and/or a need to carry actions to completeness or perfection. The data displayed in Tables 3.2 and 3.3 mirror those of many other studies (e.g., Akhtar et al., 1975; Stern and Cobb, 1978; Khanna, Kaliaperumal and Channabasavanna, 1990). Contamination fears and fears of harming oneself or others are the most common obsessional themes, while cleaning and checking are the most common compulsions. In the vast majority of instances (as noted in DSM-IV), compulsions are motivated by obsessions and aim at reducing the associated anxiety or preventing a dreaded event.

Table 3.3. Frequency of compulsive behaviors

Compulsion	Percent of patients	
	Study A[a]	Study B[b]
Checking	61	28
Cleaning/washing	50	27
Counting	36	2
Need to ask/confess	34	–
Symmetry/exactness	28	–
Multiple compulsions	58	–
Ordering	–	6
Hoarding	18	4
Repeating	–	11
Mental rituals	–	11

Notes:
[a] Rasmussen and Eisen (1992a). $N = 560$ patients meeting DSM-III or DSM-III-R criteria. Symptoms determined by structured interview. The greater frequency various compulsions derives from tabulating all symptoms, rather than patients' three primary symptoms.
[b] Foa and Kozak (1995). $N = 425$ patients meeting DSM-IV criteria. Symptoms tabulated from the patients' "three primary compulsions" from the Y–BOCS symptom checklist.

Symptom Clusters

OCD patients rarely have only one or two symptoms – multiple obsessions and compulsions are the rule (Rasmussen and Eisen, 1992b). Although an individual's symptoms often change over time, symptoms present at a given time exhibit certain understandable patterns. In a study of current symptoms drawn from patients' Y–BOCS Symptom Checklists ($n = 107$), Baer (1994) found by factor analysis that symptoms clustered into three groups. In factor 1, symmetry and exactness obsessions were strongly correlated with ordering compulsions and mildly with repeating and hoarding rituals. Hoarding obsessions, which were weakly associated with symmetry obsessions, were strongly correlated with hoarding compulsions and mildly with ordering rituals. In factor 2, contamination obsessions were strongly correlated with cleaning compulsions, as would be expected, but surprisingly, given the clinical distinction often made between cleaners and checkers, these obsessions were also mildly correlated with checking rituals. In factor 3, sexual and religious obsessions were mildly correlated, and clustered with aggressive obsessions. A study using similar methods, but examining lifetime experience of symptoms, generally confirmed these relationships, but found a fourth cluster: in this analysis aggressive, religious and sexual obsessions clustered with checking compulsions, confirming the longstanding clinical impression that patients check to be sure they have not harmed others or exposed them to risk (Leckman et al., 1997a). Rasmussen and Eisen (1992a) suggest that three core features may be more fundamental than these symptom groups: abnormal risk assessment, pathological doubt and incompleteness. To date, no phenomenological sub-grouping of OCD symptoms has been found to confer clinically important prognostic information although the individual symptoms of hoarding and obsessional slowness seem particularly difficult to treat (see pp. 72–74; 75; Hantouche et al., 1997). The patterns of obsessions and compulsions associated with comorbid Tourette's Syndrome are discussed in Chapter 7.

Cultural influences on symptom content

The same morbid themes are found in Western and non-Western cultures (Greenberg and Witztum, 1994). The frequency with which these themes are played out in life's secular and religious spheres may vary with the intensity of religious observance within a cultural group. Religious obsessions were quite common in a small series of ultra-orthodox Jewish patients (Greenberg and Witztum, 1994), and in three series of Moslem patients, one in Saudi Arabia (Mahgoub and Abdel-Hafeiz, 1991), one in Bahrain (Shooka, al-Haddad and Raees, 1998) and one in Egypt (Okasha et al., 1994), but not in a fourth (Egrilmez et al., 1997). On close examination, the morbid themes embedded in the religious obsessions and compulsions were familiar: dirt, orderliness, aggression, sex, washing, checking, repeating and slowness (Greenberg and Witztum, 1994).

Age at onset

OCD usually begins before age 25 years and often in childhood or adolescence. In individuals seeking treatment, the mean age of onset appears to be somewhat earlier in men than women. In a series of 70 children and adolescents seen at the National Institute of Mental Health (NIMH), the mean age of onset was 9.6 years for boys and 11.0 for girls (Swedo et al. 1989b). In a series of 263 adult and child patients, the mean age at onset was 21 years for men and 24 years for women (Lensi et al., 1996). In another series ($n = 514$), the means were 21 years for men and 22 years for women (Rasmussen and Eisen, 1992a). In this series, major symptoms began before age 15 years in about one-third, before age 25 in about two-thirds, and after age 35 in less than 15%.

In one series of 200 patients, 29% felt that an environmental precipitant had triggered their illness, most frequently increased responsibility, such as the birth of a child, or significant losses, such as a death in the family (Rasmussen and Eisen, 1988). Of 100 women in this study, 62% reported premenstrual worsening. In a second study (Williams and Koran, 1997), premenstrual worsening of OCD was reported by 24 of 57 women (42%). Among 38 women in this study who had been pregnant at least once, the onset of OCD was associated with pregnancy in only 5 (13%).

In community surveys, the results are mixed. The Epidemiological Catchment Area survey (ECA), which utilized lay interviewers to examine more than 18,500 individuals in five cities, reported a similar mean age of onset for men and women identified as OCD cases (22.4 and 23.0 years) (Karno et al., 1988). A similar study in Edmonton, Canada reported a slightly later median age of onset for males (age 20 years) than females (age 19 years) (Bland, Newman and Orn, 1988). Among 56 individuals in their mid-20s with obsessive–compulsive syndrome identified in a Zurich survey, the mean age of onset was 17 years for males and 19 years for females (Degonda, Wyss and Angst, 1993).

Course and prognosis

For most adult patients who come to treatment, OCD appears to be a chronic condition. In their series of 560 patients, Rasmussen and Eisen (1988, 1992a) reported that 85% had a continuous course with waxing and waning symptoms, 10% a deteriorative course and only 2% percent an episodic course marked by full remissions lasting six months or more. An Italian series reported more patients with episodic or deteriorative courses: 26% episodic, 9% deteriorative and only 64% chronic (Lensi et al., 1996). The conclusions drawn from studies that predate current diagnostic criteria, effective treatments and current patterns of health care utilization should not be applied to today's patients.

The prognosis of children and adolescents who present for treatment appears to be good for half or more. When evaluated two- to seven-years after vigorous treatment with medications, and less often with behavior therapy, a little more than half of 54 children and adolescents were only mildly affected (Leonard et al., 1993). Only six patients (11%) were symptom free, however, and only three of these were taking no medication. A 9– to 14-year follow-up study reported that 8 of 14 adolescents who had received medication treatment were medication free and did not meet OCD criteria; the other six had experienced a chronic, or a relapsing and then chronic, course (Bolton, Luckie and Steinberg, 1995). Finally, a 1.5- to 5-year follow-up of 23 children and adolescents who had received drug treatment found that four were free of OCD, eight had subclinical symptoms and the remaining 11 had chronic or episodic OCD (Thomsen and Mikkelsen, 1995). Larger studies from multiple sites are needed to establish accurately the prognosis associated with modern treatment methods.

In community-identified cases, remission, or a course marked by long, symptom-free periods, seems to be the rule (Degonda et al., 1993). The apparent frequency of this benign course is probably due to the limited diagnostic validity of interviews conducted by lay interviewers and to the large proportion of milder cases in community samples. In the ECA study, only 19% (56 of 291 subjects) meeting OCD criteria during their first lay interview met these criteria during a lay interview conducted one year later (Nelson and Rice, 1997).

Quality of life

OCD impairs patients' quality of life. Medication-free patients with moderate to severe OCD ($n = 60$) reported worse social functioning and performance in work and other activities than the general population and than patients with diabetes (Koran, Thienemann and Davenport, 1996d). The more severe the OCD, the more impaired the patients' social functioning (as measured by the MOS SF-36 – see Appendix 2), even after controlling for effects of concurrent depression. Another indicator of reduced quality of life is lower likelihood of OCD patients marrying (Rasmussen and Eisen, 1992a).

The high personal cost of OCD is mirrored in high social costs. The estimated 1990 direct costs of OCD to the United States economy were $2.1 billion, and the indirect costs (lost productivity) $6.2 billion (Dupont et al., 1995). If a greater proportion of individuals with OCD were in treatment, the direct costs would have been considerably higher. For example, among a random sample of the Baltimore ECA study participants, only 1 of 15 individuals (7%) whom a psychiatrist judged to need treatment was receiving it (Nestadt et al., 1994). The delay between symptom onset and first seeking care is often prolonged, a mean of seven years in one study (Rasmussen and Eisen, 1988) and 10 years in another (Marks, 1992). Even with much treatment foregone, OCD accounted for almost 6% of the estimated 1990 cost of all mental illness. High social costs are also reflected in the high rates of unemployment in OCD patients and receipt of disability and welfare payments (Leon, Portera and Weissman, 1995). Family members suffer as well. Patients' symptoms may create disharmony, angry or anguished demands for participating in rituals, a draining dependency, restricted access to rooms or living space, difficulty in taking holidays and interference with work obligations (Calvocoressi et al., 1995; Magliana et al., 1996; Black et al., 1998a).

Biological models

Functional neuroanatomy

Imaging studies have not consistently identified a pattern of structural brain abnormality, although two studies have reported decreased volume of the caudate nucleus (Trivedi, 1996). Functional abnormalities, on the other hand, have been repeatedly observed.

Many investigators have contributed to the hypothesis that OCD involves dysfunction in a neuronal loop running from the orbital frontal cortex to the cingulate gyrus, striatum (caudate nucleus and putamen), globus pallidus, thalamus and back to the frontal cortex. Organic insult to these regions can produce obsessive and compulsive symptoms (see Chapter 4). The results of neurosurgical treatment of OCD strongly support this hypothesis. Surgical interruption of this loop by means of cingulotomy, anterior capsulotomy or subcaudate tractotomy brings about symptomatic improvement in a large proportion of patients unresponsive to all other treatments (Insel, 1992; Trivedi, 1996). Cingulotomy interrupts this loop at the anterior cingulate cortex, thereby disrupting frontal cortical input into the Papez circuit and limbic system, which are believed to mediate anxiety and other emotional symptoms (Jenike et al., 1991a; Baer et al., 1995). (The Papez circuit involves the hippocampus, septal areas, mammillary bodies, anterior-thalamic nuclei, cingulate, and their connections.) Anterior capsulotomy (lesions within the anterior limb of the internal capsules) and subcaudate tractotomy (lesions in the substantia innominata, just under the head of the caudate nucleus) interrupt fronto-thalamic fibers, which may mediate the obsessive and compulsive components of OCD (Jenike et al., 1991a).

The results of functional imaging studies (PET, SPECT and functional MRI) and the related hypotheses and speculations are reviewed by Insel (1992) and by Trivedi (1996), who divide these studies into three types.

The first type, pretreatment studies of symptomatic patients, report increased metabolic activity or blood flow in the orbitofrontal cortex, anterior cingulate gyri and caudate nuclei. The second type, studies of symptomatic patients challenged with feared stimuli, indicate increased blood flow in these structures, the thalamus and possibly the temporal region. The third type, studies of the effects of treatment, show a decrease in regional cerebral metabolism or blood flow in various subsets of these structures. The observation that successful behavior therapy (exposure and response prevention) and successful pharmacotherapy produce the same changes in activity (Schwartz et al., 1996) is exciting, since it demonstrates the power of psychotherapy to change brain function.

Despite inconsistencies in the results of imaging studies, as a group they are supportive of the neuronal loop hypothesis. Insel (1992) points out that the inconsistencies may reflect differences in study conditions, scanner resolution, methods of analyzing scan data and comparing neuroanatomical regions, patients' anxiety levels, the medications used (clomipramine versus a selective serotonin reuptake inhibitor – SSRI), and the length of treatment before repeat scanning.

Baxter et al. (1992) hypothesized that the hyperactivity observed in this neuronal loop arises because of impaired caudate nucleus function. The impairment allows "worry inputs" from the orbitofrontal cortex to inhibit excessively the inhibitory output from the globus pallidus to the thalamus. The resulting excess in thalamic output then impinges on various brain regions involved in the experience of OCD symptoms, including the orbital frontal region, thus reinforcing hyperactivity in the neuronal loop.

Baxter et al. (1992) and Insel (1992) caution that the abnormal neurophysiology underlying OCD symptoms may involve structures as yet undetected. Decreased metabolic activity can be missed by current scanning techniques. Alternately, the metabolic hyperactivity of small neuronal fields can be missed when surrounding structures exhibit no change or mask the increase behind compensatory decreases.

Serotonin and other neurotransmitters

The hypothesis that an abnormality in serotonergic neurotransmission underlies OCD arose out of the observation that clomipramine, which inhibits both serotonin and norepinephrine reuptake, relieved symptoms, whereas noradrenergic reuptake inhibitors did not. The unique efficacy of clomipramine and the SSRIs remains the strongest support for this hypothesis. Studies of peripheral markers of serotonergic function in blood and cerebrospinal fluid have not conclusively demonstrated an abnormality (Dohlberg et al., 1996). Pharmacological challenge studies with serotonergic agonists have suggested dysregulation within the serotonin system, with behavioral hypersensitivity and neuroendocrinological hyposensitivity to the activation of serotonin receptors, but numerous inconsistencies remain to be resolved (Dohlberg et al., 1996).

The beneficial effects of enhanced serotonergic neurotransmission do not prove that abnormalities in this system are the root cause of OCD symptoms. Serotonergic neurons modulate the function of many other systems, where the primary cause or causes may lie. In patients with comorbid Tourette's syndrome, tics and schizotypal personality disorder, treatment studies (discussed subsequently) indicate a role for dopaminergic neurons.

Genetic contributions

Twin studies and family studies strongly suggest that vulnerability to OCD can be inherited (Pauls, 1992), but a positive family history is absent in many patients. Older studies of monozygotic twins show a 65% concordance for OCD, but no control groups were included. One study found an 87% concordance for "obsessional features" (OCD symptoms that may not have caused significant distress or social impairment) in monozygotic twins; the concordance of dizygotic twins was only half as large. On the other hand, none of eight monozygotic twin pairs in another study were concordant for OCD (Andrews et al., 1990). A recent review notes that in one modern study, 10% of the parents of children and adolescents with OCD themselves had the disorder, and in a second study, OCD was present in 25% of fathers and 9% of mothers (Pauls, 1992). The symptoms of parents and children usually differed, arguing against social or cultural transmission. A third study, however, found no increase in OCD prevalence in first-degree relatives of OCD patients compared to those of a control group (Black et al., 1992).

The recent finding that an antigen which is a genetic marker for rheumatic fever susceptibility is also a marker for susceptibility to an autoimmune form of childhood-onset OCD (Murphy et al., 1997; Swedo et al., 1997) will undoubtedly spur progress in unraveling genetic contributions to the pathogenesis of OCD. (See Sydenham's chorea in Chapter 6).

Assessment instruments

The Y–BOCS, a 10–item, clinician-administered scale, has become the most widely used rating scale for OCD (Goodman et al., 1989a,b). It is provided, along with suggestions for administration and rating, in Appendix 2. The Y–BOCS is designed to rate symptom severity, not to establish a diagnosis. The clinician should first ask the patient to complete the Y–BOCS Symptom Checklist (Appendix 2) and should review the completed checklist with the patient. This can be a first step in helping patients recognize all the thoughts and behaviors that are part of their illness, and allows the clinician and patient to agree on the symptoms being rated. The checklist can also be used to select target symptoms for treatment.

The Y–BOCS provides five rating dimensions for obsessions and compulsions: time spent or occupied; interference with functioning or relationships; degree of distress; resistance; and control (success in resistance). The 10 Y–BOCS items are each scored on a four-point scale from 0 = "no symptoms" to 4 = "extreme symptoms." The sum of the first five items is a severity index for obsessions, and the sum of the last five an index for compulsions. A translation of total score into an approximate index of overall severity is:

- 0–7   subclinical
- 8–15   mild
- 16–23 moderate
- 24–31 severe
- 32–40 extreme

In my estimation, patients experience a 25% decrease in a Y–BOCS score as mild to moderate improvement, and decreases of 35–50% as moderate to marked. In controlled treatment trials, a decrease of ≥ 35% is widely accepted as indicating a clinically meaningful response and translates into a global improvement rating of much or very much improved; many studies, however, have accepted a lower criterion of a ≥25% decrease.

The Y–BOCS' reliability, validity and sensitivity to change are well established (Goodman et al., 1989a,b). A computer-administered version was well received by patients (Rosenfeld et al., 1992).

Extensive reviews of alternative rating scales are available elsewhere (Pato and Pato, 1991). None is as clinically useful or as widely used in research as the Y–BOCS.

Prevalence

The two largest epidemiological studies, the ECA survey (Karno et al., 1988) and the Cross National Collaborative Group study (Weissman et al., 1994) both utilized trained lay interviewers to administer a structured diagnostic interview (the DIS). The one-year OCD prevalence rates at the five ECA sites ranged from 0.8% to 2.3% (mean = 1.6%). Excluding Taiwan, which reported a uniquely low rate (0.4%), the one-year prevalence rates in the Cross National study ranged from 1.1% (Korea) to 1.8% (Puerto Rico).

The reliability and validity of these rates have been called into question (Nelson and Rice, 1997; Stein et al., 1997a). A reanalysis of the ECA data found that less than 20% of OCD cases met diagnostic criteria when reinterviewed by lay interviewers one year later (Nelson and Rice, 1997). Since the Cross National study utilized the same methods, its results are presumably similarly affected.

Other studies also cast doubt on the ECA study's prevalence rates. In two follow-up studies, the lay interviewers' diagnoses of OCD agreed poorly with those made by physicians (Helzer et al., 1985). At the Baltimore ECA site, for example, psychiatrists using a semi-structured interview estimated a one-month OCD prevalence of 0.3% compared to the lay-administered DIS estimate of 1.3% (Anthony et al., 1985).

Stein et al. (1997a) designed a community prevalence study to overcome the problems inherent in using lay interviewers. Individuals identified by structured lay interviews as probable cases of OCD or of subclinical OCD were reinterviewed with structured instruments by a highly-experienced research nurse. The nurse reviewed her findings with the principal investigator, who assigned all diagnoses, and sought additional information when so instructed. Only 24% of individuals identified as probable OCD cases were assigned a research diagnosis of OCD. The resulting weighted one-month prevalence rate for DSM-IV OCD for the entire sample was 0.6% (95% confidence interval = 0.3%–0.8%). Since subjects who reported no obsessions or compulsions to the lay interviewers were not reinterviewed, some OCD cases may have been missed, resulting in an underestimate of the true prevalence.

We studied the prevalence rates for clinically recognized OCD in a large prepaid health plan, the Kaiser Northern California Health Plan, which has more than 1.8 million members (Koran, Leventhal, Fireman and Jacobson, 1999, unpublished data). Chart reviews on all cases with an OCD diagnosis in the Plan's computerized data base produced a one-year treated prevalence rate of 0.095% in adults aged 18 years or older. This is less than 10% of the community prevalence rates reported in the ECA and Cross National studies and only 15% of the more conservative rate reported by Stein et al. (1997a). It is far smaller than the one-month prevalence rates of 0.7% (Schulberg et al., 1985) to 2.2% (Leon et al., 1995) reported from primary care studies that utilized lay interviewers.

The OCD prevalence rates reported in community and primary care studies far exceed the clinically recognized prevalence rate in the Kaiser data base. Despite possible reasons for under-estimation in this data base, and for overestimation of clinically significant OCD in earlier studies, the difference suggests that many Kaiser members with clinically significant OCD go untreated. The proportion of untreated individuals among those with other forms of health insurance is unknown, but, given the delay in seeking treatment noted earlier, I suspect it is equally large.

Comorbidity

Patients with OCD are at high risk of having comorbid major depression and other anxiety disorders. In a series of 100 OCD patients (DSM-III-R diagnosis) who were evaluated by means of a structured psychiatric interview, the most common concurrent Axis I disorders were: major depression (31%); social phobia (11%); eating disorder (8%); alcohol abuse/dependence (8%); simple phobia (7%); panic disorder (6%); and, Tourette's syndrome (5%) (Rasmussen and Eisen, 1988). Dysthymia is also quite common (Ravizza et al., 1995).

In our Kaiser Health Plan study, 26% of patients had no comorbid psychiatric condition diagnosed during the one-year study period; 37% had one and 38% had two or more comorbid conditions (Koran, Leventhal, Fireman and Jacobson, 1998, unpublished data). These proportions did not differ substantially between men and women. The most commonly diagnosed comorbid conditions were major depression, which affected more than one-half, other anxiety disorders, affecting one-quarter, and personality disorders, diagnosed in a little more than 10%. Panic disorder and generalized anxiety disorder were the most common anxiety disorders. Bipolar mood disorder was uncommon, but schizophrenia was rare. Except for eating disorders, which were diagnosed in 1 in 20 women, the rates of specific comorbid conditions were not strikingly different between men and women.

High rates of comorbid major depression and anxiety disorders are also reported in community studies (Degonda et al., 1993). The lifetime prevalence rate for major depression in the ECA study was 32% (Karno et al., 1988) and ranged from 12% (Korea) to 60% (Munich) in the Cross National study (Weissman et al., 1994). Lifetime prevalence rates for comorbid anxiety disorders in the Cross National study ranged from 25% (Taiwan) to 70% (Munich). (Refer back to the earlier discussion of diagnostic validity in these studies.)

Only one large study has examined the prevalence of bipolar disorder in OCD patients. Among 345 outpatients with OCD, 2% had current or lifetime bipolar I and 13.6% bipolar II disorder (Perugi et al., 1997b). The bipolar OCD patients were more likely than the non-bipolar OCD patients to have a history of substance abuse or panic disorder with agoraphobia. The authors note that ascertainment bias, patient recall and medication-induced switches into hypomania or mania may have influenced their findings. Elevated rates of OCD have been reported in an inpatient group of bipolar I and II patients (Krüger et al., 1995) and in the ECA data (Chen and Dilsaver, 1995).

Reports of the lifetime rate of body dysmorphic disorder in OCD patients range from 8% (Brawman-Mintzer et al., 1995) to 37% (Phillips et al., 1995), suggesting that an accurate figure has yet to be established.

Rates of comorbid hypochondriasis have not been reported. However, Barsky et al. (1992b) found that patients with hypochondriasis had an elevated lifetime prevalence rate of OCD (9.5%) compared to medical outpatients from the same clinic.

OCD seems to be associated with a mildly increased risk for alcohol abuse and dependence. Rates of OCD observed among alcoholic patients admitted to inpatient and outpatient treatment programs exceed the rate in the general population (Schuckit and Hesselbrock, 1994), but not to the extent suggested by the ECA study, which attributed alcohol abuse or dependence to 24% of OCD subjects (Karno et al., 1988). The lifetime rate of alcohol abuse/dependence observed in carefully evaluated OCD patients (14%) is close to the general population rate (Rasmussen and Eisen, 1988).

Eating disorders may be more common in OCD patients than in the general population, but the data are sparse. A British study (Noshirvani et al., 1991) reported a history of anorexia nervosa in 9 of 77 women (12.9%) and in none of 68 men, while in an NIMH sample this diagnosis was made in 4 of 31 men (12%) and 2 of 31 women (6.5%) (Rubenstein et al., 1992). It is unclear, however, whether or not the NIMH treats representative groups of OCD patients. Flament et al. (1988) reported comorbid bulimia or atypical eating disorder in 5 of 20 adolescent cases of OCD identified in an epidemiological survey, a rate midway between the rates reported by Rasmussen and Eisen (1988) and that observed in the Kaiser Health Plan data. OCD symptoms are common in patients with anorexia nervosa, second only to depressive disorders (Rothenberg, 1990). A German study of 93 women hospitalized for anorexia nervosa or bulimia reported that 37% met DSM-III-R criteria for OCD and had (clinically significant) Y–BOCS scores of ≥ 16 (Thiel et al., 1995).

Data on comorbid trichotillomania in OCD patients are limited to reports from two convenience samples and deserve little confidence (see Chapter 11).

OCD is associated with Tourette's syndrome, both in the individual and in family pedigrees (see Chapter 7). Among 177 OCD patients drawn from two tertiary care centers, 23% met criteria for Tourette's syndrome and 9% for chronic motor tic disorder (Leckman et al., 1995). In a smaller study, 5 of 16 OCD patients (38%) met criteria for a tic disorder (1 Tourette's, 2 transient motor and 3 chronic motor) (Pitman et al., 1987). Three modern studies using structured interviews to evaluate OCD in Tourette's patients report comorbidity figures ranging from 28% to 62% (Frankel et al., 1986; Pauls et al., 1986; Pitman et al., 1987). Tic onset usually precedes OCD onset.

Methodological difficulties (discussed in Chapter 18) severely limit the validity of prevalence figures for comorbid personality disorders (PD). Some studies find that OCD patients are more likely than the general population to suffer from a PD (Torres and Del Porto, 1995), while others do not (Crino and Andrews, 1996). In three of the four studies using DSM-III-R criteria, obsessive–compulsive personality disorder (OCPD) was the most common comorbid PD, with rates ranging from 8% (Crino and Andrews, 1996) to 28% (Stanley, Turner and Borden, 1990) and 31% (Diaferia et al., 1997), but avoidant and dependent PDs were also common. These studies may suffer from a confusion of state with trait variables. For example, in one study, patients' OCPD, established by a structured clinical interview, disappeared in five of six patients whose OCD was successfully treated (Ricciardi et al., 1992); in a second study, avoidant and histrionic PDs, established by self-report, disappeared in five of eight and two of seven cases, respectively (Mavissakalian, Hamann and Jones, 1990b).

Treatment

The goals of therapy are to diminish symptoms and to ameliorate or reverse their effects on the patient's interpersonal, work place and social functioning. A modest proportion of patients will achieve freedom from significant symptoms.

The clinician can use the Y–BOCS Symptom Checklist (Appendix 2) to obtain a record of the patient's current and past symptoms. Patients may not reveal embarrassing symptoms or symptoms that they believe may suggest they are "crazy" until a trusting therapeutic relationship has been established. If completing a Y–BOCS severity rating is impractical, a useful gauge of severity is how much time obsessions and, separately, compulsions, are occupying "in an average day in the past week."

Treatment planning depends on the careful evaluation outlined in Chapter 2. As noted earlier, comorbid depressive and anxiety disorders will commonly be present. These comorbid conditions may not respond to the particular serotonin reuptake inhibitor (SRI) prescribed for the patient's OCD. Treatment approaches to such cases, including several kinds of psychotherapy, are detailed in Chapter 2. If a patient is abusing alcohol to reduce anxiety, this problem must be addressed before relying upon the patient's compliance with other elements of the treatment plan. The presence of a tic disorder, schizotypal or borderline PD, or a personal or family history of hypomania or mania should be explored, since these would influence therapy choices.

A comprehensive treatment plan evolves as one gets to know the patient. Experienced clinicians will exercise their clinical judgement in tailoring the plan to their patients' needs, preferences, capacities, situation and history. For a patient with isolated, mild to moderate OCD, a combination of an SRI and exposure and response prevention in vivo (ERP) is a reasonable initial strategy in most cases. Many such patients will respond well, however, to ERP alone. In certain situations, such as the patient with low motivation or anergia secondary to major depression, medications alone may be preferable. In still other cases, medications may be needed to decrease the intensity of symptoms so that the patient can subsequently comply with behavioral treatment. There is insufficient data to draw any conclusions about the relative efficacy of medications alone, ERP alone and their combination, but many experienced clinicians believe that the combination offers more rapid improvements and greater protection against relapse. All patients should be guided to contact the OC Foundation and other sources for educational material and access to support groups (Black and Blum, 1992a). (See Appendix 1.)

Expert Consensus Guidelines, derived from a survey of 69 specialists in the treatment of OCD, offer guidance regarding many clinical questions that have not been addressed in research studies (March et al., 1997). Like the treatment guidelines published by the American Psychiatric Association, they provide broad advice, but are not meant to determine treatment in the individual case.

With the exception of tic disorders (see Chapter 7), comorbid Axis I disorders do not seem to affect drug treatment outcome adversely, although most large, controlled clinical trials have excluded patients with comorbid conditions of marked severity. Definitive conclusions await studies of large numbers of such patients. Neither the presence of depression nor its severity (within a mild to moderate range) influences OCD response to clomipramine (DeVeaugh-Geiss et al., 1990), fluvoxamine or fluoxetine (den Boer, 1997); no data are available regarding the other SRIs, but they should be equally effective.

The literature regarding comorbid PDs is mixed, but suggests a negative effect for selected disorders. A poorer response to clomipramine was reported for patients with paranoid, schizoid or schizotypal PD (Baer et al., 1992), and a significantly lower response rate to clomipramine or fluoxetine in patients with schizotypal PD compared to those without it (20% versus 74%) (Ravizza et al., 1995). The presence of borderline PD (not unexpectedly) interfered with treatment compliance in a small case series (Hermesh, Shahar and Munitz, 1987).

The effect of a comorbid PD on behavior therapy outcome is unclear. In one study, patients with a PD ($n = 26$) were more likely to terminate behavior therapy prematurely, were rated more difficult to treat and experienced less symptom relief than patients without such a disorder ($n = 5$) (AuBuchon and Malatesta, 1994). In a second study, OCD patients with mixed schizoid, schizotypal and avoidant traits were more likely to refuse behavior therapy and less likely to benefit from it (n = 21) than those with other trait clusters ($n = 48$, 39 and 29) (Fals-Stewart and Lucente, 1993). A third study, however, found behavior therapy equally effective in 22 patients with a PD and 21 patients free of these disorders (Dreessen, Hoekstra and Arntz, 1997). Although the numbers within each Axis II category were small, no evidence of an adverse effect was found for any category. The management of avoidant and dependent personality traits and disorders is discussed in Chapter 2.

Pharmacotherapy

The efficacy of clomipramine and of five SSRIs (citalopram, fluoxetine, fluvoxamine, paroxetine and sertraline) has been established in multicenter, double-blind, placebo-controlled trials. Small, open-label trials also suggest efficacy for high doses of the serotonin/norepinephrine reuptake inhibitor, venlafaxine. Together, these studies suggest that:

- 40–60% of patients treated with an SRI will be much or very much improved.
- Treatment naive patients are more likely to respond to an SRI trial than patients who have failed a prior SRI trial.
- Patients who do not respond to one SRI often respond to another.
- In treating OCD, the effective doses of SRIs are often higher than those used to treat depressive disorders.
- Most patients do not experience substantial benefit (a Y–BOCS decrease of $\geq 35\%$) before the sixth week of treatment.
- Patients who do not respond to lower SRI doses often respond to higher ones.
- An adequate SRI trial requires 10–12 weeks, including at least six weeks at the maximum tolerated dose.
- The SSRIs are better tolerated than clomipramine, but each of these drugs is tolerated by the vast majority of patients.

Efficacy studies

Clomipramine

In two parallel, 10-week, double-blind, placebo-controlled, multicenter trials, 60% of OCD patients treated with clomipramine achieved Clinical Global Impression (CGI) ratings of much or very much improved. Y–BOCS scores in the clomipramine group fell from a baseline mean of 26.2 to 16.0. (Clomipramine Collaborative Study Group, 1991). Eight smaller double-blind, placebo-controlled studies confirm clomipramine's efficacy, although many include OCD patients with affective disorders and lack standard assessment measures (Piccinelli et al., 1995). A significant correlation between clinical outcome and plasma clomipramine levels has not been consistently observed.

Fluoxetine

In two, large, parallel, 12-week, double-blind, placebo controlled, multicenter trials, fluoxetine in fixed doses of 20, 40 and 60 mg/day was superior to placebo. About one-third in each dose group exhibited a Y–BOCS score decrease of $\geq 35\%$. Higher doses appeared to act more quickly and to cause a greater Y–BOCS score decrease (Tollefson et al., 1994a,b). Outcome was not related to plasma levels of fluoxetine, norfluoxetine or their sum (Koran et al., 1996a). A European multi-center trial produced less robust results, probably due to the short treatment period (8 weeks) (Montgomery et al., 1993). In a small, double-blind, 10-week crossover trial, fluoxetine and clomipramine produced equivalent mean decreases in Y–BOCS scores; in addition, open-label fluoxetine maintained the therapeutic response of most patients who had responded to clomipramine (Pigott et al., 1990).

Fluvoxamine

In a large, 10-week, double-blind, placebo-controlled, multicenter trial, 40% of patients treated with fluvoxamine 100–300 mg/day achieved CGI ratings of much or very much improved compared to 15% of the placebo group. The fluvoxamine group experienced a significantly greater mean decrease in Y–BOCS score (from 23.3 to 18.4) than the placebo group (Greist, et al., 1995d). Four smaller double-blind, placebo-controlled trials and one double-blind comparison with desipramine support the efficacy of fluvoxamine (see Koran et al., 1996b).

Paroxetine

In a large, 12-week, double-blind, placebo-controlled, multicenter trial, paroxetine in fixed doses of 40 and 60 mg/day for at least 10 weeks (titrated up from 20 mg/day) produced a significantly greater decrease in Y–BOCS and CGI-severity scores than placebo; paroxetine 20 mg/day did not (Wheadon, Bushnell and Steiner, 1993).

Sertraline

In a large, 12-week, double-blind, placebo-controlled multicenter trial, sertraline in fixed doses of 50, 100 and 200 mg/day produced significantly greater improvement than placebo on one, but not all outcome measures (Greist et al., 1995a). In the dose group with the best response (200 mg/day), the mean Y–BOCS score decreased from 23.5 to 17.3; 44% achieved CGI ratings of much or very much improved. The high early dropout rate in the 100 mg/day dosage group probably explains the group's failure to separate from the placebo group. Overall, 39% of sertraline patients and 30% of placebo patients achieved CGI ratings of much or very much improved. (This is an unusually high placebo response rate for OCD patients.) Clinical outcome was not correlated with sertraline plasma levels. A 10-week, double-blind, placebo-controlled trial comparing flexible doses of sertraline (50–200 mg/day) also found sertraline superior to placebo (Chouinard et al., 1990).

Citalopram

In a European multicenter, double-blind, placebo-controlled trial, citalopram in doses of 20, 40 and 60 mg/day was more effective than placebo (abstract, Montgomery, 1998). A randomized, single-blind, 10-week trial comparing citalopram (mean dose = 50 mg/day) with paroxetine (mean dose = 53 mg/day) and fluvoxamine (mean dose = 290 mg/day) in 30 OCD patients found no significant difference in outcome as measured by Y–BOCS scores. Mean Y–BOCS scores of the citalopram group dropped from 29.3 to 19.8 (Mundo, Bianchi and Bellodi, 1997). In a 24-week, open pilot study of citalopram, 22 of 29 patients (76%), most receiving 40 or 60 mg/day, had a clinically significant response (Koponen et al., 1997). An open-label, 10-week trial in 23 children and adolescents reported that 75% had "a marked improvement" (Thomsen, 1997). Citalopram was released in the United States in September 1998 and the European study, mentioned above, demonstrates its efficacy.

Venlafaxine

In a 12-week, open trial, 3 of 10 patients experienced a decrease of ≥35% in Y–BOCS scores; all were treated with 375 mg/day (Rauch, O'Sullivan and Jenike, 1996). An additional patient, treated with 225 mg/day was rated much improved despite a minimal increase in Y–BOCS score. In an eight-week, double-blind, placebo-controlled trial of venlafaxine titrated up to 225 mg/day, neither the venlafaxine group ($n=23$) nor the placebo group ($n=19$) showed a statistically significant mean decrease in Y–BOCS score (Yaryura-Tobias and Neziroglu, 1996, and unpublished data on file, Wyeth Laboratories, 1996). Case reports describe responses to 150 mg/day (Ananth et al., 1995), 225 mg/day (Grossman and

Hollander, 1996) and 375 mg/day (Zajecka, Fawcett and Guy, 1990). Taken together, these results suggest that if a venlafaxine trial is undertaken, the target dose should be at least 225 mg/day. At this dose, about 7% of patients will have to discontinue the drug or lower the dose because of sustained hypertension; above 300 mg/day, about 13% of patients are affected (Medical Economics Company, 1998).

Comparison studies

Two meta-analyses of clomipramine versus SSRI treatment of OCD have suggested that clomipramine has a greater therapeutic effect, although the analyses included no parallel-group comparison studies (Greist et al., 1995c; Piccinelli et al., 1995). Meta-analyses may reach erroneous conclusions because of differences in study designs (e.g., fixed versus flexible dosing, lengths of treatment and outcome measures) and in patient populations (e.g., illness severity, previous exposure to treatment). For example, the clomipramine study utilized in the Greist et al. (1995c) meta-analysis enrolled only SRI-naive patients, whereas a large proportion of patients in the comparison studies had failed one or more SRI trials. None of the randomized, double-blind, parallel-group studies described subsequently has found clomipramine superior to an SSRI. None of these studies, however, has had a sample size sufficient to detect with 80% power the 17% difference in mean CGI improvement scores reported in the meta-analysis of Greist et al. (1995c) (See Koran et al., 1996b for a discussion.) Thus, differences of this magnitude may exist. In general, the parallel-group comparison studies have found the SSRIs to be better tolerated than clomipramine.

A double-blind comparison of *clomipramine* 150 mg/day to *fluoxetine* 40 mg/day in 55 patients found equivalent mean changes in Y–BOCS scores, mean CGI-improvement scores and in the proportion of each group achieving a $\geq 35\%$ decrease in Y–BOCS scores (López-Ibor et al., 1996).

Three 10-week, double-blind studies comparing flexible doses of *clomipramine* and *fluvoxamine* in study groups of 66 (Freeman et al., 1994), 79 (Koran et al., 1996b) and 26 patients (Milanfranchi et al., 1997) found no significant difference in outcome.

A 12-week, double-blind comparison of flexible doses of *clomipramine* and *sertraline* (after 4 weeks of 50 mg/day for either drug) found greater efficacy for sertraline in the intent-to-treat group, e.g., a mean Y–BOCS decrease of 51% versus 43%. But the differences were "almost wholly" due to the larger dropout rate among clomipramine patients (Bisserbe et al., 1997). Patients receiving at least four weeks of double-blind study medication exhibited no statistically significant differences in outcome.

A 12-week, double-blind comparison of flexible doses of *clomipramine, paroxetine* and *placebo* found both active drugs superior to placebo and equivalent to one another (e.g., 55% of both active drug groups achieved a ≥25% decrease in Y–BOCS scores (Zohar et al., 1996).

Predictors of outcome

Patients who fail to respond to one or more SRI trials may be less likely than treatment naive patients to respond to the next SRI trial. Among more than 450 OCD patients participating in double-blind, placebo-controlled, sertraline trials, only 33% of those who had failed one or more SRI trials benefitted compared to 53% of those who were treatment naive (Rasmussen, Baer, Eisen and Shera, unpublished data, 150th Annual Meeting, American Psychiatric Association, May 17–22, 1997). A reanalysis of data from a multicenter fluoxetine trial has also reported that SRI-naive patients were more likely to respond than SRI-experienced patients (Ackerman et al., 1998). Analyses of other large data sets are needed to confirm or refine these observations. Meanwhile, clinicians should not burden patients with negative expectations based on these reports. In my clinical experience, most patients who have failed to respond to one SRI respond to another or to an augmenting strategy, although it may take several trials to identify the SRI or augmenting drug that is effective for the patient. There are no clinically useful predictors of which SRI will be effective for a given patient (Ackerman et al., 1994).

OCD patients with a comorbid tic disorder usually require combined treatment with a dopamine blocking agent and an SRI (see Chapter 7). A retrospective case-controlled analysis comparing OCD patients with and without a comorbid tic disorder found that only 21% of those with, compared to 52% of those without the comorbid disorder had a clinically meaningful response to fluvoxamine (McDougle et al., 1993a). In a double-blind, placebo-controlled study, eight of eight patients with a comorbid tic disorder, having failed to respond to eight weeks of fluvoxamine monotherapy, responded to the addition of haloperidol (mean dose = 6 mg/day) within two weeks; of the seven similar patients assigned to added placebo, none responded (McDougle et al., 1994a). In my experience, good results can also be obtained by adding risperidone. The place of risperidone and other novel neuroleptics in these cases remains to be defined.

OCD patients with schizotypal PD may benefit from the addition of haloperidol or pimozide to an SSRI, but the number of reported cases is very small (McDougle et al., 1990; McDougle, Goodman and Price, 1994b). Risperidone or olanzapine would be equally reasonable choices and have benefitted a number of my patients. Expert opinion does not support monotherapy with neuroleptics for any patient with OCD (March et al., 1997).

Dosing

Since the prevention and management of side effects play a large role in treating chronic disorders like OCD, Chapter 4 is devoted to an extensive treatment of this

Table 3.4. Dose regimens for primary anti-OCD drugs

Medication (brand name)	Daily dose[a]		
	Usual starting (mg)	Average target (mg)	Usual maximum (mg)
Citalopram (Celexa in USA)	20	40–60	60
Clomipramine (Anafranil)	25–50	100–250	250
Fluoxetine (Prozac)	20	40–60	80
Fluvoxamine (Luvox)	50	200	300
Paroxetine (Paxil)	20	50	60
Sertraline (Zoloft)	50	150	225

Note:

[a] Daily doses shown for fluoxetine, fluvoxamine, paroxetine and sertraline are those recommended by the Expert Consensus Guideline for Treatment of OCD (March et al., 1997).

Table 3.5. Dose regimens for additional drugs used in treating OCD

Medication (brand name)	Daily dose[a]		
	Usual starting (mg)	Average target (mg)	Usual maximum (mg)
Buspirone (Buspar)[a]	20	60	90
Clonazepam (Klonopin)	0.5	1–3	4
Gabapentin (Neurontin)	300	1800–2400	3600
Haloperidol (Haldol)[a]	0.25	0.25–6	6
Inositol (Inositol)	6	18	18
Lorazepam (Ativan)[a]	0.5	1–6	6
Lithium (various)	300	[b]	[b]
Pimozide (Orap)[a]	0.5	1–6	6
Risperidone (Risperdal)	0.5	0.5–5	6
Tryptophan	2[c]	4–6[c]	8[c]
Venlafaxine (Effexor)	37.5	225–375	375

Notes:

[a] Doses recommended by the Expert Consensus Guideline for Treatment of OCD (March et al., 1997).

[b] Adjust the dose to achieve a serum level of 0.6–1.2 mEq/l.

[c] grams.

topic. The Chapter also includes tables of drug pharmacokinetics and of potential drug interactions, which may be important in deciding which SRI and which augmenting agents to prescribe for a particular patient.

The usual starting doses, target doses and maximum doses for medications utilized in treating OCD are shown in Tables 3.4 and 3.5. In elderly patients, those with comorbid panic disorder, and those who are anxious about taking medications, initial doses lower than those shown are often advisable. In particular, elderly patients metabolize all of the SSRIs except fluoxetine more slowly. Before starting clomipramine or an SSRI, I inform the patient that:

• A trial of 10–12 weeks at the maximum tolerated dose will be needed to determine whether the medication brings substantial benefit.
• Symptoms may not improve until six or more weeks after reaching the maximum tolerated dose. Lack of improvement in this period should not be taken as a discouraging sign.
• Predicting which drug will be effective for a given patient is not yet possible. Therefore, a number of trials may be needed to find a medication that works for the patient.
• Certain side effects commonly associated with the medication may occur. If they are not transient or manageable, we have many other approaches to explore.

Since clomipramine and the SSRIs appear to be equally effective on a population basis, the more benign side effect profile of the SSRIs (Chapter 4) gives them an advantage over clomipramine as an initial therapy.

My usual practice in patients who accept medications easily is to increase the dose of clomipramine or an SSRI every five to seven days to the maximum tolerated dose and then wait six to eight weeks for signs of a response. This pattern of dose increases allows steady state to be achieved between dose increments for all of the SRIs except fluoxetine and clomipramine, and usually allows acute side effects to become apparent. For many patients, this approach achieves response more rapidly than the alternative preferred by some experts: target an intermediate dose, wait six weeks to observe the response, and increase the dose to maximum levels only if an inadequate response is observed (March et al., 1997). Since I increase the dose only if side effects are not troubling, the rapid pursuit of maximum doses does not often cause noncompliance or unwillingness to continue a drug trial.

Plasma levels of clomipramine can be measured in cases of questionable compliance, severe adverse events at low doses or lack of response despite maximum doses (to investigate whether the patient is a particularly slow or rapid metabolizer of the drug). Clomipramine reaches steady state plasma levels in about two weeks and desmethylclomipramine in three weeks at constant dosing (Medical Economics Company, 1998).

Several months after the patient has achieved substantial therapeutic benefit, I begin tapering the drug dose by about 15–20% every two months to reach the lowest dose that will maintain the patient's therapeutic response. This rate is slow enough to allow signs of relapse to appear (Pato et al., 1988).

Maintenance treatment and discontinuation

Clomipramine and the SSRIs remain effective in long-term treatment. Patients continue to improve modestly between months 4 and 12 of treatment. Of 70 responders to fluoxetine, only 5% relapsed in the ensuing six months; most patients continued to improve (Tollefson et al., 1994a). Of 96 responders to sertraline, only 9% relapsed in the ensuing nine months (Greist et al., 1995b). Mallya et al. (1992) report continued improvement during one year of fluvoxamine treatment.

Sertraline's safety, tolerability and continued efficacy over a two-year treatment period is supported by an open-label, one-year extension study of 51 patients who were responders after one year of double-blind treatment (Rasmussen et al., 1997). There was no increase in incidence or severity of side effects and only three patients (6%) discontinued because of adverse experiences. OCD symptoms continued to improve during this second year of treatment with sertraline.

Discontinuation of medication carries a high risk of relapse. Sixteen of 18 patients (89%) who discontinued clomipramine double-blind after 5 to 27 months of successful treatment relapsed by the end of the seven-week placebo period (Pato et al., 1988). Maintenance studies are consistent with these results. Fontaine and Chouinard (1989), however, reported an anomalous result: only 8 of 43 patients (23%) who had responded to fluoxetine for 12 months relapsed during the year after drug discontinuation. Implementing ERP therapy during the drug treatment period may prevent or delay relapse (Foa and Kozak, 1996), but this has not been firmly established. The decision to discontinue medication should be taken cautiously. In one study, about 20% of patients who had discontinued medication and relapsed failed to respond when the initially effective medication was restarted (Ravizza L. et al. Presented at the American Psychiatric Association, 151st Annual Meeting, Toronto, Canada, May 30–June 4, 1998).

Patients can be successfully maintained on SRI doses substantially lower than those used during acute treatment. Ravizza et al. (1996a) studied maintenance treatment in 130 patients who had responded for six months to clomipramine 150 mg/day, fluoxetine 40 mg/day or fluvoxamine 300 mg/day. About one-quarter to one-third of those randomly assigned to continuing full- or half-dose treatment relapsed over a two-year period compared to at least three-quarters of those assigned to discontinue medication. A 14-week maintenance study divided 30 responders to at least 10 weeks of clomipramine 160 mg/day or fluvoxamine 260 mg/day into three groups: full dose, two-thirds dose and one-third dose (Mundo et al., 1997). No significant difference in relapse rates was observed (10–30%). The small sample size (4 or 5 patients in each drug-dose group), however, limits the accuracy of these relapse risk estimates. Pato, Hill and Murphy (1990) reported that 10 patients treated with clomipramine (mean dose = 270 mg/day) tolerated a gradual dose reduction of about 40% (mean final dose = 165 mg/day) over

1.5–2 years with no relapse during a mean follow-up period of six months (minimum = 2 months).

Pharmacological augmentation strategies

Many patients will require the addition of an augmenting drug. The double-blind, placebo-controlled studies that established the efficacy of clomipramine and the SSRIs reported that 40–60% of patients treated with one drug alone failed to achieve an adequate response (Greist et al., 1995c). When the patient has experienced some benefit, but this falls short of a substantial decrease in symptom frequency and discomfort and a substantial increase in ability to perform the ordinary tasks of daily living, the response is inadequate. In this circumstance, a number of strategies should be considered, including initiating ERP if this has not already been done.

When the patient's first SRI or SSRI trial brings a partial but inadequate response, the clinician must choose between trying a different drug or an augmentation trial. No controlled comparisons of these alternate strategies are available. If side effects are mildly or moderately troubling, trying another drug is the more attractive option. If side effects are minimal, then a few augmentation trials are in order, and, if successful, may bring about improvement more rapidly than starting a new SRI trial. Drugs that can be considered include:

- buspirone;
- clonazepam;
- fenfluramine;
- gabapentin;
- inositol;
- lithium;
- L-tryptophan;
- the addition of clomipramine to an SSRI.

No single augmentation strategy is uniformly effective, perhaps because the pathophysiological basis of OCD is heterogeneous. Although controlled trials have been generally disappointing, the case report literature and my clinical experience are consistent with a modestly hopeful attitude in the individual case.

Buspirone

Buspirone is a 5-HT$_{1A}$ receptor partial agonist that gradually enhances 5-HT neurotransmission. Controlled 4- to 10-week trials of buspirone augmentation (Pigott et al., 1992a; Grady et al., 1993; McDougle et al., 1993b) failed to confirm the positive results reported in case studies and uncontrolled series (Markovitz, Stagno and Calabrese, 1990; Jenike, Baer and Buttolph, 1991b). However, many patients enrolled in the controlled trials may have been treatment-resistant

(McDougle et al., 1993b) rather than partial responders. In one controlled trial, 4 (29%) of 14 patients experienced a clinically meaningful improvement (Pigott et al., 1992a).

I begin buspirone at 10 mg twice daily and increase the dose by 10 mg every third day as tolerated, to a target dose of 60–90 mg/day in three divided doses. At 60 mg/day or above, irritability and forgetfulness have been dose-limiting side effects. The trial should be continued for six weeks at the maximum tolerated dose. My experience and the literature suggest that perhaps one in five or six patients has a significant response.

Clonazepam

Clonazepam is an unusual benzodiazepine in that it affects serotonergic systems and upregulates 5-HT$_1$ and 5-HT$_2$ receptor binding sites in the frontal cortex (Hewlett, Vinogradov and Agras, 1992). Clonazepam has been beneficial alone (Bodkin and White, 1989; Bacher, 1990; Hewlett, Vinogradov and Agras, 1990) and as an augmenter (Leonard et al., 1994). A complex, double-blind crossover trial of four drugs, each given for six weeks, found clonazepam, 4–10 mg/day, as effective as clomipramine 175–250 mg/day (Hewlett et al., 1992). Twelve of 25 clonazepam subjects (48%) and 14 of 26 clomipramine subjects (54%) experienced $\geq$25% decreases in Y–BOCS scores. Clonazepam response was not correlated with changes in anxiety. The side effects associated with these doses of clonazepam were notable: five patients discontinued the drug because of suicidal depression, irritability or intoxication; others were troubled by ataxia, dysarthria, disinhibition or mood alteration.

My usual practice is to add clonazepam beginning at 0.5 mg once or twice daily and increase the dose weekly or every other week by 1 mg/day to a maximum of 4 mg/day as needed. A four-week trial at the maximum tolerated dose is adequate. Patients with high levels of anxiety, agitation, insomnia or comorbid panic or bipolar disorder are good candidates for clonazepam augmentation; depressed patients are not. Case reports of benefit from alprazolam monotherapy exist (e.g., Tollefson, 1985), but its shorter half-life, more difficult withdrawal and smaller database make it less attractive than clonazepam. Double-blind, placebo-controlled, parallel-group, trials are needed to determine the role of clonazepam in treating OCD.

Fenfluramine

Fenfluramine, marketed as an anorectic agent, is a serotonin releaser and reuptake inhibitor. Doses of 20–60 mg/day were beneficial within one to four weeks of initiating augmentation treatment in two small case series (Hollander et al., 1990; Judd et al., 1991). Fenfluramine has been withdrawn from the United States market because of concerns about cardiac valvular damage observed in individuals who took fenfluramine in combination with phentermine for weight loss. If these concerns prove groundless, the case reports suggest that a reasonable trial can consist of increments of 20 mg/day every one to two weeks to a maximum dose of 60 mg/day for one month. In my experience, fenfluramine seemed helpful in about 10–15% of trials; an expert panel ranked it below lithium and above L-tryptophan as an augmentation choice (March et al., 1997).

Gabapentin

Gabapentin is a well-tolerated, easily titrated anticonvulsant whose mechanism of action is unknown. It is largely excreted unchanged in the urine and does not interfere with hepatic metabolism of other drugs (Medical Economics Company, 1998). Communications among clinicians via the internet suggest that gabapentin monotherapy relieves generalized anxiety and chronic low grade depression, both of which may complicate OCD. In ongoing studies at the NIMH, gabapentin added to an SRI has produced mild to moderate improvement in anxiety, depression and OCD symptoms (Corá-Locatelli et al., 1998). After abrupt discontinuation of gabapentin, however, five patients quickly experienced return of symptoms with greater intensity.

The handful of patients with severe OCD for whom I have added gabapentin to a stable SRI regimen have reported moderate decrease in anxiety and in the frequency of obsessions. They note a resultant modest increase in their ability to dismiss obsessions and resist compulsions. I usually begin with 300 mg twice daily and increase the dose by 300 mg/day every few days to a target dose of 1800–2400 mg/day for a two- to four-week observation period. In a few cases, doses of 3600 mg/day were well tolerated, but did not bring added benefit. The bioavailability of gabapentin decreases as the dose increases (Medical Economics Company, 1998); an individual dose should not exceed 1200 mg.

Inositol

Inositol is a normal constituent of the diet and is the precursor of the second messenger (phosphatidylinositol) for several neurotransmitter systems, including several serotonin receptor subtypes. In a double-blind, placebo-controlled, six-week per phase, crossover trial of inositol 18 g/day, 6 of 13 patients completing the trial experienced a $\geq 25\%$ decrease in Y–BOCS score after inositol monotherapy, compared to none during the placebo phase (Fux et al., 1996). The only side effects appear to be flatus, nausea and diarrhea. The investigators administered inositol as two teaspoonfuls (about 6 g) in juice three times daily. In the United States, inositol is available in health food stores as a water-soluble, sweet powder. I have observed modest improvement within a month when adding inositol to an SRI in several patients who were partial responders; however, the majority of my patients given inositol have experienced little or no benefit. Patients start with one teaspoonful three times daily for a few days to confirm tolerability and then move to the full dose. Inositol deserves study both as a monotherapy and as an augmenting agent.

Lithium

Lithium enhances serotonergic transmission by several mechanisms as well as affecting norepinephrine and dopamine neurotransmission and the G-protein second messenger system (Schatzberg, Cole and DeBattista, 1997). The positive results reported in OCD case series (e.g., Ruegg et al., 1992) have not been mirrored in controlled trials. In sequential, four-week, double-blind crossover periods, neither lithium (mean serum level 0.54 mEq/l) nor triiodothyronine (25 μgm/day) produced clinically meaningful benefit in patients who were partial responders to at least six months of clomipramine treatment (Pigott et al., 1991b). In two- and four-week double-blind, placebo-controlled trials of lithium augmentation of ongoing fluvoxamine treatment in nonresponders, only 2 of 11 (18%) and none of 5 patients randomized to lithium (mean serum level = 0.77 mEq/l) had a "moderately clinically meaningful" response (McDougle et al., 1991). Overall, the literature suggests that lithium augmentation is only occasionally beneficial, although it can be effective for comorbid depression. The combination of lithium and an SSRI can induce a troubling degree of tremor, and occasional cases of neurotoxicity have been reported, with and without elevated serum lithium levels (Ciraulo et al., 1995).

L-Tryptophan

The amino acid precursor of serotonin, L-tryptophan was removed from over-the-counter distribution in the United States because of cases of associated eosinophilia myalgia syndrome – some fatal. A contaminant introduced by one manufacturer was later suspected and tryptophan is now available by prescription from pharmacists in some cities in the United States. L-tryptophan 6 gm/day added to clomipramine was reported beneficial in one case (Rasmussen, 1984), and in doses of 3–9 gm/day, combined with nicotinic acid, 1000 mg and pyridoxine HCl 200 mg twice daily (to promote serotonin synthesis), was reported beneficial in a series of seven cases (Yaryura-Tobias and Bhagavan, 1977). In a recent open trial, seven of nine patients receiving an SRI and pindolol 2.5 mg three times daily exhibited clinically significant improvement (Y–BOCS score decrease of ≥ 5) after four weeks of added L-tryptophan 2 g twice daily (Blier and Bergeron, 1996). Pindolol, a 5-HT$_{1A}$ and β-adrenergic receptor antagonist, blocks midbrain 5-HT$_{1A}$ autoreceptors, which decrease neuronal firing, but not limbic forebrain post-synaptic 5-HT$_{1A}$

receptors. As a result, pindolol may facilitate serotonergic neuronal activity in patients given SRIs (Blier and Bergeron, 1996). Subsequently, doses up to 8 gm/day were well tolerated and were associated with further improvement. Caution is in order since L-tryptophan combined with fluoxetine has resulted in the serotonin syndrome (Steiner and Fontaine, 1986). The safety and efficacy of L-tryptophan augmentation, with and without concomitant pindolol administration, require more study.

Adding clomipramine (CMI) to an SSRI

Expert opinion, but no well-controlled trials, support the addition of CMI to an SSRI in patients with an inadequate response (March et al., 1997; Figueroa et al., 1998). Ravizza (8th Annual Congress of the European College of Neuropsychopharmacology, Venice, Italy, September 30–October 4, 1995) reported that "about 50%" of a small series of patients who had failed either fluoxetine 40 mg/day or sertraline 200 mg/day became "responders" within a month when CMI 75 mg/day was added. Since CMI 75 mg/day may itself be effective for some patients, and the SSRIs may have raised plasma CMI levels, these results may simply reflect the effectiveness of CMI. Ravizza et al. (1996b) randomly assigned patients who had failed to respond adequately to six months of CMI 150 mg/day to eight weeks of either increasing the dose to 250 mg/day ($n = 11$) or adding sertraline 50 mg/day ($n = 13$). Adverse events and the rate of drop out for side effects were significantly higher in the CMI group. Although the proportion of responders (Y–BOCS decrease of $\geq$ 35% and CGI much or very much improved) in the two groups was not significantly different, 38.5% of the sertraline group were responders compared to 18.2% of the CMI group. Since 50 mg/day of sertraline by itself is an effective anti-OCD regimen, these results may reflect the effectiveness of sertraline.

In a randomized, open-label, 90-day trial in patients who had failed adequate trials of CMI and fluoxetine, nine of nine patients assigned to CMI 150 mg/day plus citalopram 40 mg day experienced a $\geq$ 35% decrease in Y–BOCS scores compared to only one of seven assigned to citalopram alone (Pallanti et al., 1998). CMI plasma levels were not measured, but citalopram does not strongly inhibit the hepatic enzymes that metabolize CMI (see Chapter 4).

If a trial of combining CMI and an SSRI is elected, plasma levels of CMI and desmethylclomipramine (DCMI) should be assayed and pulse rates and blood pressure should be monitored; obtaining a screening ECG may be advisable, especially in patients suspected of having heart disease or over the age of 40. On the basis of the results of our work with intravenous CMI (discussed below), I attempt to bring the plasma CMI level to 225 ng/ml or more, while keeping the total plasma concentration of CMI and DCMI below 450 ng/ml to avoid cardiac and central nervous system toxicity (see Chapter 2). I usually utilize a combination of fluvoxamine 75–150 mg/day and CMI 100–150 mg/day to achieve these plasma levels. Fluvoxamine inhibits the conversion of CMI to DCMI, raising plasma CMI levels about four-fold while keeping DCMI levels low (Szegedi et al., 1996). When adding CMI to fluvoxamine (or another SSRI), I lower the fluvoxamine dose to 100 mg/day. After allowing five days for steady state to occur, I add CMI 50 mg/day and increase the dose weekly by 25–50 mg/day to the target dose, measuring plasma levels two to three weeks after a dose of 100 mg/day is reached. The combination is usually well tolerated and has been effective in patients who have failed or been intolerant of CMI alone or multiple SSRIs alone. Double-blind, placebo-controlled trials are needed to evaluate the efficacy of adding CMI to an SSRI in patients who are either partial responders or treatment refractory.

Pharmacological treatment of refractory cases

Estimates of the proportion of patients whose OCD does not respond satisfactorily after several medication trials range from 20% (Jenike and Rauch, 1994) to 40% (Rasmussen, Eisen and Pato, 1993; Piccinelli et al., 1995). Alternative strategies include the *augmentation approaches* described earlier; alternative agents such as monotherapies, and alternative routes of administration as well as behavioral and neurosurgical approaches, are discussed subsequently. The most promising pharmacotherapy interventions in treatment-refractory patients appear to be the addition of *risperidone* and the use of *intravenous clomipramine*, which is experimental in the United States. Other approaches include *phenelzine monotherapy*, *clonazepam monotherapy*, and the use of *intermittent oral morphine*.

Risperidone

Risperidone is a potent and selective 5-HT$_2$ receptor antagonist as well as an antagonist at α_1, α_2, histamine-1 and dopamine D$_2$ sites; it is a weak antagonist at the dopamine D$_1$ site blocked by older neuroleptics. The addition of risperidone to an SRI in treatment-refractory OCD has been strikingly effective in reports totalling more than 50 patients (Jacobsen, 1995; McDougle et al., 1995b; Ravizza et al., 1996b; Saxena et al., 1996; Stein et al., 1997a). In one open study, seven of eight patients with comorbid schizoaffective disorder ($n=4$), schizophrenia ($n=2$) or schizotypal PD ($n=2$) and 7 of 14 patients with other comorbid conditions improved within two to three weeks after risperidone 0.5–8 mg/day (mean $=2.75$ mg/day) (Saxena et al., 1996) was added to an SSRI. In the second open trial, risperidone 3 mg/day added for eight weeks to clomipramine 250 mg/day ($n=7$) or clomipramine 150 mg/day plus sertraline 50 mg/day ($n=7$) was associated with statistically significant decreases in Y–BOCS scores (20% and 28% in the two groups) (Ravizza et al., 1996b). Akathisia, drowsiness and weight gain may be intolerable side effects.

My usual practice is to begin risperidone at 0.5 mg daily for one week and increase the dose by 0.5–1.0 mg weekly to a maximum dose of 6 mg/day, although in nonpsychotic patients I have never reached that dose before benefit or intolerable side effects interrupted the progression. A four-week trial at the maximum tolerated dose should be adequate to determine efficacy. Because fluoxetine, paroxetine and sertraline inhibit the CYP 2D6 hepatic isoenzyme that metabolizes risperidone, careful attention to side effects is in order when risperidone is added to these drugs. Whether olanzapine, which has a somewhat different profile of receptor blockade, will prove as effective as risperidone remains to be seen.

Phenelzine

A 12-week, double-blind comparison of the MAOI (monoamine oxidase inhibitor) phenelzine 75 mg/day ($n = 14$) and clomipramine 225 mg/day ($n = 16$) found the two drugs equally effective (7 responders in each group) (Vallejo et al., 1992). However, a 10-week, placebo-controlled comparison of phenelzine 60 mg/day and fluoxetine 80 mg/day found phenelzine no more effective than placebo (Jenike et al., 1997). Noting that 7 of 20 phenelzine-treated patients (35%) were responders and six of these patients had symmetry obsessions, the authors suggested that a phenelzine trial might be considered for patients with symmetry obsessions who have failed several SRI trials. In contrast to case reports of positive OCD response to MAOIs, high anxiety did not predict a response to phenelzine. Additional controlled trials are needed to establish phenelzine's place in the treatment of OCD.

Intravenous clomipramine (CMI)

Although available in Europe and Canada, intravenous CMI is experimental in the United States and is only available at a few institutions. Data from case series and a double-blind, controlled trial suggest that intravenously administered CMI reduces OCD symptoms much more quickly than oral CMI and is better tolerated. Warneke (1984, 1985, 1989) reported moderate to marked improvement in nine patients toward the end of 14 daily infusions or shortly thereafter, and stated that about half of his 30 patients experienced "moderate to marked improvement." Fallon et al. (1992) reported a 39% mean decrease in symptom scores in three of five patients after 14 consecutive weekday infusions. Patients unable to tolerate adequate doses of oral CMI easily tolerated intravenous CMI.

In an open trial, five patients treated with gradually increased doses of intravenous CMI improved to a marked degree within four weeks, i.e., almost twice as fast as is usual in trials of oral CMI (Koran, Faravelli and Pallanti, 1994). In a double-blind trial of pulse loaded intravenous versus oral CMI, six of seven patients given intravenous but only one of eight given oral CMI responded to the drug (Koran, Sallee and Pallanti, 1997). After eight weeks of oral CMI, four of the six intravenous responders continued their improvement, but patients who had responded to pulse loading did not improve statistically significantly by endpoint more than those who had not. Additional controlled trials are needed to determine whether intravenous pulse loading of CMI is a valuable new treatment for treatment-refractory patients.

Oral Morphine

Warneke (1997) reports that oral morphine in doses of 20–40 mg every five to eight days brought marked benefit to five "end-stage" OCD patients. None of the patients became euphoric, and the intermittent dosing schedule minimizes a risk of physiological addiction or dependence. In one patient, pentazocine and propoxyphene had had no effect. On the basis of Warneke's observations, I administered oral codeine 30 mg twice daily to two patients in a double-blind crossover trial with two-week phases, using lorazepam 1 mg twice daily as the comparison agent. One patient responded and has continued to benefit from this regimen, but must discontinue codeine for three to five days after a week of use because tolerance develops. The therapeutic effect, marked diminution in obsessions and a markedly increased ability to discard hoarded items, persists for three to four hours after each dose. Warneke (1997) notes that opioid receptors are found in the striatal system (particularly the caudate nuclei). (See the earlier section 'Biological models'.) Complementing Warneke's observation is the report that double-blind, placebo-controlled administration of intravenous naloxone (0.3 mg/kg) produced an acute exacerbation of OCD symptoms in two patients (Insel and Pickar, 1983). However, in a subsequent study of 13 patients, double-blind infusion of naloxone 0.175 mg/kg exacerbated OCD symptoms in only three patients (Keuler et al., 1996). These observations support proceeding with very carefully controlled trials of intermittent oral morphine in treatment-refractory patients.

Clozapine

None of 10 treatment refractory patients, including two with chronic motor tic disorder, responded to a 10-week, open-label trial of clozapine (mean dose = 462.5 mg/day) (McDougle et al., 1995a).

Adding desipramine

In a six-week, double-blind, placebo-controlled trial involving 33 SSRI-refractory patients, desipramine added in doses sufficient to produce plasma levels ≥ 125 ng/ml produced no clinically meaningful reduction in OCD or depressive symptoms (Barr et al., 1997). The data suggest that inhibition of norepinephrine reuptake is not critical to clomipramine's effectiveness in OCD. This study also raises questions about the effectiveness of tricyclic antidepressants in treating comorbid depression in treatment-refractory OCD (See Chapter 2). A study in a less selected group of patients, however, found that comorbid depression responded to imipramine (Foa et al., 1992).

Trazodone

Although case reports have suggested efficacy for trazodone, especially in doses of 500 mg/day (Hermesh, Aizenberg and Munitz, 1990), a double-blind, placebo controlled 10-week trial of trazodone (mean dose = 235 mg/day) found no difference in OCD or depression ratings in the two treatment groups (Pigott et al., 1992b). Given the availability of many effective agents with more tolerable side effect profiles than high-dose trazodone, there seems little reason to pursue trials of this strategy.

Neurosurgical interventions

Expert opinion reserves consideration of neurosurgical intervention to treatment-refractory, severely and chronically ill patients who have not responded to all conventional pharmacological and behavioral treatments (Baer et al., 1995; March et al., 1997). Stereotactic neurosurgical procedures, described earlier, include anterior cingulotomy, anterior capsulotomy, subcaudate tractotomy and limbic leukotomy (tractotomy plus anterior cingulotomy). No well-controlled, parallel group comparisons of safety and efficacy are available.

Follow-up studies in the 1960s and 1970s suggested that half to two-thirds of patients were much or very much improved (Mindus and Jenike, 1992). This improvement rate may be spuriously high; many patients were probably not treatment-refractory by current standards. None of the neurosurgical procedures just listed seemed clearly superior. Retrospective reviews suggest that the risks of acute surgical complications, post-operative epilepsy, adverse personality change and suicide are quite small.

In the United States, a retrospective follow-up of 33 treatment-refractory patients who underwent cingulotomy at the Massachusetts General Hospital between 1965 and 1986 found that 25%–30% benefitted substantially (Jenike et al., 1991a). None had serious, persistent, neurological, intellectual, personality or behavioral deficits attributable to the surgery. These investigators recently performed a prospective follow-up of 18 additional patients undergoing cingulotomy (Baer et al., 1995). Five of 18 patients (28%) were responders (decrease in Y–BOCS score of ≥ 35% and a CGI score of much or very much improved, not attributable to any intervening treatment) when evaluated a mean of 27 months later. Seven patients had undergone two cingulotomies and one patient three cingulotomies. Again, few serious adverse effects were noted, in particular, there were no instances of epilepsy or suicide.

A retrospective follow-up of 16 patients who underwent ventromedial frontal leukotomy involving several lesion sites found that most subjects' OCD symptoms were substantially improved (Irle et al., 1998). However, 8 of 11 subjects with lesions in the ventral striatum developed substance dependence postoperatively.

To date, ethical considerations surrounding the risks associated with opening the skull have prevented controlled trials comparing the efficacy of sham and actual neurosurgical procedures. The introduction of the gamma knife, a radiosurgical device that creates destructive lesions by focussing gamma rays from more than 200 cobalt[60] emitting sites, will ameliorate the ethical dilemma (Rasmussen and Eisen, 1997). Unpublished pilot data suggest that 40%–50% of treatment-refractory patients receiving gamma knife capsulotomy benefitted without experiencing significant side effects (Rasmussen and Eisen, 1997).

Clinicians wishing to refer an apparently treatment-refractory patient for neurosurgical intervention should consult the review by Mindus and Jenike (1992) for information regarding selection guidelines, indications, contraindications, probable outcome, risks and preoperative workup. The next step would be to contact the multidisciplinary review committee at an institution that is well experienced with these procedures in order to learn about contemporary eligibility criteria, risks and benefits. These institutions include: Massachusetts General Hospital in Boston, MA and Rhode Island Hospital in Providence, RI in the United States; Karolinska Institute in Stockholm, Sweden; Priory Hospital in London, England; The Prince Henry Hospital, Little Bay, Sydney, Australia; and, the Department of Neurosurgery, University of Göttingen, Göttingen, Germany.

Inpatient treatment and partial hospitalization

Inpatient treatment and partial hospitalization programs encompassing weeks or months of treatment have reportedly been helpful for patients with severe, treatment-refractory OCD, and should be considered for such cases (Megens and Vandereycken, 1988; Calvocoressi et al., 1993; Bystritsky et al., 1996). Few such programs exist, however. Patients described in published series often suffered from noncompliance with outpatient treatment, impaired self-care ability, potentially self-injurious behavior or severe disruption of the home environment as a result of symptomatic behavior (Calvocoressi et al., 1993). These programs are multimodal, combining careful physical, neurological, psychological and social assessments with medication management, cognitive-behavioral therapy, education about OCD, and interventions aimed at dependency or control issues, social skill deficits and family issues. Detailed program descriptions are provided in the references just cited. The cost-effectiveness of such programs deserves study before they are choked off by arbitrary limitation of insurance benefits.

Special symptoms

Clinicians should be aware of the management of certain less common symptoms of OCD.

Bowel obsessions

Bowel obsessions center on fears of fecal incontinence; urinary incontinence is an alternative focus. Patients with these obsessions often spend long hours on the toilet and may avoid leaving home or interacting socially because they fear public humiliation or fear that public bathrooms will not be readily available. Case reports note successful treatment of bowel obsessions with ERP (exposure and response prevention) (Hatch, 1997), as well as pharmacotherapies that include imipramine (Jenike et al., 1987), trazodone (Ramchandani, 1990), nortriptyline (Lyketsos, 1992) and clomipramine (Kahne and Wray, 1989; Sharma, 1991). The response to drugs other than SRIs suggests that this symptom is not always a manifestation of OCD.

Moral or religious scrupulosity

Ciarrocchi (1995) has defined scrupulosity as "seeing sin where there is none." Fallon et al. (1990) define it as "excessive observance of moral or religious teachings" compared to the expectations of the person's peers and to realistically achievable observance. Their series of 10 patients suggests that scrupulosity responds as well as other OCD symptoms to pharmacotherapy, although in my experience and that of others (Markowitz, 1994), the patient may obsess about whether taking medication is morally acceptable. Ciarrocchi (1995) has written a very useful clinical guide for sufferers and clinicians. The book describes historical cases of scrupulosity including the "case" John Bunyan; provides detailed instructions, aids and clinical examples aimed at helping patients identify and overcome symptoms; and, analyzes moral reasoning to assist patients in reviewing moral teachings without becoming lost in obsessions.

Hoarding

Hoarding behavior can be defined as collecting and being unable to discard excessive quantities of goods or objects that are of limited value or worthless. Greenberg (1987) describes four compulsive hoarders who came to psychiatric attention because of family members' complaints. All strenuously resisted attempts to change their behavior or to discard any hoarded materials. Hoarding behavior has also been described in the context of autism (McDougle et al., 1995c), schizophrenia (Greenberg, Witzum and Levy, 1990; Luchins et al., 1992), dementia (Greenberg et al., 1990), anorexia nervosa (Frankenburg, 1984), Prader–Willi syndrome (Hellings and Warnock, 1994) and the frontal lobe syndrome (Sebit, Acuda and Chibanda, 1996).

Frost and Gross (1993) studied 32 respondents to an advertisement for "pack-rats or chronic savers." Hoarding behavior was ego-syntonic in most cases, although most individuals had tried unsuccessfully to stop because of problems such as inability to invite people to their homes and conflicts with relatives. Most began hoarding in childhood or adolescence. Examining an additional 20 respondents, Frost et al. (1995) suggested that the most important motives for hoarding were indecisiveness, concerns about discarding useful items, excessive concern about future needs and sentimental attachment to possessions.

DSM-IV mentions hoarding behavior only as a criterion for OCPD. Nonetheless, hoarding is a common symptom in OCD (Table 3.3). Hoarding is not limited to Anglo-American cultures: "hoarding/saving obsessions" were present in 25% of a series of Egyptian OCD patients (Okasha et al., 1994).

We utilized semi-structured interview methods to gather data from 9 women and 11 men with hoarding compulsions (Winsberg, Cassic and Koran, 1999). Hoarding began over a wide age range: from age 5 to age 46 years (mean age = 20 years); hoarding began before other OCD symptoms in 11 patients. The most commonly hoarded items were newspapers and magazines, junk mail, old clothes, notes or lists and old receipts. Hoarded material occupied from one room and all closets to more than one room together with all closets, the garage and yard. Seven patients rented additional storage space for hoarded items. A striking 80% of these patients grew up in a household where someone else hoarded. The most frequent primary motives for hoarding were the fear of discarding something useful or something that would be needed in the future. Lifetime prevalence of major depression and of impulse control disorders, especially compulsive shopping, were high; only three patients met DSM-IV criteria for OCPD.

For the vast majority, hoarding substantially impaired social relationships and caused substantial distress. Family members were angry at having to live amid clutter and at being embarrassed when friends visited. Some patients invited no one to their homes and because of embarrassment, would not let their children invite friends in. Some did not date because they felt no one would understand. Some could not work because collecting items took so much of their time.

Response of hoarding to SRI treatment was less robust than is expected for OCD. ERP combined with medication seemed more effective. I use the following general approach:

- Assess the magnitude of the problem. Ask the patient to bring photographs of the rooms or spaces cluttered with hoarded material so that you can together plan a gradual attack. Failing this, ask for a very detailed room-by-room description of the hoard.
- Assess and strengthen the patient's motivation for treatment. Ask the patient to list and analyze with you the advantages and disadvantages of hoarding.

- Pick a starting point. The patient should select a room in which to begin, and within the room, a class of items or an area with which to start, e.g., papers, boxes, clothes, or gifts. Adhere to the ERP principle of starting with items low on the anxiety hierarchy.
- Obtain a specific commitment. Ask the patient to commit either to spending an agreed upon length of time or to discarding an agreed upon quantity of material each day (or nearly every day) until the next visit.
- Bring order to chaos. Encourage the patient to sort items into "keep," "discard/recycle/give away," and "cannot decide." This last pile must be small. The "discard" pile is to be dealt with daily or every few days if at all possible.
- Prevent continued accumulation. Enjoin the patient not to accumulate more material during the debulking process. This may mean dealing with the incoming mail daily, terminating newspaper or magazine subscriptions, and avoiding stores or shopping malls unless accompanied by a family member aware of the treatment process.
- Empower the family. When a supportive family member shares the patient's living space, make that person a part of the treatment team. Empower the family member to discard an agreed upon amount of material daily if the patient fails to keep his bargain. This is highly motivating, since patients usually prefer to decide which items will be discarded.
- Document progress. Periodically request new photographs or descriptions, praise the patient generously for progress made and acknowledge repeatedly how difficult it is to confront these decisions.

  Cognitive therapy, e.g., teaching the patient decision-making skills, reframing junk mail as "someone is trying to sell you something," helping the patient realistically estimate how much of an item can be used in a reasonable amount of time, and so on, can be helpful. Many patients who lack and do not develop insight respond nonetheless to the program outlined above. Patience is essential; the process of debulking may take more than a year.

Intrusive music

Pupko (1997) has reviewed the literature regarding this unusual symptom. The patient experiences repetitive phrases, tunes or complex musical pieces that originate inside the head, i.e., are pseudohallucinations, for periods lasting from seconds to days. Advertising jingles or popular tunes are common triggers. Organic causes of musical hallucinations should be ruled out, including unilateral or bilateral deafness (Gordon, 1994) and temporal lobe epilepsy (Erkwoh, 1993). Treatment with clomipramine (Cameron and Wasielewski, 1990) or an SSRI may be helpful. One of my patients experienced a substantial, sustained response when taking fluoxetine 40 mg/day.

Obsessional slowness

Veale (1993) reviewed the literature concerning obsessional slowness and noted that it was originally described as "a meticulous concern for orderliness." The patient takes hours to complete ordinary self-care tasks such as dressing or grooming because each task must be performed correctly, in sequence and "just right," or because of a need to concentrate intently on suppressing or neutralizing obsessional thoughts. Veale believes obsessional slowness is a result of the patient's compulsion to avoid disorder, inexactness and lack of meticulousness, but others regard it as an independent symptom because it persists after other OCD symptoms have improved (Takeuchi et al., 1997). Behavioral treatment with pacing, prompting and modelling produces only transitory change. Veale (1993) recommends gradual exposure to disorder and inexactness, with response prevention. In the absence of data, trials of this approach and of standard pharmacotherapies are reasonable.

Psychotherapy

Among the psychotherapies, only ERP in vivo has been found in multiple trials to be effective in treating OCD. Both components, exposure to feared situations or thoughts and the prevention of rituals, whether physical or mental, are necessary to maximize treatment response (Foa, Steketee and Ozarow, 1985). Clinicians who have not been trained in this approach can readily learn the basic principles and apply them for their patients' benefit. Detailed instruction is available elsewhere (see Baer and Minichiello, 1990; Riggs and Foa, 1993; and excellent self-help books listed in Appendix 1, e.g., Baer, 1991; Foa and Wilson, 1991; Steketee and White, 1990). In addition, the OC Foundation (Appendix 1) sponsors training courses for clinicians. As noted earlier, educating the patient and the family regarding the nature and treatment of OCD is always a first step in therapy and precedes attempts to engage the patient in ERP (see educational materials in Appendix 1).

A meta-analysis of 16 studies of ERP conducted between 1974 and 1992 reported that an average of 76% of patients (range 50%–100%) were still responders at a mean follow-up time of 29 months (range 6–72 months) (Foa and Kozak, 1996). (The means are weighted by the number of subjects in each study.) Most "responders" were much or very much improved, and some experienced complete freedom from symptoms. Most studies involved 10–15, one- to two-hour treatment sessions conducted over 3 to 12 weeks, but the range of treatment intensity (session number, frequency, duration, assignment of homework, therapist and family involvement in exposure, and inpatient/outpatient setting) was wide.

Several caveats are in order before accepting these encouraging outcome figures uncritically. First, few of these studies included a control group that did not receive ERP. Second, each study was small (20 or fewer patients in half the studies). Third, the vast majority of patients in these studies, and in other studies investigating ERP treatment for OCD (Ball, Baer and Otto, 1996), suffered from cleaning and/or checking compulsions. Whether these results can be transferred to patients with multiple types of compulsions, or compulsions such as hoarding, ordering, repeating, counting and seeking "just right" sensations, is unknown. Moreover, ERP is more difficult to apply to patients with obsessions alone, and cognitive-behavioral interventions are still in an early stage of development (Van Oppen and Arntz, 1993; Freeston, Rhéaume and Ladouceur, 1996). Fourth, some patients received treatments during the follow-up periods and some provided no information regarding intervening treatments. Fifth, experienced investigators estimate that 20%–30% of OCD patients are unresponsive to ERP and an additional 20% drop out of treatment before attaining much benefit (Emmelkamp, 1982; Jenike, 1992). Finally, the likelihood that ERP or other forms of behavior therapy will benefit patients unresponsive to medications is unknown.

These caveats notwithstanding, ERP is an effective treatment for many OCD patients and should be strongly considered in treatment planning for the vast majority. Most studies (Foa et al., 1985; Keijsers et al., 1994), but not all (Foa et al., 1992) suggest that the presence of major depression adversely affects the outcome of ERP, perhaps because exposure does not produce extinction of the patient's anxiety.

Acute treatment

One begins by obtaining a description of the patient's obsessions and compulsions and their relationship to provoking cues, situations or events. The clinician should explore with the patient the obsessive thoughts, images and urges eliciting the anxiety that induces the patient's compulsions. The patient is likely to believe that (Freeston et al., 1996):

- He is primarily or mostly or even totally responsible for events whose occurrence he fears.
- Thoughts are extremely important and powerful ("if I think it, it will happen"), i.e., magical thinking is present.
- The probability of negative or feared events occurring is (unrealistically) high.
- Uncertainty is intolerable.
- Perfect order, control or completeness is necessary (in order to avoid some feared outcome).
- Anxiety is unacceptable or dangerous.

The clinician should ascertain the patient's degree of insight into the irrationality of his doubts, fears and rituals, since this may influence willingness to cooperate in ERP. Several studies, however, report that patients with little or no insight or with overvalued ideas are as likely to respond to ERP as those with insight intact, once they consent to treatment (Lelliott et al., 1988; Hoogduin et al., 1989). The clinician must also determine in what ways and to what extent the patient's family members are facilitating his symptomatic behavior. For example, a family member may be repeatedly providing requested reassurances or agreeing to wash excessively or carry out the patient's bedtime checking routine so that the patient "can get some rest." In these cases, it will be necessary to intervene with the family as well as the patient.

After obtaining a good understanding of the symptoms, the clinician should guide the patient in creating a list of target symptoms (using the Y–BOCS Symptom Checklist, for example). The list is then divided into two, one list containing items or situations that are avoided because they provoke obsessions or compulsions, and the other containing the provoked compulsions or rituals. The clinicians should ask the patient to rearrange each list in a hierarchy, with the least anxiety-provoking items at the top and the most anxiety-provoking at the bottom. Exposure, planning and review sessions can then be scheduled from daily (e.g., in a partial hospitalization program) to weekly or less often, but often enough to keep up pressure for behavioral change. During each session the clinician can proceed as follows:

- Ask the patient to choose a cue that provokes mild to moderate anxiety for a trial of exposure in vivo coupled with refraining, for one to two hours, from performing the usual anxiety-relieving compulsion. In very severe cases, it may be necessary to start with shorter periods of refraining, perhaps lasting only a few minutes.

- Prepare a written, detailed, ERP homework assignment and discuss with the patient how he will carry it out, what rationalizations will tempt him to postpone exposure, and how these will be dealt with. In some cases, engaging the patient's family member in the behavioral change process may be necessary or desirable.

- Explain that daily ERP, preferably several times daily, is needed in order to break the connection between the stimulus or cue and the provoked anxiety. I tell the patient that he will actually feel worse, i.e., more anxious or distressed, during the first few exposures and must be willing to tolerate this increased anxiety without performing a ritual in order for the anxiety to dissipate on its own. It seems helpful to phrase the situation: "Your body must learn that nothing terrible will really happen; with repeated exposures, the intensity of the fear will gradually decrease to little or none."

- Inform the patient that it may take a week or somewhat more for the anxiety associated with the exposure situation to be reduced to mild levels. Explain that one must change behavior first; anxiety or distress will change about a week later; and, obsessions or thoughts concerning the exposure situation will fade significantly after about a month (Baer and Minichiello, 1990).

- Move on to a more anxiety-provoking cue or situation only after the current one has been successfully treated.

The literature concerning ERP treatment, albeit composed mostly of uncontrolled observations or studies with little statistical power to identify even large differences between groups, suggests that the therapist need not model the desired behaviors, that prolonged exposure with response prevention (i.e., an hour or more) is more effective than the same total time divided into multiple brief exposure periods, and that each feared item and compulsion must be treated specifically (benefits do not generalize across symptoms) (Foa et al., 1985). Nonetheless, in beginning treatment with patients who are severely anxious, the clinician may initially have to accompany the patient in the exposure exercise, e.g., accompanying the patient to a "contaminated" site or store.

Enhancing long-term outcome

Expert behavioral therapists urge the use of relapse prevention procedures once the acute treatment has been completed. For a fully recovered patient, experts favor monthly visits for the next three to six months; for the partially recovered patient, weekly or monthly visits for three to six months are equally favored (March et al., 1997).

Foa and Kozak (1996) believe that supplementing ERP with exposure in imagination to feared consequences enhances long-term outcome. In addition, they recommend: teaching patients to distinguish between a lapse and a relapse; encouraging them to engage in posttreatment exposure and in analysis of distorted cognitions; engaging the family in supportive activities; and, contacting the patient periodically by telephone to check on continued response.

Treating patients with obsessions only

Pharmacotherapy with an SRI is likely to be effective, but pursuing augmentation strategies may be necessary. If a cognitive therapy approach is elected, case reports or small series suggest several options, but none has been demonstrated effective in large, well-controlled trials.

Satiation involves exposing the patient to obsessional thoughts for prolonged periods until they loose their power to elicit anxiety. A convenient way to do this is to ask the patient to prepare a written script of his obsessions and then record it on an endless loop tape. Then instruct the patient to listen to the tape for a specified period each day. Similarly, in imaginal flooding, the clinician encourages the patient to bring his obsessional material to mind in daily sessions, intensify its terribleness or repugnance and dwell on it for periods of minutes to an hour or more. This technique is not recommended for patients with defective reality testing, e.g., schizotypal patients (Baer and Minichiello, 1990).

Thought stopping involves teaching the patient to shout "STOP!" mentally whenever he begins to obsess. The clinician begins by asking the patient to relax

Table 3.6. Obsessive–compulsive disorder: treatment planning guidelines

- Assess the patient's degree of insight and motivation for treatment.
- Assess and treat comorbid mood, anxiety and substance use disorders.
- Assess for comorbid tic disorder and schizotypal personality disorder. If either is present, successful pharmacotherapy may require a neuroleptic combined with a serotonin reuptake inhibitor (SRI).
- Identify and explore OCD symptoms (e.g., with the Y–BOCS Symptom Checklist).
- Measure baseline severity of OCD (Y–BOCS).
- Educate the patient and concerned others about OCD and its treatment.
- Consider a trial of exposure and response prevention (ERP), an SRI, or combined ERP and SRI treatment (depending on the patient's needs, preferences, capacities, situation and history). An adequate SRI trial requires 10–12 weeks, and at least six weeks at maximum tolerated dose.
- Maintain effective pharmacotherapy long-term, but consider tapering the dose slowly after stable improvement has been achieved.
- For patients with a partial response to pharmacotherapy, consider augmentation with ERP or an augmenting agent.
- For patients with a partial response to ERP, consider adding an SRI and/or more intensive or modified ERP, including cognitive techniques.
- Consider the need for couple or family therapy to address complicity.
- Institute psychotherapy for functional deficits and life issues.
- For treatment-refractory patients, consider augmentation as above, inpatient treatment, clonazepam monotherapy, phenelzine, intravenous clomipramine (experimental), other augmenting or experimental agents and, after exhausting options, neurosurgery.
- Arrange for maintenance treatment and utilize relapse prevention strategies.

Note:
Y–BOCS: Yale–Brown Obsessive–Compulsive Scale.

and then signal when obsessions or anxious rumination begins. The clinician then loudly says, "STOP!" The procedure is repeated some number of times and the patient is encouraged to take over the responsibility for the verbal command, audibly at first, and later simply in the mind.

Postponement involves encouraging the patient to respond to the start of an obsession with an internal agreement that he will deal with it later, e.g., in the last 10 minutes of every hour, or from 4 p.m. to 6 p.m.

Schwartz (1996), in a book written for patients, recommends four cognitive steps which he terms the "brain lock" approach. These techniques are designed to complement ERP. Patients are taught: to relabel the obsessive or compulsive experience as symptomatic of OCD rather than reflecting their essential selves; to recognize that the symptom is occurring because of brain activity rather than because of real, external threats; to refocus their attention on something other than the immediate obsession or compulsion; and, to devalue the obsessive ideation as "worthless garbage." The book can be recommended to patients, but appears to overestimate the proportion who can do without short- or long-term pharmacotherapy.

Finally, Freeston et al., (1996) and Freeston and Ladouceur (1997) provide detailed, creative interventions for the categories of distorted beliefs described earlier. They utilize logical analysis to attack magical thinking, or may demonstrate the irrationality of magical thinking by asking the patient to use thoughts alone to make an appliance break or kill a goldfish. They challenge the assumption that thoughts are morally equivalent to actions. They invite the patient to examine his degree of responsibility by alternately playing the prosecuting and defending attorneys arguing about the evidence. They help the patient analyze the advantages and disadvantages of perfectionism. Their clinical examples are intriguing and encouraging. Clinicians can try their suggested approaches while awaiting the results of controlled trials.

Table 3.6 summarizes the pharmacotherapy and behavioral treatment approaches described in this chapter.

4

Managing the side effects of serotonergic drugs

For in diseases of the mind, as well as in all other ailments, it is an art of no little importance to administer medicines properly.

Philippe Pinel (1745–1826). *A Treatise on Insanity.*

The side effects of selective serotonin reuptake inhibitors (SSRIs) are generally more easily tolerated than those of earlier generations of antidepressants. Nonetheless, SSRI side effects can cause noncompliance or reluctantly prescribed changes in pharmacotherapy. This chapter aims at minimizing these undesirable outcomes and is divided for this purpose into seven sections:
- General principles of side-effect management.
- Managing side effects of specific drugs.
- Interactions of SSRIs with other drugs.
- Managing the serotonin syndrome.
- Managing SSRI sexual side effects.
- Use of psychotropic drugs in pregnancy and the puerperium.
- Managing SSRI withdrawal symptoms.

Because few controlled trials of side-effect management strategies have been published, the suggestions that follow are derived largely from uncontrolled published observations and my clinical experience. Their rates of efficacy are unknown. Before adding a medication to an SRI (serotonin reuptake inhibitor) in order to manage side effects, the clinician should consult this chapter's section describing the interactions of SSRIs with other drugs. Interactions may occur that have not been documented in the case reports of successful side-effect management.

General principles

Despite the plethora of possible drug side effects, the clinician can apply certain general principles to their prevention and management (McElroy, Keck and Friedman, 1995). Like principles pertinent to treatment planning, these generalities must be artfully tailored to the individual circumstance.

- Educate patients and concerned family members about the medication's most frequent side effects to prevent anxiety-provoking surprises. This will usually enhance compliance.
- Educate patients about common sense strategies to minimize side effects, such as taking certain medications with meals to decrease stomach upset, taking stimulating medications in the morning and soporific drugs at bedtime, and dividing total daily doses into two or more portions.
- Inform patients that we cannot predict who will experience a given side effect, and encourage them to telephone if questions arise before the next scheduled visit. This usually prevents patients from ill advisedly discontinuing medications.
- Elicit patients' concerns about the medication, such as whether it is "addicting," must be taken "for the rest of my life," or can be taken during pregnancy.
- At each visit, ask whether the patient is experiencing any side effects. Always listen to the answer, even when it is unwelcome. The patients' complaint may be a genuine side effect, even if the physician has never before heard of its association with the prescribed drug. Since rare events do occur, I like to consult various sources, e.g., the *Physicians' Desk Reference* (Medical Economics Company, 1998), *Drug Interactions in Psychiatry* (Ciraulo, Shader, Greenblatt and Creelman, 1995), and on-line medical literature searches before reaching a conclusion. Of course, the patient's complaint may stem from the underlying psychiatric condition, from anxiety about taking medications, from a comorbid psychiatric or medical condition or from a placebo effect.
- One can try slowly increasing the dose, reducing the dose, or switching drugs to prevent or manage almost any side effect. These strategies are not repeatedly mentioned, but should be kept in mind.

Side effects of individual drugs

The side effects of each medication are considered within an alphabetized list of organ systems and are discussed in alphabetical order. Table 4.1 provides a guide. For side effects shown in boldface type in the Table, management suggestions are provided in the text; for those shown in standard typeface in the Table, literature citations only are given in the text. For more extensive lists of side effects, the reader is referred to the latest edition of the *Physicians' Desk Reference* (Medical Economics Company, 1998) or a comparable source. Both common and uncommon side effects are considered. The common ones were selected because management by strategies other than slowly increasing the dose, reducing the dose or switching medications may be effective; the uncommon ones are clinically important or of interest.

Side effects are defined as "common," if they are reported to affect 5% or more of patients, or occur substantially more often than in placebo control groups, i.e.,

Table 4.1. Guide to side effects discussed in association with particular drugs

Body system	Drug				
	Clomipramine	Fluoxetine	Fluvoxamine	Paroxetine	Sertraline
Body as a whole	**weight gain**				
Cardiovascular	**hypotension**	bradycardia hypertension			
Digestive	**constipation dry mouth nausea**	**bruxism** nausea			**diarrhea**
Endocrine		**hyponatremia**		hyponatremia	breast tenderness
Hemic, lymphatic		bleeding bruising		**bleeding**	
Musculoskeletal	**myoclonus**				
Nervous	**blurred vision drowsiness** seizures **tremor**	**agitation restlessness apathy** extrapyramidal symptoms **headache insomnia myoclonus mania memory impairment**	extrapyramidal symptoms mania	dystonia	**akathisia** dystonia speech blockage

Table 4.1 (*cont.*)

Body system	Drug				
	Clomipramine	Fluoxetine	Fluvoxamine	Paroxetine	Sertraline
Nervous (*cont.*)		sedation			
		stuttering			
Respiratory	yawning	yawning			
Skin, appendages		**hair loss**	hair loss		hair loss
Urogenital	**difficulty urinating**	**frequent urination**			

Notes:

Management suggestions are provided in the text for side effects shown in bold typeface.

Only literature citations are provided in the text for side effects shown in ordinary typeface.

at least 1.5 times as often. This information is taken from the *Physicians' Desk Reference* (Medical Economics Company, 1998). The specific rates reported there, however, do not reflect accurately the rates to be expected in clinical practice, since they are based on clinical trials in which patients are carefully selected and side effects are not systematically investigated. Naturally, elderly patients and patients with concomitant medical disorders are at higher risk for many common and uncommon side effects. When prescribing for such patients, greater caution, more vigorous patient education and greater vigilance are required.

The prevalence of "uncommon" side effects is unknown, since knowledge of their existence often comes from case reports. Causality is usually less than certain in these reports, but I have tried to balance skepticism with a sensitivity to early warnings. Rather than repeatedly discussing an uncommon side effect associated with more than one SSRI, it is discussed with the SSRI for which the most cases have been reported; citations are provided for cases associated with other SSRIs. Given the SSRIs' shared mechanism of action, case reports linking one SSRI to a metabolic, endocrine or central nervous system side effect indicate the possibility of its occurring with each of the others, although differences in receptor selectivity preclude identical side effect profiles. Patients intolerant of one SSRI may easily tolerate another (Brown and Harrison, 1995).

Since many side effects are related to plasma levels or to the effects of active metabolites and usually appear by the time steady state levels are attained, pharmacokinetic information is provided for the SSRIs and for other medications that are likely to be utilized in treating patients with OCD or OCD spectrum disorders (See Tables 4.2, 4.3 and 4.4).

Buspirone

The most common side effects occurring substantially more often with buspirone than placebo are dizziness, drowsiness, nervousness, nausea and headache.

Citalopram

Citalopram, an SSRI long available in European and other countries for the treatment of depressive disorders (Noble and Benfield, 1997) and OCD (Koponen et al., 1997) has recently been approved in the United States as an antidepressant. When a drug is released in Europe before the United States release, a physician with a United States medical license can legally obtain it from Swiss pharmacies using a prescription blank filled out for an individual patient; the patient's written informed consent to take the "experimental" drug should be documented in the medical record. In European Phase II and III studies, citalopram's most common side effects, occurring substantially more often than in the placebo group, were nausea, dry mouth, somnolence, increased sweating and tremor (Muldoon, 1996).

Table 4.2. Pharmacokinetic comparison of selective serotonin reuptake inhibitors

| | Drug | | | | |
Drug	Citalopram[a]	Fluoxetine	Fluvoxamine	Paroxetine	Sertraline
T_{max} (hours)	2–4	6–8	3–8	5.2	4.5–8.4
Dose-proportional plasma level?	Yes	No	No	No	Yes
$T_{1/2}$ (hours)	33	24–72[b]	15.6	21	26
Metabolite activity	<10%	norfluoxetine (equal)	<10%	<2%	desmethyl-sertraline 6–15%
Metabolite $T_{1/2}$	–	4–16 days	–	–	62–104 hours
Steady state plasma level	~1 week	4–5 weeks	~1 week[c]	10 days[c]	~1 week[c]
Oral dosages available	20 mg 40 mg	10 mg, 20 mg 20 mg/5 ml liquid	25 mg, 50 mg, 100 mg	10 mg, 20 mg, 30 mg, 40 mg	25 mg, 50 mg, 100 mg

Notes:

[a] Noble and Benfield (1997)

[b] After acute administration; 4–6 days after chronic administration.

[c] Elderly patients clear the drug more slowly.

Source: *Physicians' Desk Reference* (Medical Economics Company, 1998).

Table 4.3. Pharmacokinetic comparison of selected antidepressants

	Drug				
	Bupropion	Bupropion-SR (Sustained release)	Mirtazapine	Nefazodone	Venlafaxine
Dose-proportional plasma level?	Yes	Yes	Yes	No	Yes
$T_{1/2}$ (hours)	8–24	21±9	37 (females) 26 (males)	2–4	5±2
Metabolite activity	Several active[a]		Negligible	OH-N[b]	O-DV[c]
Metabolite $T_{1/2}$ (hours)	>24		–	1.5–4.0	11±2
Steady state plasma level	4–8 days	8 days	5 days	4–5 days	3 days
Dosages available	75, 100 mg	100, 125 mg	15, 30 mg	100, 150, 200, 250 mg	25, 37.5, 50, 75, 100 mg

Notes:

[a] Although active metabolites are present at greater concentration than bupropion, their contribution to therapeutic and side effects has not been determined.

[b] OH-nefazodone (OH-N) is pharmacologically similar to nefazodone. The triazoledione metabolite is a 5-HT$_{2A}$ antagonist of uncertain significance. The metabolite, meta-chlorophenylpiperazine (mCPP), is present in low concentration and its actions are antagonized by nefazodone and OH-N.

[c] O-desmethylvenlafaxine (O-DV) is pharmacologically similar to venlafaxine.

Source: Physicians' Desk Reference (Medical Economics Company, 1998).

Table 4.4. Pharmacokinetic comparison of selected anxiolytics

	Drug			
	Buspirone	Alprazolam	Lorazepam	Clonazepam
T_{max} (hours)	0.6–1.5	1–2	2	1–4
Dose-proportional plasma level?[a]	No	Yes	Yes	Yes
$T_{1/2}$ (hours)	2–3	6.3–15.8[b]	12	18.7–39
Metabolite activity	Probably unimportant	Probably unimportant	No	No
Dosages available	5, 10, 15 mg	0.25, 0.5, 1, 2 mg[c]	0.5, 1, 2 mg	0.5, 1, 2 mg

Notes:

[a] Plasma levels and clinical effects of benzodiazepines correlate poorly for a number of reasons, e.g., individual variation in sensitivity; indirect effects on other neurotransmitter systems; tolerance.

[b] 9.0–26.9 hours in the elderly.

[c] also available as 2 mg/ml and 4 mg/ml for IM or IV use.

Source: Physicians' Desk Reference (Medical Economics Company, 1998).

Table 4.5. Clomipramine side effects occurring substantially more often than with placebo

Side effects affecting >50% of patients	
Dizziness	
Dry mouth	
Somnolence	
Tremor	
Other common side effects	
Anxiety	Micturition disorder
Blurred vision	Myoclonus
↓ Concentration	Nausea
Constipation	Paresthesia
Dyspepsia	Postural hypotension
Fatigue	Sexual disorder
Flatulence	↑ Sweating
Flushing	Twitching
Insomnia	Vomiting
Memory impairment	Weight gain

Source: Physicians' Desk Reference (Medical Economics Company, 1998).

Clomipramine

Table 4.5 displays the side effects occurring substantially more often with clomipramine than placebo.

Since clomipramine at doses up to 300 mg/day carries a higher seizure risk than the SSRIs (about 0.6% at 90 days and 1.4% at one year versus 0.1% to 0.2%, (Medical Economics Company, 1998), it should be avoided in patients with risk factors for seizures, and prescribed in doses no greater than 250 mg/day.

Body as a whole

Weight gain may be difficult to manage; increased appetite and craving for sweets are powerful motives. Monitoring weight and advising dietary discretion and increased exercise can be tried, but in my experience are not usually effective. Lowering the clomipramine dose may help, but usually trials of other SRIs are necessary.

Cardiovascular system

Cardiac toxicity, especially arrhythmias, may occur in hyperthyroid patients or those receiving thyroid replacement therapy.

Orthostatic hypotension, with attendant dizziness or light headedness, results from α_1 adrenergic receptor blockade and rarely abates with time. To minimize contributing factors, patients should be cautioned to rise slowly from chairs or bed, and avoid large meals and alcohol. Some patients benefit from wearing support hose, but made-to-measure hose are expensive and often poorly tolerated. Salt tablets can be prescribed to bring the daily salt intake to 3–4 g per day, but one should check for fluid overload and monitor the patient's supine blood pressure. Fluorohydrocortisone can be started in doses of 0.1–0.5 mg/day and gradually raised to as much as 0.5 mg three times daily, but potassium supplementation may be needed. The patient's supine blood pressure must be monitored for hypertension.

Digestive system

Constipation, resulting from anticholinergic effects on bowel smooth muscle, may respond to increased intake of bran and adequate fluid, to natural laxatives such as prune and fruit juices, or to preparations that keep water in the bowel, such as a bulking agent, powdered psyllium seed (Metamucil® or Fibercon®), one to two tablespoonfuls in a glass of water daily, or the surfactant, docusate sodium 500 mg one to three times daily. Effects are seen within one to three days. Stimulating laxatives should be avoided because of the danger of dependency, although occasional use may be necessary.

Clomipramine's anticholinergic effects decrease saliva production. The resulting dry mouth promotes dental caries. Patients should be advised to brush their teeth after meals, floss regularly, avoid foods containing sugar, and schedule dental visits for plaque removal every six months. Salivation can be stimulated with sugarless gum or lozenges, and artificial saliva preparations can be used. Parasympathomimetic agents are effective in more severe cases: a 1% solution of pilocarpine, taken three to four times daily; pilocarpine 5 mg three to four times daily; or, bethanecol 10–30 mg two to three times daily, but sweating, abdominal cramping and diarrhea may occur. These agents are contraindicated in patients with some forms of pulmonary or cardiac disease.

Elevated liver enzymes occur in 1% (serum glutamic-oxaloacetic transaminase, SGOT; now termed aspartate transaminase) to 3% (serum glutamic-pyruvic transaminase, SGPT) of patients and are indications for discontinuing clomipramine.

Nausea may respond to taking clomipramine with meals or at bedtime. When this strategy fails, the dose should be lowered for one to two weeks before a second attempt at dose escalation.

Musculoskeletal system

Myoclonus, often occurring at night, can interfere with sleep. Clonazepam 0.5–1.0 mg at bedtime, or another benzodiazepine, may abolish this symptom.

Nervous system

Blurred vision, resulting from anticholinergic-induced pupillary dilation and sluggish ciliary muscle response, may respond to a 1% solution of pilocarpine eye drops two to three times per day, oral bethanechol 10–30 mg three to four times daily, or require corrective lenses. In patients with increased intraocular pressure or a history of narrow angle glaucoma, paroxetine, the most anticholinergic SSRI, would be the least suitable.

Drowsiness or daytime sedation may respond to nighttime dosing or increased caffeine intake, but the patient may still find sensations of mental slowing, "fogginess" or "being in a fishbowl" intolerable.

Tremor, which can interfere with writing, eating or drinking, may respond to a beta-blocker. One can prescribe propranolol 10–20 mg twice daily and gradually increase the dose as needed to 80–120 mg daily. Bradycardia, fatigue, nausea, diarrhea or skin rash occasionally occur. Metoprolol 100–200 mg per day in divided doses or nadolol can also be used; nadolol is preferred when renal excretion rather than hepatic metabolism is desired. Beta-blockers are contraindicated in patients with heart failure, second or third degree heart block, asthma, impaired lung function or insulin dependent diabetes.

Respiratory system

Frequent yawning, with concomitant sexual urges or orgasm, has been reported (McLean, Forsythe and Kapkin, 1983).

Urogenital system

Difficulty initiating urination results from anticholinergic effects on the detrusor muscle and can lead to bladder enlargement and infections. Bethanecol may be useful. In patients with a history of urinary retention or difficulty with urination, paroxetine's anticholinergic activity makes it the least suitable SSRI.

Fluoxetine

Table 4.6 displays the common side effects occurring substantially more often with fluoxetine than placebo.

Cardiovascular system

Sinus bradycardia, with faintness and syncope, and separately, hypertension, have been reported rarely and may necessitate discontinuing fluoxetine (Ellison, Milofsky and Ely, 1990; Feder, 1991). In patients with left bundle branch block (Drake and Gordon, 1994) or coronary artery disease (Walley et al., 1993) who are taking propranolol or metoprolol, fluoxetine may produce severe bradycardia. However, in patients free of heart disease and other contraindications, propranolol (20–120 mg/day) may be used to treat fluoxetine-induced tremor.

Table 4.6. Fluoxetine side effects occurring substantially more often than with placebo

Anxiety or nervousness	Dyspepsia
Diarrhea	Excessive sweating
Dizziness	Insomnia
Drowsiness	Nausea
Dry Mouth	Tremor

Source: Physicians' Desk Reference (Medical Economics Company, 1998).

Digestive system

Nocturnal and daytime bruxism may present with complaints of jaw muscle tension, pain or headaches on awakening. It may respond to dose reduction or to the addition of buspirone from 5 mg at bedtime to 10 mg three times daily (Ellison and Stanziani, 1993). Diazepam 2–5 mg/day and propranolol 10–20 mg/day have also been reported helpful.

Nausea usually occurs early and is mild; patients often complain of "queasiness" rather than true nausea. The symptom often abates in one to two weeks, and the patient can be asked to tolerate it temporarily or to try home remedies such as mint or ginger. Severe nausea has responded within two to three days to cisapride 5 mg twice daily (Bergeron and Blier, 1994) and 10 mg twice daily. (Russell, 1996). Cisapride can be tapered and discontinued within several weeks. Since cisapride can can cause cardiac arrhythmias and is contraindicated in patients taking drugs that inhibit cytochrome P450 3A4 (e.g., nefazodone), the U.S. Food and Drug Administration has warned that it should be used only as a last resort (Ault, 1998).

Endocrine system

Hyponatremia, with the syndrome of inappropriate secretion of antidiuretic hormone (SIADH), has been rarely reported, especially in geriatric patients (Cohen, Mahelsky and Adler, 1990; Staab et al., 1990). Renal, thyroid and adrenal dysfunction should be evaluated as possible causes, and concomitant medications reviewed. In one reported case, the patient tolerated rechallenge with fluoxetine (Staab et al., 1990). SIADH may recur when a second SSRI is tried (Jackson et al., 1995). Fluid restriction may permit SSRI treatment to continue.

Hemic and lymphatic system

Easy bruising and bleeding (e.g., epistaxis; bleeding from internal hemorrhoids) may occur after weeks or months of treatment (Yaryura-Tobias et al., 1991; Skop and Brown, 1996). These symptoms remit with drug discontinuation. (For vitamin C treatment, see 'Bleeding', under 'Paroxetine')

Nervous system

Agitation or "jitteriness," restlessness or anxiety occur early, but may abate within one to two weeks at constant doses. Rapid dose escalation and higher doses seem to be risk factors. Propranolol 10–20 mg twice or three times daily for several weeks may help. Alprazolam 0.5–4.0 mg/day for two weeks, followed by a two-week taper, was effective in patients who continued to receive fluoxetine 20 mg/day (Amsterdam, Hornig-Rohan and Maislin, 1994), but fluoxetine may modestly increase alprazolam blood levels.

Apathy, or loss of motivation, drive and interest, can occur without drowsiness, low energy or sad mood (Hoehn-Saric, Lipsey and McLeod, 1990). It does not remit unless the fluoxetine dose is reduced or the drug is discontinued.

Extrapyramidal symptoms, including dyskinesia, dystonia, opisthotonos, severe akathisia, and marked tremor occur very rarely and are reversible when fluoxetine is discontinued. Co-administration of fluoxetine with neuroleptics or metoclopramide may increase the risk (Lipinski et al., 1989; Black and Uhde, 1992; Arya, 1994; Coulter and Pillans, 1995; Sandler, 1996). Fluoxetine-induced akathisia disappeared in two patients switched to paroxetine (Bauer, Hellweg and Baumgartner, 1996a).

Headache is often due not to fluoxetine, but to comorbid tension, depression, or caffeine withdrawal. Hypertension and neurologic conditions must also be considered. Stress management, hot or cold compresses, nonprescription analgesics and scalp massage to loosen tight muscles are mainstays of treatment. For migraine headaches worsened by fluoxetine, sumatriptan (Blier and Bergeron, 1995b), amitriptyline, 25–100 mg/day, or valproate in doses producing plasma levels of 50–100 ng/ml (McElroy et al., 1995) may be effective.

Insomnia, with frequent, brief awakenings often remits after several weeks. Morning dosing can be tried, or trazodone, 25–100 mg at bedtime for persistent or troubling insomnia. Others suggest sedating tricyclic antidepressants such as amitriptyline or clomipramine 25–75 mg at bedtime (McElroy et al., 1995). The newer antidepressants with sedating side effects, such as nefazodone and mirtazapine, may ultimately prove useful, although fluoxetine (and other SSRIs inhibiting hepatic isoenzyme CYP2D6) can increase the plasma levels of the anxiogenic metabolite of nefazodone, meta-chlorophenylpiperazine (mCPP). Because benzodiazepines can produce dependency and rebound insomnia, other interventions for insomnia take precedence. The clinician should consider whether akathisia, hypomania or myoclonus underlies the insomnia complaint. Myoclonus will usually respond to clonazepam 1–2 mg at bedtime (Pollack and Rosenbaum, 1987).

Mania or hypomania can be precipitated by any antidepressant medication, especially in patients with a personal or family history of the disorder (Achmallah and Decker, 1991). For hypomania, one can add valproate in doses producing plasma levels of 50–100 ng/ml. In treating manic episodes, fluoxetine should be discontinued, while treatment proceeds with valproate and haloperidol as needed. Once the mania remits, SSRI treatment can be added to valproate. Lithium or other mood stabilizers should work as well in treating SSRI-induced mania.

Memory impairment affects short-term memory (where items have been put, appointments, items on mental lists) and learning (Mirow, 1991). In my experience, it requires dose reduction or discontinuation of fluoxetine, and may reappear with the next SSRI prescribed.

Sedation may be ameliorated by administering fluoxetine at bedtime or by increased consumption of coffee or tea. The addition of stimulating drugs such as bupropion 75–150 mg once to twice daily, or dextroamphetamine 5–30 mg once to twice daily, is a more aggressive strategy.

Stuttering has been reported (Guthrie and Grunhaus, 1990).

Respiratory system

Frequent yawning in the absence of drowsiness may trouble the patient. In my experience, it disappears after several weeks. Modell (1989) reports a case in which yawning was associated with multiple, spontaneous orgasms.

Skin and appendages

Hair loss occurs rarely, more often in women than in men, and presents as an increased rate of loss of hair while grooming, or as alopecia (Jenike, 1991). The hair loss may begin in the first week of treatment (Ogilvie, 1993) or after several months (Ananth and Elmishaugh, 1991), and occurs at doses as low as 20 mg/day. It usually reverses within months of discontinuing fluoxetine, but in one case did not (Gupta and Major, 1991). Scalp disease and hypothyroidism should be considered as alternative explanations. The patient may tolerate another SSRI without hair loss (Bhatara, Gupta and Freeman, 1996). Clinicians recommend 25–100 µg/day of selenium or 10–50 mg/day of zinc for hair loss, but no data on the efficacy of these mineral supplements are available.

Urogenital system

If frequent urination with urgency occurs, dose reduction may help.

Fluvoxamine

Table 4.7 displays the most common side effects occurring substantially more often with fluvoxamine than placebo.

Endocrine system

For hyponatremia, see Baliga and McHardy (1993).

Table 4.7. Fluvoxamine side effects occurring substantially more often than with placebo

Anorexia	Nervousness
Asthenia (weakness)	Sweating
Diarrhea	Sexual dysfunction
Dizziness	Somnolence
Dyspepsia	Tremor
Insomnia	Vomiting
Nausea	

Source: Physicians' Desk Reference (Medical Economics Company, 1998).

Nervous system

Extrapyramidal symptoms including akathisia, dyskinesias and dystonia are reported (Arya and Szabadi, 1993; George and Trimble, 1993; Chong, 1995). The extrapyramidal symptoms associated with SRIs may result from serotonergic inhibitory influences on dopaminergic neurons in the basal ganglia (Arya and Szabadi, 1993).

Cases of mania (Burrai, Bocchetta and Del Zompo, 1991; Jefferson et al., 1991) and disinhibition and aggression (possibly hypomania) are reported (Diaferia et al., 1994).

Skin and appendages

For hair loss, see Parameshwar (1996).

Mirtazapine

Mirtazapine antagonizes α_2 adrenergic autoreceptors and presynaptic α_2 hetero-receptors on 5-HT neurons (leading to increased norepinephrine and serotonin output), the 5-HT$_2$ (leading to antianxiety effects) and 5-HT$_3$ receptors (leading to antinausea effects). The most common side effects occurring substantially more often with mirtazapine than placebo are somnolence, dry mouth, increased appetite, weight gain, constipation, asthenia and dizziness. The somnolence and increased appetite may be the result of the drug's antagonist activity at the histamine (H$_1$) receptor. In my experience, somnolence usually diminishes or disappears at doses above 15 mg/day, perhaps because the drug's effects on serotonergic and noradrenergic function then outweigh its antihistaminic action. In premarketing trials, agranulocytosis was reported in 3 of 2796 patients (Medical Economics Company, 1998); I am unaware of any additional case reports.

Table 4.8. Paroxetine side effects occurring substantially more often than with placebo

Asthenia (weakness)	Insomnia
Constipation	Nausea
Decreased appetite	Nervousness
Diarrhea	Somnolence
Dizziness	Sweating
Dry mouth	Tremor
Impaired male sexual functioning	

Source: Physicians' Desk Reference (Medical Economics Company, 1998).

Paroxetine

Table 4.8 displays the most common side effects occurring substantially more often with paroxetine than placebo.

Digestive system

Management of dry mouth is discussed under 'Clomipramine'.

Endocrine system

Hyponatremia is reported by Chua and Vong (1993).

Hemic and lymphatic system

Bleeding is described by Ottervanger et al., (1994). One case of easy bruising and excessive menstrual bleeding responded after three weeks to vitamin C, 500 mg/day (Tielens, 1997). Bleeding recurred when the patient was switched to fluvoxamine, but again responded to vitamin C. This benign treatment can be tried with any SSRI while the results of controlled trials are awaited.

Nervous system

Dystonias may begin within a few days of starting treatment, but remit within days of discontinuing the drug (Committee on Safety of Medicines, 1993).

Sertraline

Table 4.9 displays the most common side effects occurring substantially more often than in placebo control groups.

Digestive system

Diarrhea may respond within a few days to taking twice daily capsules of lactobacillus acidophilus, a bacterium used in making yogurt; the capsules are available

Table 4.9. Sertraline side effects occurring
substantially more often than with placebo

Diarrhea/loose stools	Insomnia
Dizziness	Male ejaculatory delay
Dry mouth	Nausea
Dyspepsia	Somnolence

Source: Physicians' Desk Reference (Medical
Economics Company, 1998).

in health food stores (Kline and Koppes, 1994). In my experience, this intervention
works in about half of all cases.

Endocrine system

Breast tenderness and enlargement occur very rarely, and disappear with drug discontinuation (Hall, 1994).

Hyponatremia associated with SIADH may occur within days of starting sertraline (Crews et al, 1993). In patients unresponsive to other antidepressants, continuing sertraline may be possible if strict fluid restriction is observed (Thornton and
Resch, 1995).

Nervous system

Akathisia and dystonias have been reported at doses as low as 25 mg/day, associated
with a "crawling skin sensation" and increased sensitivity to touch (Altshuler et al.,
1994). The symptoms resolve within days of discontinuing sertraline, during which
time low doses of lorazepam or clonazepam may be helpful (LaPorta, 1993).

Speech blockage, with 3- to 6-second delays between words, and stuttering have
been reported at doses of 50 and 100 mg/day, resolving within days of drug discontinuation (Makela, Sullivan and Taylor, 1994; McCall, 1994; Christensen, Byerly
and McElroy, 1996). Interestingly, clomipramine has been reported to be beneficial
in the treatment of stuttering (Gordon et al., 1995).

Skin and appendages

Hair loss is reported by Bourgeois (1996).

Venlafaxine

The most common side effects occurring substantially more often with venlafaxine
than placebo are anxiety, anorexia, asthenia, blurred vision, constipation, dry
mouth, dizziness, insomnia, nausea, nervousness, sexual dysfunction, somnolence,
sweating, tremor and vomiting. Sustained diastolic hypertension ($\geq$90 mm Hg or

more) occurs in more than 5% of patients taking 225 mg/day or more of venlafax-ine (Danjou and Hackett, 1995; Medical Economics Company, 1998). Blood pressure should be monitored regularly in patients receiving these doses. The dose should be lowered or the drug discontinued if sustained hypertension is observed.

SSRI interactions with other drugs

Patients will often require treatment with more than one psychotropic agent, either because they suffer from more than one condition, or because they are unresponsive to one agent alone. In addition, patients will often be taking medications for comorbid medical conditions. Under these circumstances, the clinician contemplating pharmacotherapies must take into account numerous potential drug interactions. Table 4.10, pp. 100–2 arrays interactions caused by the SSRIs' inhibition of liver metabolic pathways. Although many of the interactions shown are derived from in vitro data and have not yet been reported to cause clinically significant adverse events, the clinician should be aware of the potential for such events.

Certain concepts help to organize one's thinking about drug interactions, which may be pharmacokinetic or pharmacodynamic or both. The term, "pharmacokinetics," refers to the time course of drug absorption, distribution, transport to and away from receptors, and to metabolism and excretion. Pharmacokinetics reflects what the body does to a drug. The term, "pharmacodynamics," refers to drug activity at receptors and to receptor effects on physiology, in other words, to the effects of the drug on the body. Pharmacodynamic interactions can take place because two drugs have additive or opposing effects at the same receptor, or because their effects at different receptor sites produce adverse consequences, e.g., the interaction of SSRIs and MAOIs (mono-amine oxidase inhibitors). The drug interactions considered here are primarily pharmacokinetic and reflect mainly the effects of SSRIs upon the metabolism of other drugs. The clinician undertaking well-motivated polypharmacy should consider the various other factors that influence the likelihood and severity of pharmacokinetic and pharmacodynamic drug interactions. These factors include the patient's age, gender, diet, comorbid medical conditions and concomitant prescription and nonprescription medications.

Most drug metabolism is carried out by the P450 isoenzyme system, located in the endoplasmic reticulum of hepatocytes. This enzyme system metabolizes foreign substances, making them more useful, or less toxic, as well as more water soluble and easily excreted. Eleven gene families producing these enzymes have been identified in humans, of which three (families 1, 2 and 3) are the locus of most drug metabolism (Preskorn and Magnus, 1994). These families are notated as CYP (for **c**ytochrome **P**450), followed by an arabic numeral for family (meaning partially shared amino acid sequences), a capital letter for subfamily (more closely shared amino acid sequences) and an arabic numeral for gene (coding the amino acid sequences), e.g., CYP2D6. The isoenzymes now known to be affected by SSRIs are: CYP1A2, CYP2C9, CYP2C19, CYP2D6 and CYP3A3/4. Of these, the last two are involved in the greatest number of potential interactions.

The degree to which one drug interferes with another's metabolism depends on the activity of the enzyme metabolizing the target drug, each drug's affinity for this enzyme, drug concentrations, the availability of alternative metabolic pathways, and their robustness. About 5% to 10% of Caucasians possess little or no CYP2D6 activity, and hence are slow metabolizers of the many drugs this enzyme metabolizes; an equal percentage have high levels of CYP2D6 activity and metabolize these drugs more rapidly than the general population (Nemeroff, DeVane and Pollock, 1996). Similarly, about 3% to 5% of Caucasians, 18% of Japanese, 19% of African Americans and 8% of Africans possess little or no CYP2C19 activity and are slow metabolizers of the smaller group of drugs this isoenzyme is known to metabolize (Nemeroff et al., 1996). Even within the majority of the population who are not slow metabolizers, however, the range in drug metabolism rates is wide. If knowing a drug's plasma level in an individual patient is important, it can only be determined by an assay, not by extrapolating from average figures.

Certain substances are P450 isoenzyme inducers and thereby increase rates of drug metabolism. Alcohol, for example, induces increased activity in all of the isoenzymes involved in psychotropic drug metabolism. Cigarette smoke induces the CYP1A2 and CYP3A3/4 isoenzymes.

The clinical evidence for SSRI effects on drug metabolism is generally limited to case reports, which are simply signals for caution. Preskorn (1996b) points out that case reports do not control for compliance in medication dosing, dietary influences on drug levels, assay validity or the timing of samples, and by definition, do not include representative samples of patients. In addition, all patients with equally elevated plasma drug concentrations will not experience side effects (DeVane, 1996). Controlled studies are needed to establish risk factors, dose relationships and the relative potential of different SSRIs to cause clinically significant interactions. A summary of data concerning the magnitude of SSRI effects on CYP isoenzymes, derived largely from in vitro studies, can be found in Preskorn (1996a).

Combining any SSRI (or bupropion, mirtazapine, nefazodone, or venlafaxine) with an MAOI is contra-indicated; pharmacodynamic interactions have produced the serotonin syndrome, occasionally with fatal results. At least 14 days should elapse between stopping citalopram, fluvoxamine, paroxetine or sertraline and starting an MAOI; because fluoxetine and norfluoxetine have prolonged half-lives after chronic administration (4–6 days, and 16 days, respectively), at least five weeks should elapse between the last fluoxetine dose and starting an MAOI. If larger daily

Table 4.10. Cytochrome P450 isoenzymes and their relationship to potential drug interactions

Isoenzyme	Isoenzyme-inhibiting drug	Drugs whose metabolism may be inhibited
CYP 2D6	*Strong inhibition:* fluoxetine norfluoxetine paroxetine quinidine thioridazine *Moderate inhibition:* sertraline	*Antiarrhythmics* encainide flecainide mexiletine propafenone *Antidepressants* tricyclics clomipramine N-desmethyl-clomipramine N-desmethyl-citalopram paroxetine venlafaxine *Antipsychotics* clozapine fluphenazine haloperidol perphenazine risperidone thioridazine *Beta Blockers* alprenolol metoprolol propranolol timolol *Opiates* codeine oxycodone *Others* dextromethophan verapamil
CYP3A3/4	*Moderate Inhibition:* fluvoxamine norfluoxetine	*Antiarrhythmics* lidocaine propafenone quinidine

Table 4.10 (*cont.*)

Isoenzyme	Isoenzyme-inhibiting drug	Drugs whose metabolism may be inhibited
CYP3A3/4	*Strong Inhibition:* nefazodone erythromycin ketoconazole ritonavir saquinavir	*Anticonvulsants* carbamazepine *Antidepressants* amitriptyline clomipramine imipramine nefazodone sertraline venlafaxine *Antihistamines* astemizole terfenadine *Benzodiazepines* alprazolam midazolam triazolam *Calcium Channel Blockers* diltiazem felodipine nifedipine verapamil *Others* acetaminophen cisapride cyclosporine erythromycin ethinyl estradiol tamoxifen
CYP1A2	*Strong inhibition:* fluvoxamine grapefruit juice	*Antidepressants* amitriptyline clomipramine imipramine *Antipsychotics* clozapine

Table 4.10 (*cont.*)

Isoenzyme	Isoenzyme-inhibiting drug	Drugs whose metabolism may be inhibited
CYP1A2		*Beta Blockers* propranolol *Others* acetaminophen caffeine tacrine theophylline R-warfarin
CYP2C9	*Important inhibition:* fluoxetine fluvoxamine sertraline	*Nonsteroidal anti-inflammatories* diclofenac ibuprofen mefenamic acid naproxen piroxicam *Others* phenytoin tolbutamide S-warfarin
CYP2C19	*Strong Inhibition:* fluvoxamine *Moderate Inhibition:* fluoxetine	*Antidepressants* citalopram clomipramine imipramine *Barbiturates* hexobarbital mephobarbital S-mephenytoin *Beta Blockers* propranolol *Others* diazepam

Sources: Nemeroff, DeVane and Pollock (1996); Preskorn (1995); Reisenman (1995).

doses of fluoxetine have been taken, e.g., 40 mg/day or more, a longer washout period is advisable. After an MAOI is discontinued, a washout period of 14 days should elapse before starting an SSRI.

Citalopram: metabolic interactions

Citalopram is a weak inhibitor of P450 isoenzyme CYP2D6 and does not inhibit isoenzymes CYP1A2 or CYP3A4. As a result, it appears to have a low potential for pharmacokinetic drug interactions.

Fluoxetine: clinically reported metabolic interactions

Because fluoxetine has been available longer than the other SSRIs, it has been the subject of more drug interaction reports.

Fluoxetine 20 mg/day can increase *tricyclic antidepressant* plasma levels two- to six-fold (Nemeroff et al., 1996; Preskorn, 1996b).

Fluoxetine 20 mg/day may increase *haloperidol* plasma levels by 20%, but the clinical significance is uncertain (Riesenman, 1995).

Substantial increases in *alprazolam* and *diazepam* plasma levels have been reported, as well as toxic levels of *phenytoin* (Nemeroff et al., 1996). Clonazepam plasma levels are not affected (Greenblatt et al., 1992).

Carbamazepine plasma levels have been increased in several case reports, but one study reported no important effect (Gidal et al., 1993).

Fluoxetine added to *terfenadine* (Seldane®) apparently caused nonfatal cardiovascular toxicity (Swims, 1993). The combination should be avoided. Other nonsedating antihistamines, such as cirtirizine (Zyrtec®) or loratadine (Claritin®), can be used safely. The type 1C antiarrhythmics (*encainide, flecainide* and *propafenone*) have narrow therapeutic indices. Because fluoxetine, sertraline and paroxetine inhibit their metabolism by CYP2D6, these SSRIs should not be given to patients receiving these antiarrhythmics. Adding fluoxetine to the beta blocker, *metoprolol,* has been associated with significant bradycardia (Riesenman, 1995).

The rate at which competitive inhibition of drug metabolism decreases is related to the inhibiting drug's elimination half-life. The long half-lives of fluoxetine and norfluoxetine imply that for five weeks or more after stopping fluoxetine, these agents may significantly inhibit the metabolism of competitively metabolized drugs.

Fluvoxamine: clinically reported metabolic interactions

Fluvoxamine increases plasma concentrations of *imipramine, amitriptyline* and *clomipramine* (Szegedi et al., 1996), probably by virtue of inhibiting CYP1A2, 3A4 and the 2C family (Nemeroff et al., 1996). Fluvoxamine has a small, but not negligible, inhibitory effect on CYP2D6.

Fluvoxamine has been associated with substantial increases in *haloperidol* and *clozapine* plasma levels (Nemeroff et al., 1996). Since clozapine-related seizures and orthostatic hypotension appear to be related to plasma levels, careful monitoring is advised (Medical Economics Company, 1998).

Fluvoxamine elevates *alprazolam* plasma levels and should probably be avoided in patients taking *triazolam* or requiring *midazolam* as a component of anesthesia (Nemeroff et al., 1996). Co-administration of *diazepam* is contraindicated because fluvoxamine markedly decreases the clearance of the parent drug and its active metabolite, N-desmethyldiazepam (Medical Economics Company, 1998). Benzodiazepines without active metabolites, such as lorazepam, oxazepam and clonazepam, can be prescribed safely.

Because fluvoxamine's inhibition of CYP3A4 can produce elevated plasma levels of *terfenadine* (Seldane®), *astemizole* (Hismanal®) or *cisapride* (Propulsid®), with fatal cardiac toxicity, these combinations are contraindicated (Medical Economics Company, 1998). The non-sedating antihistamines, cirtirizine (Zyrtec®) or loratadine (Claritin®) can be prescribed.

Propranolol levels increased 2- to 17-fold in normal volunteers administered fluvoxamine 100 mg/day, with mild effects on heart rate and blood pressure (Medical Economics Company, 1998). Since atenolol is eliminated primarily by renal excretion, it can be co-administered with fluvoxamine.

Diltiazem combined with fluvoxamine has induced significant bradycardia (Medical Economics Company, 1998).

Fluvoxamine can produce toxic plasma levels of *theophylline* (Nemeroff et al., 1996). Theophylline doses should be decreased by two-thirds if fluvoxamine is co-administered (Medical Economics Company, 1998).

The half-life of *caffeine* is markedly increased by fluvoxamine. Some patients taking fluvoxamine complain of unpleasantly increased stimulation from their usual intake of coffee.

Case reports of increased *carbamazepine* levels were not confirmed in a controlled study, but caution is still advised (Nemeroff et al., 1996).

Because fluvoxamine increases active levels of *S-warfarin*, with increases in prothrombin time, this laboratory result should be monitored and the warfarin dose adjusted as necessary (Medical Economics Company, 1998).

Because *lithium*, L-*tryptophan* (Steiner and Fontaine, 1986) and *sumatriptan* affect the serotonin system and could result in the serotonin syndrome when combined with fluvoxamine or any other SSRI, caution is in order. Lithium has been well tolerated, however, in combination with fluoxetine (Bauer et al., 1996b).

Mirtazapine: clinically reported metabolic interactions

Mirtazapine is metabolized by CYP2D6, CYP1A2 and CYP3A4, but is not a potent inhibitor of these isoenzymes. As a result, it appears to have a low likelihood of metabolic interaction with drugs metabolized by these isoenzymes.

Paroxetine: clinically reported metabolic interactions

Paroxetine inhibits CYP2D6, but has little effect on CYP3A4. As a result, combining paroxetine with any drug metabolized by CYP2D6 should be approached with caution.

In healthy volunteers, paroxetine 20 mg/day increased *desipramine* plasma levels two- to four-fold (Nemeroff et al., 1996).

Paroxetine 20 mg/day administered to a patient taking 50 mg/day of *trazodone* resulted in the serotonin syndrome (Reeves, 1995).

Theophylline levels are increased by paroxetine (Medical Economics Company, 1998).

Propranolol plasma concentrations do not appear to be influenced by paroxetine (Medical Economics Company, 1998).

Cimetidine, which inhibits many P450 enzymes, may elevate paroxetine plasma levels, whereas *phenobarbital* and *phenytoin*, which are P450 enzyme inducers, may lower these levels (Medical Economics Company, 1998).

Sertraline: clinically reported metabolic interactions

Sertraline inhibits CYP2D6, but has little effect on CYP3A4. As a result, combining sertraline with any drug metabolized by CYP2D6 should be approached with caution (Medical Economics Company, 1998).

At doses of 50 mg/day, sertraline has increased *tricyclic antidepressant* plasma levels from 50–150%. In doses of 100–150 mg/day, the increase has generally ranged from 5–66% (Preskorn, 1996b), but has been as high as 200–300% (DeVane, 1996).

Tolbutamide and *diazepam* clearance are decreased by sertraline (Nemeroff et al., 1996; Medical Economics Company, 1998).

Managing the serotonin syndrome

The serotonin syndrome (agitation, excitability, confusion, delirium, fever, sweating, nausea, diarrhea, ataxia, myoclonus and muscle rigidity) can be precipitated by any SRI taken within two weeks of stopping a MAOI, e.g., phenelzine (Nierenberg and Semprebon, 1993; Ruiz, 1994). A similar drug-free period should be maintained between stopping an MAOI and starting one of the newer serotonergic drugs, venlafaxine (Heisler, Guidry and Arnecke, 1996; Gitlin, 1997), nefazodone (John et al., 1997) and mirtazapine. Although usually self-limiting, the syndrome can be fatal. Case reports suggest that symptoms disappear within 24 hours if all serotonergic drugs are discontinued and supportive care is provided. When symptoms are severe, nonspecific serotonin receptor antagonists can be administered (Lane and Baldwin, 1997). Cyproheptadine 4–8 mg, for example, can be administered followed by 4 mg every two to four hours, with a total dose of 0.5

mg/kg/day. Methysergide 2–6 mg/day can be given instead. Propranolol and chlorpromazine are less regularly effective and carry more side-effect risks. Benzodiazepines and dantrolene are useful for reducing muscular rigidity, which can cause dangerous hyperpyrexia (Lane and Baldwin, 1997).

Managing sexual side effects of SSRIs

Usually the clinician will have to inquire about sexual side effects, since patients are often reluctant to mention them. Sexual side effects can be divided into four categories: diminished or absent desire; decreased genital sensitivity; male erectile dysfunction; and, delayed, less pleasurable or absent orgasm. Sexual dysfunction can also be due to an organic cause other than medication or to comorbid anxiety, depression, interpersonal conflict or a history of sexual abuse. In taking the history, the clinician should explore the onset and whether the symptom is situational or global. Does the problem relate to the start of drug treatment, to medical problems such as diabetes, to other psychotropic (Gitlin, 1994) or nonpsychiatric medications (Medical Letter, 1992), to substance use, or relationship problems? When the complaint is not clearly related to starting the medication, a physical examination may reveal signs suggesting an endocrine, vascular or neurological cause. Men may exhibit signs of excess estrogen secondary to alcohol-induced liver impairment (palmar erythema, spider angiomata), to a prolactinoma (gynecomastia), or to vascular disease (diminished pedal pulses). Physical examination of women is not likely to be helpful unless the complaint is dyspareunia, which is not recognized as a medication side effect. Assaying plasma testosterone, follicle stimulating hormone and thyroid hormone levels can establish the presence of primary or secondary hypogonadism.

The prevalence of sexual side effects associated with each SRI is unknown, but a reasonable estimate is that 25–35% of patients are affected (Jacobsen, 1992; Patterson, 1993; Gitlin, 1994). Clomipramine induces sexual side effects much more frequently than do the SSRIs (Monteiro et al., 1987). Delayed orgasm may begin at clomipramine doses of 25 mg/day and anorgasmia at 100 mg/day; the symptom remits within days of drug discontinuation (Monteiro et al., 1987).

Balon (1994) reports a unique case of the onset of sexual obsessions in a woman treated for depression with fluoxetine; they quickly resolved when the drug was discontinued.

First approaches to management of sexual side effects include decreasing the SRI dose, trying drug holidays, i.e., skipping a day's medication, and waiting for the body to accommodate to the medication. Switching to a different SRI runs the risk of losing the therapeutic effect, with no assurance of avoiding sexual dysfunction. In my clinical experience, only a minority of patients can reduce their drug dose sufficiently to avoid sexual side effects while maintaining the therapeutic effect. About one-third note a shift over several months from anorgasmia to delayed orgasm, or from delayed to normal orgasm. With all SSRIs except fluoxetine, patients' sexual problem may respond to taking one drug holiday per week by skipping a day's medication, then taking the second day's medication just after sexual intercourse (Rothschild, 1995). This approach is not effective, however, in cases of reduced desire.

Anecdotal case reports and small case series support the exploration of a number of pharmacological interventions. Because negative case reports are rarely published, one should expect only a minority of patients to respond to any particular intervention.

Reduced desire may respond to:
- bupropion, 75–150 mg/day (Labbate and Pollack, 1994);
- buspirone, 30–60 mg/day (Norden, 1994);
- cyproheptadine, an antihistamine with antiserotonergic activity, 4–8 mg/day (Aizenberg, Zemishlany and Weizman, 1995);
- stimulants such as dextroamphetamine 10 mg twice daily, pemoline 18.75 mg/day or methylphenidate 5–25 mg/day (Bartlik, Kaplan and Kaplan, 1995; Gitlin, 1995b);
- yohimbine, a presynaptic alpha-2 blocker, 5.4 mg three times daily (Jacobsen, 1992);

Impaired arousal or erection may respond to:
- amantadine 100 mg/day or twice daily (Balogh, Hendricks and Kang, 1992);
- yohimbine (Jacobsen, 1992);
- the role of sildenafil, released in the United States at the time of writing, is unclear.

Delayed orgasm and anorgasmia may respond to:
- amantadine 200–400 mg daily for 48 hours before coitus (Shrivastava et al., 1995) or 100 mg/day to 200 mg twice daily (Balogh et al.,1992);
- buspirone, 30–60 mg/day (Norden, 1994);
- cyproheptadine, 4–12 mg taken one to two hours before coitus (McCormick, Olin and Brotman, 1990; Arnott and Nutt 1994; Aizenberg et al., 1995);
- granisetron, an antinausea 5-HT_3 antagonist, 1 mg, one hour before coitus (Nelson, Keck and McElroy, 1997);
- nefazodone 150 mg about an hour before coitus (Reynolds, 1997);
- yohimbine 5.4–16.2 mg, two to four hours before coitus (Hollander and McCarley, 1992) or 5.4 mg three times daily. Jacobsen, 1992).

Colleagues are anecdotally reporting response of anorgasmia to mirtazapine 15–30 mg, or nefazodone 50–150 mg, one hour before coitus. This effect may be related to 5-HT_2 or 5-HT_3 receptor blockade (Nelson, et al., 1997). The "antidotes" I try first are bupropion, buspirone and amantadine because of their favorable side-effect profiles. Mirtazapine and nefazodone, however, appear quite promising. The other "antidotes" have disadvantages: cyproheptadine often causes drowsiness or fatigue during the following day and can reverse SSRI antidepressant effects; granisetron has only been reported successful in one case; and, yohimbine may cause anxiety, jitteriness, insomnia, excessive sweating and fatigue. Fine dose adjustments may be needed to balance yohimbine's therapeutic and side effects.

Psychotropic medications during pregnancy and the puerperium

Deciding whether to start or continue an SRI or other psychotropic drug during pregnancy or the puerperium is difficult. It requires both a risk-benefit calculation constrained by imperfect information, and a carefully documented informed consent, regardless of the decision. The clinician, the patient and the patient's concerned others must consider the risks to fetal and infant well-being if the mother's mental illness goes untreated alongside the risks of medication. When prescribing for a nursing mother, the clinician should use the minimum effective dose, and prefer a medication to which the mother has previously responded, one which does not require a second drug to treat side effects, and is rapidly metabolized.

SRIs in pregnancy

For fluoxetine, the available data suggest that the risks of administration during pregnancy are small. The risks for clomipramine and for SSRIs other than fluoxetine are much less studied, but animal studies do not suggest that these drugs are teratogenic or fetotoxic in clinical doses (Robert, 1996; Medical Economics Company, 1998). Current information regarding toxic fetal effects of drugs can be obtained from two telephone hotlines in the United States: the Pregnancy Environmental Hotline, Teratogen Information Service, National Birth Defect Center, in Massachusetts (telephone 1–800–322–5014), or, in California, the Teratogen Information Service (telephone 1–800–532–3749). These numbers are toll free in the United States only.

Information on 783 pregnancies occurring during fluoxetine use, collected through mid-1994 by the manufacturer, suggests that the rates of major anomalies, spontaneous abortion or stillbirth and premature delivery are no higher than those in the general population (Chambers et al., 1996). A study of 109 infants whose mothers took fluoxetine during pregnancy (Rosa, 1994) and a study of 128 pregnancies in which fluoxetine exposure was limited to the first trimester (Pastuszak et al., 1993) both found no excess rate of major anomalies.

Chambers et al. (1996) compared the outcome for 228 pregnant women taking fluoxetine to that for 254 women who called the same teratogen information service. Women taking fluoxetine experienced an excess proportion of infants with three or more minor anomalies and, for infants exposed in the third trimester, higher rates of premature delivery, admission to special care nurseries and poor neonatal adaptation. This study has been criticized for not controlling for coexisting diseases, not correcting for the more severe depression affecting the women taking fluoxetine throughout pregnancy, and because 30% of the fluoxetine-treated women took other psychoactive drugs (Robert, 1996). Moreover, the presence of a psychiatric disorder may itself be associated with perinatal problems (Robert, 1996).

The pregnancy outcomes for 267 women who took fluvoxamine, paroxetine or sertraline during pregnancy and contacted a teratology information service were compared prospectively to those of 267 women who had taken nonteratogenic drugs (Kulin et al., 1998). No significant differences were observed in the rates of miscarriage, stillbirth, premature delivery, or major fetal malformations. Outcomes for the women who took the SSRI in the first trimester did not differ from those of women who continued the drug throughout the pregnancy.

Doses of tricyclic drugs necessary to maintain therapeutic antidepressant response are increased in the second half of pregnancy (Wisner, Perel and Wheeler, 1993) because of increased metabolism and increased volume of distribution. Whether analogous dose increases are needed when administering SSRIs during this period has not been determined.

Reducing the dose of clomipramine in the weeks before delivery is sound practice. Clomipramine is strongly anticholinergic, and anticholinergic tricyclics have been associated with occasional cases of neonatal tachyarrhythmias, urinary retention and intestinal obstruction. The taper rate should be slow enough (50–75 mg/day per week) to prevent withdrawal effects, which in the neonate can take the form of irritability, tremor, hyperreflexia, hypotonia, tachypnea, poor suckling and temperature instability (Misri and Sivertz, 1991). No neonatal withdrawal symptoms have been reported in infants born to women taking SSRIs.

SSRIs and nursing mothers

Psychotropic drugs accumulate in breast milk, but suggestions of harm to the nursing infant are rare. Fluoxetine and its metabolite, norfluoxetine, can accumulate in newborns continuously exposed through breast milk, whereas sertraline and clomipramine apparently do not accumulate (Wisner, Perel and Findling, 1996) and have not been reported to cause acute adverse effects. The American Academy of Pediatrics Committee on Drugs (1994) considers clomipramine compatible with breast-feeding. Like adults, infants clear these drugs primarily through hepatic metabolism. One case of colic possibly associated with fluoxetine accumulation has been reported (Lester et al., 1993), suggesting that problems related to its accumulation are very rare.

Sertraline in doses of 50 to 100 mg/day taken by three nursing mothers caused no acute adverse effects through ages 11, 12 and 19 months in their infants (Mammen et al., 1997). Infant plasma levels of sertraline and norsertraline (which is only 10% as potent as sertraline in blocking serotonin reuptake but has a much longer half-life) were less than 2 ng/ml alone and combined. Stowe et al. (1997) also reported an absence of adverse effects in 11 nursing infants of mothers taking sertraline 25–200 mg/day. Sertraline and norsertraline levels below the detection limit of most commercial laboratories were observed in the infants' plasma.

Parents may also be legitimately concerned about the effects of SSRI exposure during pregnancy or through breast feeding on a child's long-term development. The limited data available regarding fluoxetine are reassuring. Nulman et al. (1997) utilized well validated instruments to study the language development, global IQ and behavioral development of 55 children whose mothers had received fluoxetine during pregnancy and compared these children to 80 exposed to a tricyclic antidepressant and 84 not exposed to any known adverse agent. The data analysis controlled for maternal factors known to affect these outcomes. When evaluated between 16 and 86 months of age, the three groups of children exhibited no significant differences on any measure. Similar data for other SSRIs are not available.

Other psychotropic drugs during pregnancy and the puerperium

Women suffering from the disorders discussed in this book or from comorbid conditions may require treatment with psychotropic drugs from any class. While a complete review of their use in pregnancy and the puerperium is beyond the scope of this chapter, a brief overview can be offered. More detail can be found in the reviews by Stowe and Nemeroff (1995) and Altshuler et al. (1996).

Antidepressant drugs

Administration of tricyclic antidepressants during pregnancy has not been associated with morphologic or behavioral teratogenicity (Misri and Sivertz, 1991; Nulman et al., 1997). As noted earlier, the clinician should be alert to anticholinergic side effects in the fetus or neonate, and if a taper-off drug is elected, the taper rate should be moderate. Because of an increased volume of distribution and changes in drug metabolism, a higher dose may be required during the second half of pregnancy (Wisner et al., 1993). Like all psychotropics, tricyclic antidepressants are excreted in breast milk, but the resultant blood levels in infants are likely to be low. The clinical significance of this exposure is unknown, but substantive risk has not been documented. Since nortriptyline and desipramine have favorable side-effect profiles and measurable serum levels, they are good choices when a tricyclic antidepressant is needed during pregnancy or periods of breast-feeding.

The newer antidepressants, including bupropion, mirtazapine, nefazodone and venlafaxine, have not yet been the subject of large-scale studies in pregnant or nursing women and for this reason must be assumed to carry more risk.

Anxiolytics

Recent studies of benzodiazepines do not support earlier reports of an association between first trimester use and cleft lip and palate (McElhatton, 1994). Two poorly controlled studies (Laegreid, Hagberg and Lundberg, 1992; Viggedal et al., 1993) suggested that neonatal exposure to benzodiazepines can cause motor and intellectual immaturity, but concomitant exposure to alcohol and other substances may have been the actual explanation (Bergman et al., 1992). A case report suggests that neonates can experience withdrawal symptoms after prolonged in utero exposure to benzodiazepines (Mazzi, 1977). As a result, these drugs should be slowly tapered as delivery approaches; a drug without active metabolites, such as lorazepam, is preferred (Whitelaw, Cummings and McFadyen, 1981). If benzodiazepines are administered to a nursing mother, shorter half-life drugs and low doses would be prudent.

The risks of exposure to buspirone during pregnancy and the neonatal period have not been determined.

Neuroleptic drugs

High potency neuroleptics, such as haloperidol and the piperazine phenothiazines (trifluoperzine, perphenazine and fluphenazine), appear unlikely to be associated with morphologic or behavioral teratogenicity and are less likely than low potency drugs to cause anticholinergic fetal side effects (Stowe and Nemeroff, 1995). The safety of in utero exposure to the atypical antipsychotic drugs such as clozapine, risperidone and olanzapine has not been studied. Since prolonged in utero exposure to antipsychotic drugs has occasionally been reported to induce withdrawal dyskinesias (Sexson and Barak, 1989), the clinician should consider tapering these drugs in the weeks before delivery. Breast-fed infants of mothers taking neuroleptic drugs should be observed for sedation and irritability (McElhatton, 1992).

Mood stabilizing drugs

Lithium use during the first trimester is associated with an increased risk of Epstein's anomaly (displacement of the tricuspid valve into the right ventricle), which is often fatal. However, the risk level, estimated at about 1/700 exposed infants (Cohen et al., 1994), is considerably lower than the risk of spina bifida, about 1/100, estimated for infants exposed in utero to valproate (McElroy and Keck, 1995). Cohen et al. (1994) also provide risk estimates derived from various data bases for lithium induction of at least one congenital abnormality. Lithium has been associated with a slightly increased likelihood of premature labor (Troyer et al., 1993), but appears to be free of behavioral teratogenicity (Schou, 1976) as does carbamazepine (van der Pol et al., 1991; Scolnik et al., 1994). The American Academy of Pediatrics Committee on Drugs (1994) considers lithium a contraindication to breast feeding, but others believe it may be used by careful, trustworthy patients who are educated regarding the dangers (Schou, 1990).

Exposure in utero to carbamazepine carries the risk of craniofacial defects, spina bifida and developmental delay. Exposure in utero to valproate carries the risk of neural tube defects (Lindhout, Meinardi and Meijer, 1992). The American Academy of Pediatrics Committee on Drugs (1994) considers both carbamazepine and valproate compatible with breast feeding.

Counseling before and during pregnancy

In counseling the pregnant woman (and her spouse or parents), or the woman wishing to become pregnant, about the advisability of starting or continuing a drug during pregnancy or while nursing, the physician should provide clear summaries of the available data, and the original studies if requested. The woman and the concerned others together with the clinician must weigh several factors:

- The probability that the psychiatric disorder will relapse or recur without medication.
- The disorder's effect on the patient and on her ability to successfully manage the pregnancy and puerperium.
- The availability and effectiveness of nonpharmacologic treatments.
- The available data regarding the drug's effects on the pregnancy, the fetus and the developing child.

Should the couple decide to start or continue drug treatment, the physician should ask both the patient and her spouse or parents to sign a "hold harmless" letter drafted by a knowledgeable attorney. The letter should spell out the information provided, the individuals' agreement to accept full responsibility for the decision to treat, and their decision to hold the physician harmless should the pregnancy have a less than satisfactory outcome. This process of education and documentation of the decisions will prevent most litigation. Nonetheless, a child born with a defect can initiate a suit in many jurisdictions at any time before reaching age 21.

Managing SSRI withdrawal symptoms

The risk factors for SSRI withdrawal symptoms are higher doses, longer treatment and shorter drug half-life. The symptoms are usually mild, but occasionally quite troubling. No large-scale, well controlled studies have established the frequency of these symptoms. Anecdotal case reports, spontaneous reports to health authorities and clinical studies all suggest that discontinuation of paroxetine elicits the highest rate of withdrawal symptoms and fluoxetine the lowest (Haddad, 1997). Paroxetine's relatively high rate may reflect its short half-life (21 hours), its auto-inhibition of metabolism (the elimination rate increases as the plasma level falls), and its muscarinic-receptor blockade (Haddad, 1997).

The most common SSRI withdrawal symptoms are anxiety, irritability and symptoms suggestive of flu (malaise, myalgia, rhinorrhea, nausea, vomiting, diarrhea and chills) (Lejoyeaux and Adès, 1997). Dizziness is also common and is frequently worsened by movement. Patients complain of feeling unsteady, uncertain of balance or position in space, and "spacey" or "spaced out." Paresthesias (especially "electric shock-like" sensations, vivid or abnormal dreams, insomnia and headache are also frequent elements of the syndrome (Zajecka, Tracy and Mitchell, 1997). The relative frequency of various symptoms when different SSRIs are discontinued has not been determined. However, the more commonly reported symptoms for each drug are described subsequently. Literature reviews are provided by Lejoyeux and Adès (1997) and by Zajecka et al. (1997).

Clomipramine withdrawal symptoms include dizziness, nausea, malaise, insomnia, headache and irritability. Doses should be tapered by 50 to 75 mg/day weekly and from 50 mg/day to zero by 25 mg steps over 10 to 14 days.

Fluvoxamine discontinuation has been associated in one small study with dizziness/incoordination, headaches, irritability and nausea (Black, Wesner and Gabel, 1993b); another study reported additional symptoms of confusion, memory problems, low energy and weakness (Mallya, White and Gunderson, 1993). The symptoms may appear within 24 hours of stopping the drug, seem to peak at about day 5 and disappear within two weeks (Mallya et al., 1993). Fluvoxamine should be tapered by 25–50 mg/day every four to seven days.

Paroxetine withdrawal symptoms may occur even after tapering the dose weekly by 10 mg/day (Coupland, Bell and Potokar, 1996). They resemble those described for sertraline, except that electric shock-like paresthesias, dizziness and feelings of incoordination are mentioned more often (Zajecka et al., 1997). The symptoms usually begin within two to three days after drug discontinuation, do not respond to benzodiazepines, may last three weeks, and remit within 24 hours of resuming the drug. They may be severe enough to prevent the patient from going to work (Barr, Goodman and Price, 1994; Kethuen et al., 1994). If withdrawal symptoms occur, a very slow taper over many weeks should be initiated, with weekly or biweekly dose reductions of as little as 5 mg/day. A second SSRI trial can be initiated concomitantly. Fluoxetine doses as low as 10 mg/day may abolish paroxetine withdrawal symptoms (Kethuen et al., 1994).

Sertraline withdrawal symptoms, including flu-like symptoms (aching, headaches, chills without fever), abdominal distress, nausea, malaise, tremulousness, impaired short-term memory, insomnia and increased dreaming, may occur after abrupt discontinuation of 100 mg/day or more and may last for more than a month (Louie, Lannon and Ajari, 1994). Brief, electric-like shocks, occurring every few minutes, may persist for many weeks; this troubling symptom is also seen in the withdrawal syndromes associated with paroxetine and fluoxetine (Frost and Lal, 1995). In patients troubled by withdrawal, tapering the sertraline dose over six weeks or more may permit discontinuation with mild or no symptoms. My usual practice is to taper sertraline by 25–50 mg every four to seven days.

Although venlafaxine is not an SSRI, in that it also inhibits norepinephrine reuptake, it appears capable of inducing a similar withdrawal syndrome. After a 4- to 14-day taper from doses of 150 to 375 mg/day, four of nine patients treated for OCD experienced flu-like symptoms including muscle aches, fatigue, headache, nausea and dizziness (Rauch, O'Sullivan and Jenike, 1996). The symptoms were relieved by resuming venlafaxine and tapering at a slower rate. The manufacturer recommends a slow taper because discontinuation symptoms, including asthenia, dizziness, headache, insomnia, nausea and nervousness, occurred in 5% or more of patients participating in premarketing studies (Medical Economics Company, 1998).

A washout period between the administration of different SSRIs is probably not necessary, except when switching from fluoxetine, which has a long half-life. In my experience, allowing a several-day washout of fluoxetine reduces the likelihood of adverse events. In addition, several cases of the serotonin syndrome have been reported with immediate switching from fluoxetine to a second SSRI (Lane and Baldwin, 1997). However, in a double-blind, randomized study, patients switched from fluoxetine 20–40 mg/day to paroxetine 20 mg/day with no washout period did not have significantly more side effects than those switched after a two-week placebo washout (Kreider et al., 1995). Whether immediate switches among all the other SSRIs are easily tolerated has not been established. With patients who are not greatly concerned about medication side effects, my general practice is to taper an ineffective SSRI by 25% every three to five days while substituting equivalent doses of the next SSRI. During crossover periods, the clinician should be alert for withdrawal symptoms, since one SSRI may not completely substitute for another.

5

Obsessive–compulsive symptoms in schizophrenic disorders

That he is mad, 'tis true: 'tis true 'tis pity;
and pity 'tis 'tis true.

Shakespeare, Hamlet

In patients with schizophrenia and related disorders, obsessions and compulsions may preexist, emerge spontaneously, or be precipitated or exacerbated by neuroleptics.

Clinical picture

The content of the obsessions and compulsions in schizophrenic patients differs little from the content in patients with OCD. OCD rituals, however, can interfere with the treatment of schizophrenia when they complicate the taking of medications (Eales and Layeni, 1994).

Obsessions and compulsions and schizophrenic symptoms may assume various relationships (Porto et al., 1997). In some cases the symptoms remain distinct; insight into the irrationality of the obsessions and compulsions is preserved, and they are experienced as ego-alien. In other cases, the obsessions and compulsions become the subject of delusional elaboration during periods of active psychosis. For example, a schizophrenic patient believed he was controlling world events by means of ordering rituals involving his clothing (Fenton and McGlashan, 1986). In still other cases, the OCD symptoms are inseparable from delusional beliefs, as for example, when the patient believes that sexual or aggressive obsessions are present because of thought insertion by a spiritual or an alien being.

The presence of obsessive–compulsive symptoms in patients with schizophrenia is associated with a much poorer long-term outcome (Fenton and McGlashan, 1986; Berman et al., 1995a).

Novel neuroleptics that simultaneously block serotonergic 5-HT$_2$ and dopamine receptors have been associated with both new onset and exacerbated obsessions and compulsions in schizophrenic patients, but a causal link has not always been firmly demonstrated. More than a dozen cases have been reported with clozapine

(Baker et al., 1996) and a lesser number with risperidone (Kopala and Honer, 1994; Remington and Adams, 1994; Alzaid and Jones, 1997; Dodt et al., 1997; Mahendran, 1998). The numbers are small given the tens of thousands of patients treated with these drugs. The obsessive–compulsive symptoms may start or worsen within weeks of initiating the antipsychotic medication (Alzaid and Jones, 1997) or emerge after six months or more of treatment (Baker et al., 1992). The frequency of this adverse reaction is probably less than 1% (Ghaemi et al., 1995), although no careful large-scale studies have been published. Whether olanzapine and other novel neuroleptics will also cause obsessive–compulsive symptoms, remains to be seen (Baker et al., 1996).

Some patients with OCD lose insight into the irrationality of their obsessions and compulsions in the course of their illness and become delusional (see Chapter 3). They can be distinguished from schizophrenic patients with comorbid OCD by the absence of the other signs and symptoms of schizophrenia.

Prevalence

Modern studies report a prevalence of obsessions and compulsions in patients with schizophrenia ranging from 8% (Eisen et al., 1997) to 46% (Porto et al., 1997). Eisen et al. (1997) administered structured interviews, conducted chart reviews and spoke to the therapists of outpatients with schizophrenia or schizoaffective disorder at two mental health centers. Five of 25 (20%) patients with schizoaffective disorder and 1 of 52 (2%) patients with schizophrenia met DSM-III-R criteria for obsessive–compulsive disorder; all had both obsessions and compulsions including symmetry, contamination and aggressive obsessions and touching, ordering, arranging, washing and checking rituals.

Berman et al. (1995a), studying 108 patients at a mental health center, utilized chart reviews and interviews with the patients' therapists. These investigators reported a 25% prevalence of obsessive–compulsive symptoms, but did not establish cases of OCD meeting DSM-IV diagnostic criteria. An earlier study, limited to chart review of patients who had been hospitalized at one facility, reported a 13% prevalence of obsessive–compulsive symptoms (Fenton and McGlashan, 1986).

Porto et al. (1997) utilized structured interviews to assess 50 chronically ill schizophrenic patients at a day treatment center. Comorbid DSM-IV OCD, distinct from schizophrenia, was present in 26%; an additional 20% had obsessions and compulsions variously intertwined with their psychotic symptoms.

All of these studies attempted to exclude ruminations, preoccupations with upsetting thoughts and delusional symptoms of schizophrenia, although the investigators noted that these distinctions can be difficult to make.

Treatment

Schizophrenic patients with concomitant OCD symptoms pose a difficult challenge. Only limited data are available to guide treatment decisions. Adding a serotonin reuptake inhibitor (SRI) carries a small risk of exacerbating the schizophrenic symptoms. Sasson, Bermanzohn and Zohar (1997) recommend that anti-obsessional drugs be used only in stable patients taking a stable maintenance dose of a neuroleptic, and that potential adverse drug interactions be carefully considered. These recommendations are sound.

In patients with comorbid, idiopathic obsessions and compulsions, the results of adding an SRI to conventional neuroleptics (phenothiazines or butyrophenones) are mixed. Adding clomipramine 250–300 mg/day brought about a moderate to marked response within four to six weeks in a small, double-blind placebo-controlled crossover trial (Berman et al., 1995b) and in an open-label case series (Zohar, Kaplan and Benjamin, 1993). Signs and symptoms of schizophrenia often improved concurrently, but worsened in one case (Zohar et al., 1993). The OCD symptoms recurred when clomipramine was withdrawn (Sasson, Bermanzohn and Zohar, 1997). In another case, schizophrenia worsened when clomipramine was added to a phenothiazine (Bark and Lindenmayer, 1992).

The OCD symptoms of 12 schizophrenic patients did not improve significantly when fluvoxamine 100–150 mg/day was added for eight weeks to stable regimens of conventional neuroleptics (Reznik and Sirota, 1996).

Supplemental fluoxetine benefitted one patient with comorbid OCD (Hwang et al., 1993), but in doses of 20–60 mg/day, made two patients rapidly worse (Lindenmayer, Vakharia and Kanofsky, 1990; Baker, 1992). In another case, fluoxetine 20 mg/day, added to haloperidol 15 mg/day, markedly reduced the frequency of a patient's compulsive masturbation within one month (Kornreich et al., 1995).

Equally variable outcomes have been reported for obsessive–compulsive symptoms induced by the novel neuroleptics that simultaneously block 5-HT_2 and dopamine receptors. The induced OCD symptoms have remitted spontaneously (Patil, 1992), responded to neuroleptic dosage reduction (Remington and Adams, 1994), responded to an added selective serotonin reuptake inhibitor (SSRI) after one to two months (Allen and Tejera, 1994; Baker et al., 1996; Suppes and Rush, 1996; Dodt et al., 1997) and persisted unless the neuroleptic was stopped (Baker et al., 1992; Buckely, Sajatovic and Meltzer, 1994; Eales and Layeni, 1994). Given the spontaneous remission observed after 1½ to 3 weeks in two cases (Patil, 1992), adding an SRI can be delayed for that long when obsessions or compulsions appear to be neuroleptic-induced.

Note that fluvoxamine can interfere with the hepatic metabolism of haloperidol and clozapine (Hiemke et al., 1994; Nemeroff et al., 1996); in one study, fluvoxamine 50 mg/day raised serum levels of clozapine and N-desmethylclozapine three-fold (Wetzel et al., 1998), albeit with improvement in negative schizo-phrenic symptoms and depression, and without clinically important side effects. This dose of fluvoxamine, however, would be unlikely to benefit OCD symptoms. The increases in clozapine serum levels associated with other SSRIs are smaller: fluoxetine, 20–75%; sertraline 20%; and, paroxetine 20 mg/day, insignificant (Wetzel et al., 1998). Since clozapine-related seizures (and weight gain) appear to be related to serum levels, careful monitoring is advised (Medical Economics Company, 1998).

When adding an SSRI to a neuroleptic, vigilance should be maintained for addi-tive side effects such as postural hypotension, drowsiness and anticholinergic side effects, especially when clomipramine is co-administered (Baker et al., 1997). Clomipramine should not be combined with pimozide because of the potential for additive cardiac side effects.

6

Medical conditions associated with obsessive and compulsive symptoms

. . . we are not ourselves
When nature, being oppress'd, commands the mind
To suffer with the body.

Shakespeare, *King Lear*

A variety of medical disorders have induced full-fledged OCD or phenomena resembling obsessions and compulsions. In general, the underlying lesions involve the caudate nuclei, putamen, globus pallidus, cingulate gyrus or frontal lobes. These same regions exhibit hyperactivity or increased blood flow in imaging studies (PET, SPECT and functional MRI) of OCD patients (Baxter, 1994; Schwartz et al., 1996; Breiter et al., 1996). This concordance lends strong support to the neuroanatomical models that have been proposed for the disorder (Modell et al., 1989; Baxter et al., 1992; McGuire et al., 1994; Trivedi, 1996). How these models will relate to cases associated with temporal lobe epilepsy and cases induced by drugs remains to be seen.

On the motor side, the phenomena swept within the penumbra of the concept, "compulsion," have included: repetitive, involuntary, discrete motor acts such as moving a limb; feeling compelled to stare at something; repetitive speech (palilalia); and, episodes of stereotyped complex behaviors, such as drinking glasses of water. These "compulsions" differ from those of OCD in that they are not purposeful. They are simply experienced as unwanted, forced or irresistible, stereotyped actions. On the psychological side, the content of the intrusive, repetitive, ego-alien thinking may or may not resemble the content of the obsessions seen in OCD. Atypical content has most often been associated with temporal or frontal lobe partial complex seizures and with oculogyric crises afflicting survivors of encephalitis lethargica. The duration of the "obsessions" has usually been brief.

The medical conditions associated with induced obsessions and compulsions can be organized according to traditional etiological categories (Table 6.1). Only rarely will the clinician need to investigate whether an adult presenting with symptoms of OCD has an occult medical disorder. When such a disorder is present, ordinary history-taking and clinical observation will uncover obvious incriminating

119

Table 6.1. Medical conditions associated with obsessive and compulsive symptoms

---

Genetic disorder
Tourette's syndrome

Infection
Encephalitis lethargica (Von Economo's encephalitis)
Human immuno-deficiency virus (HIV)

Autoimmune disorder
Sydenham's chorea

Seizure disorders
Partial complex seizures
Frontal lobe seizures
Tonic–clonic seizures (grand mal)

Brain tumor

Head trauma

Cerebrovascular accident

Neurodegenerative disorder
Parkinson's disease and Levodopa
Huntington's disease
Creutzfeldt-Jakob disease
Pick's disease and other frontal lobe degenerations
Neuroacanthocytosis

Endocrine/metabolic disorder
Hypoparathyroidism
Acute Intermittent Porphyria
Diabetes Insipidus, Vasopressin and Oxytocin

Toxin or drug
Carbon monoxide poisoning
Anoxia
Wasp venom
Manganese poisoning

Clozapine
Risperidone
Nefazodone
Stimulants

---

symptoms and signs. An underlying medical condition should be seriously considered, however, in cases with:

- onset after age 40;
- onset linked to new neurological symptoms;
- atypical symptoms (unusual content);
- a history of seizures or recent head trauma with loss of consciousness;
- a family history of tics or Tourette's syndrome.

Unfortunately, in some cases due to head injury or inapparent small strokes, focal neurological signs may be absent (Berthier et al., 1996). The discussion of medical conditions associated with OCD or partially similar signs and symptoms is organized by etiological category. Chapter 7 is devoted to Tourette's syndrome.

Most case reports concerning organically induced OCD or related phenomena are silent regarding treatment, many because they predate the era of effective treatments. As discussed subsequently, OCD phenomena related to Sydenham's chorea and epilepsy may respond to treatment of the inciting condition or its biological effects, while those related to head trauma have a variable response to selective serotonin reuptake inhibitors (SSRIs). Whether treatment with serotonin reuptake inhibitors (SRIs) ameliorates OCD phenomena associated with cerebrovascular accidents, neurodegenerative disorders or other conditions that permanently damage structures thought to be related to OCD is unknown and deserves study.

Infection

Encephalitis lethargica (Von Economo's encephalitis)

The early twentieth-century (1916–1917) epidemics of encephalitis lethargica left many survivors with neurological sequelae, although a causative agent was never isolated. Cases with intermittent "obsessions" or "compulsions" or both, some associated with post-encephalitic Parkinsonism, others with periods of oculogyric crises, are described by many authors and summarized by Jelliffe (1929; 1932) and by Brickner, Rosner and Munro (1940). Symptoms in post-encephalitic Parkinson's patients included: counting; palilalia; intrusive, repetitive thoughts; invariable, ego-alien thoughts elicited by encountering certain individuals; and, repetitive, stereotyped movements such as clapping, rubbing one's nose or pushing the tongue against the cheeks (Brickner et al., 1940).

Only a small percentage of encephalitis patients went on to suffer oculogyric crises. In such cases, the crises were usually preceded by brief periods of anxiety and often by forced thoughts or by patterns of thought that the individual could not change (Brickner et al., 1940). The attacks themselves, which could last from minutes to days and could occur from daily to once every several months, were frequently accompanied by intense anxious or depressive affect, and a few cases of resultant suicide are recorded (Jelliffe, 1929). The forced thought content rarely mimicked the focus on contamination, responsibility for harm or fears of errors that typify idiopathic OCD, but a few cases of ego-alien urges to harm relatives were reported (Jelliffe, 1929). Since the oculomotor circuit involves portions of the caudate nucleus and globus pallidus, the pathological process inducing oculogyric crises conceivably could have damaged the adjacent areas now thought to be related to OCD, particularly those participating in the lateral orbitofrontal and anterior cingulate circuits (Cummings, 1993).

Schilder (1938), who is often cited as an observer of medically induced cases of OCD, describes the case of a woman who was "worrisome" since childhood, developed encephalitis at age 15 and obsessions and compulsions at age 27, following childbirth. When examined at age 30 she exhibited Parkinsonian symptoms and palilalia. The connection between the organic insult and the much later onset of OCD is postulated, but not demonstrated.

Human immunodeficiency virus (HIV)

McDaniel and Johnson (1995) describe two patients with HIV who developed OCD about five years after becoming HIV positive. In both cases, the onset of OCD was closely associated with the onset of major depression, and in both, the OCD and depression responded well to fluoxetine. One patient had no signs of central nervous system involvement and was taking no HIV-related medications. The other had mild cortical atrophy, a low CD4 count, a Mini-Mental State Examination score of 26 of 30 and was receiving treatment with acyclovir, zalcitabine (dideooxycytidine), ethambutol and clarithromycin. Whether the OCD bore any relation to HIV infection is unknown, but the authors note that HIV encephalopathy may preferentially affect the basal ganglia.

Autoimmune disorder

Sydenham's chorea

Sydenham's chorea, an autoimmune disease affecting children and adolescents and triggered by a Group A ß-hemolytic streptococcal (GABHS) infections, is named after the English physician who described it in 1686 (Moore, 1996). Rheumatic fever develops in 2–3% of children with streptococcal pharyngitis, and 10–30% of rheumatic fever patients develop Sydenham's chorea; its presence is sufficient to establish a diagnosis of rheumatic fever (Swedo, 1994). The most common manifestations of rheumatic fever are carditis and polyarthritis. Less common manifestations are erythema marginatum and subcutaneous nodules (Moore, 1996). While most signs and symptoms of rheumatic fever begin about 10 to 20 days after the pharyngitis, Sydenham's chorea occurs one to six months later, making diagnosis difficult, since antistreptococcal antibody titers may no longer be elevated (Swedo, 1994). A number of other causes of chorea must be considered, including stimulant abuse, hyperparathyroidism, hyperthyroidism, collagen vascular disease, Wilson's disease and syphilis (Moore, 1996).

In Sydenham's chorea, choreiform movements most often affect the face, arms and hands, and develop over several weeks. The child notices "jumps" or "twitches" and may exhibit clumsy gait, drop objects, spill liquids and manifest dysarthric speech (Swedo, 1994). Muscular weakness and inability to sustain tetanic contractions produce a limp handshake termed "milkmaid's grip." Teachers may notice deterioration of the child's handwriting. Psychological symptoms, including nervousness, separation anxiety, irritability, emotional lability and hyperactivity, usually appear two to four weeks before the chorea (Swedo, 1994).

Swedo and her colleagues have established that obsessive–compulsive symptoms are present in over 70% of children with Sydenham's chorea, and that Sydenham's chorea is a risk factor for later development of OCD (Swedo, 1994; Swedo, Leonard and Kiessling, 1994). Unlike the symptoms of idiopathic OCD, obsessions and compulsions associated with Sydenham's chorea tend to begin suddenly and have an episodic course. The development of both the chorea and OCD symptoms has been linked to the presence of antibodies directed against the cytoplasm of cells in the caudate and subthalamic nuclei. Symptom severity correlates over time with antineuronal antibody titers (Swedo, 1994).

A B lymphocyte cell surface antigen recognized by the D8/17 monoclonal antibody is a genetic marker for susceptibility to rheumatic fever. This marker is significantly more common in children with OCD or tic disorders, with or without associated Sydenham's chorea, than in matched controls (Murphy et al., 1997; Swedo et al., 1997). Thus, this antigen is also a genetic marker for susceptibility to childhood-onset OCD related to GABHS infection. Swedo et al. (1998) have identified a set of diagnostic criteria that isolate prepubertal children who have OCD or tic disorders that have been triggered by GABHS infection in the absence of Sydenham's chorea or rheumatic fever. The children's symptom severity follows an episodic course, exacerbated by exposure to GABHS infection and, less often, other infections. Studies of this autoimmune form of OCD may shed light on the pathogenesis of other forms of the disorder. Whether autoimmune factors play a role in adult-onset OCD remains to be elucidated.

The treatment implications of these findings are several. First, children with rapid onset of OCD should be examined for possible carditis, since they may be suffering from an autoimmune manifestation of rheumatic fever. Second, children with Sydenham's chorea should be watched carefully for the development of OCD. Third, while the chorea may respond to valproate or neuroleptic drug treatment, the OCD does not (Swedo, 1994; Moore, 1996). Treatment trials are underway to determine whether plasmapheresis or intravenous immunoglobulin are safe and effective treatments for the OCD and chorea and whether penicillin prophylaxis diminishes the likelihood of subsequent episodes, as it does for Sydenham's chorea (Swedo, 1994).

Seizure disorders

Partial complex seizures

"Obsessional" thinking associated with partial complex seizures has occurred as an aura, an ictal phenomenon and postictally – in the first two instances, it is often termed "forced thinking." Cascino and Sutula (1989) describe the case of a 39-year-old woman with the onset of tonic–clonic seizures at age 11 and partial complex seizures at age 21. The latter were associated with an ictal, irresistible urge to drink large amounts of water, without any accompanying dry mouth, dry throat or other oral or pharyngeal discomfort. Right temporal lobectomy removed all the symptoms. The authors cite 20 similar cases reviewed by Remillard et al. (1981).

A 26-year-old man had partial complex seizures, undiagnosed for six years. They were characterized by a vacant stare, twitching of the shoulder and arm, a visual hallucination, occasional olfactory hallucinations and an increase in intrusive, repetitive, ego-alien thoughts and associated anxiety concerning fears he would harm his mother, other women or babies. Although the patient was previously diagnosed incorrectly as having paranoid schizophrenia, his obsessions and seizure disorder remitted throughout six months of carbamazepine treatment (Kroll and Drummond, 1993).

An 11-year-old girl had the onset of complex partial seizures some years before developing DSM-III-R OCD at about age 8 (Levin and Duchowny, 1991). Her case is unusual in that the seizure focus was located in the anterior cingulate gyrus (right-sided). Cingulotomy cured her seizures. Fifteen months later, her OCD was significantly improved and many symptoms had remitted. Since OCD may have a waxing and waning course, a causal connection between the surgery and the improvement cannot be presumed. The authors note that cingulate epilepsy presents as prolonged, treatment-resistant, partial complex seizures that are often associated with prominent, lateralized asymmetries in the EEG. They recommend that individuals with this diagnosis be carefully evaluated for comorbid OCD.

Kettl and Marks (1986) describe a 12-year-old whose OCD began six months after the onset of temporal lobe epilepsy, but the causal link is not well established here nor in the two cases reported by Pacella, Polatin and Nagler (1944), where OCD began a few months before the start of petit mal seizures.

Interictal "obsessionalism," characterized by excessive orderliness and attention to detail, has been described in patients with long-standing temporal lobe epilepsy (Bear and Fedio, 1977), along with hypergraphia (the keeping of extensive notes or diaries or autobiographical writings). The hypergraphia, however, differs from compulsive behavior in that it is ego-syntonic and is not aimed at warding off or undoing unwanted events. Pronounced conscientiousness, resembling the trait criterion adduced in diagnosing obsessive–compulsive personality disorder, is common in patients with chronic temporal lobe epilepsy caused by left-sided lesions (Bear and Fedio, 1977).

Frontal lobe seizures

Chauvel et al. (1995) mention "forced thinking," with content atypical of OCD, as a symptom of frontal lobe seizures in 8 of 39 patients. In four cases, the forced thinking was an isolated manifestation of seizure activity, and in two it progressed to automatisms. The ideational content did not continue during motor seizures. Ward (1988) describes two patients whose frontal seizure activity was associated with "a feeling of compulsion," e.g., to move or shake a body part, but without overt action. Within a few months, both patients were found to have frontal lobe glioblastomas. Other cases of forced thinking associated with frontal seizures are reported by Mulder (1953) and by Penfield and Jasper (1954).

Tonic–clonic seizures (Grand Mal)

Fixation of gaze is occasionally experienced as the aura to tonic–clonic, generalized seizures; fixation of thought or forced thinking of a sequence of thoughts are rarer auras (Brickner et al., 1940).

Brain tumors

Some of the epileptic cases mentioned earlier were associated with brain tumors (Brickner et al., 1940; Ward, 1988). A few cases of tumors seemingly associated with typical OCD have been published. Moriarty, Trimble and Hayward (1993) describe a 9-year-old girl whose OCD was apparently the presenting manifestation of a brain stem astrocytoma extending into the left cerebellum. After surgery and radiation treatment, her OCD symptoms remitted, only to recur five years later with tumor recurrence. A second operation coupled with radiation again led to remission, but her OCD subsequently recurred without evidence of tumor regrowth. Her family history was positive for OCD.

Paradis, Friedman and Hatch (1992) describe a woman who developed germ phobias and acquired immunodeficiency syndrome (AIDS) fears along with compulsive hand washing during post-surgical rehabilitation. Removal of a non-malignant, right parietal vertex tumor had been associated with perioperative damage to the right frontoparietal area. She improved with exposure and response prevention.

A 40-year-old man had the onset of fears of contamination about three months into X-ray therapy for a left fronto-temporal xanthoastrocytoma (Rogers and Mendoza, 1994). Trials of clomipramine, fluoxetine and clonazepam were unsuccessful; he improved slightly with sertraline.

A case marked by repetitive questioning, compulsion to repeat parts of conversations and the keeping of a verbatim notebook of conversations, all beginning at age 51, bears a tenuous relationship to a right frontal dural lesion diagnosed during work-up (Seibyl et al., 1989). The patient's OCD symptoms improved within a month of starting treatment with tranylcypromine augmented by lithium, without surgical removal of the meningioma; the improvement was maintained during a 12-month follow-up period. The authors believe that the late onset and the presence of severe affective blunting and emotional lability argue for a probable association between the meningioma and the OCD.

Head injury

Loss of consciousness, for minutes to days, has characterized almost all cases of head injury with subsequent OCD (McKeon, McGuffin and Robinson, 1984; Donovan and Barry, 1994; Kant et al., 1996; Childers et al., 1998). OCD has begun from within 24 hours of awakening to as long as six months later, although the longer the interval, the less persuasive the argument for a causal connection. Neurodiagnostic tests, including EEG, MRI, SPECT, PET and CAT scans, may be normal.

Closed head injury often causes diffuse frontal lobe injury, with orbitofrontal damage, which may be related to the appearance of OCD symptoms. Alternatively, checking rituals may conceivably be induced by the anxiety or subtle memory impairments caused by the head injury. When a frontal lobe syndrome is present, the patient may exhibit apathy rather than anxiety concerning the obsessions and compulsions (Donovan and Barry, 1994).

Checking, counting and cleaning rituals are the most common compulsive symptoms in head injury cases, and comorbid major depression is frequently seen. Insight is usually, but not always, preserved. Response to SSRIs is as variable as in idiopathic OCD. Recovery, without treatment, occasionally occurs after several years (McKeon et al., 1984).

Drummond (1988) reports a case in which a blow to the head at the work place, with brief loss of consciousness, led to a 6-month period of disability leave followed by onset of OCD symptoms on return to work. The symptoms included having to do things perfectly, washing, checking and obsessions about harm coming to the patient's family. Exposure and response prevention were not helpful, but the symptoms markedly improved once a workman's compensation claim was settled. The possible contributions of stress exacerbating induced or idiopathic OCD and of secondary gain magnifying the symptoms cannot be disentangled.

Cerebrovascular accident

A 62-year-old man, who had always been anxious and perfectionistic but without OCD, suddenly developed need-to-know compulsions, starting with the need to know the name of an actor in a television commercial (Swoboda and Jenike, 1995). The compulsion rapidly spread to newspaper items and random bits of information and became all consuming. Three years later a CT revealed an old right frontal infarct. His symptoms were refractory to trials of 35 medications, including all SSRIs.

In another patient, a right frontal infarct and left subfrontal contusion resulting from a motor vehicle accident were associated with counting, chewing, numerical and reading rituals which began when the patient awakened after a three-week coma (Donovan and Barry, 1994).

In the case of a 56-year-old woman, compulsive skin scraping and forced counting of books and other objects began after sequential, unilateral infarcts damaged the heads of both caudate nuclei (Croisile et al., 1989). Like many patients with basal ganglia lesions, the patient was apathetic and had decreased initiative. She did not become anxious when ordered to stop counting.

Daniele et al. (1997) describe a Parkinsonian patient who developed fears of harm coming to her children and repetitive behaviors, including repeating sentences and coprolalia, within days of a stroke damaging the left anterior putamen.

A 48-year-old woman began purposeless hand movements, resembling typing, a year after becoming depressed over her mother's death (Williams, Owen and Heath, 1988). She could inhibit the movements, but found them comforting. CT scan revealed cavitations of unknown etiology, although possibly ischemic, in both caudate nuclei and the right putamen.

Neurodegenerative disorders

Parkinson's disease and levodopa

As ingested levodopa begins to relieve akinesia, some Parkinsonian patients experience a period of several minutes of stereotyped, involuntary limb movements (Hardie, Lees and Stern, 1984). Most patients recognize these movements as early signs of the return of mobility, but in some cases patients incorporate the involuntary movements into a complex mannerism such as "stretching" or "yawning" or believe that the movements are necessary to regaining mobility. In that the movements are involuntary rather than intentional, and are not performed in response to obsessions, their resemblance to symptoms of OCD is modest. Perseverative repetition of stereotyped phrases and stereotyped actions (e.g., picking, tapping, banging) are described in levodopa-induced delirium in three moderately demented Parkinsonian patients (Sacks et al., 1970).

More typical obsessions and compulsions have been described in a few cases of postencephalitic Parkinsonism (Jelliffe, 1932). Wexberg (1937) describes two Parkinsonian patients with no history of encephalitis who experienced episodes of forced mental content, not typical of OCD, in conjunction with oculogyric crises.

Huntington's disease

Huntington's disease, named after the nineteenth-century American physician who described it, is an autosomal dominant disorder with a prevalence of 4–8 per 100,000 persons. It is marked by atrophy of the caudate nuclei and putamen associated with choreiform movements and progressive dementia. Only two cases of OCD linked to this disorder have been described (Cummings and Cunningham, 1992). The first patient developed socially inappropriate, severe cleaning compulsions at an unspecified point in his illness. Haloperidol was without effect. The second patient developed a socially inappropriate smoking compulsion, increasing his daily smoking from half a pack to five or more packs per day. His fingers were burned from compulsively smoking each cigarette to its end. Both patients became belligerent if their compulsive behaviors were interfered with.

Creutzfeldt–Jakob disease

A 65-year-old man exhibited compulsive exercising, constant talking to himself about his life and children and repetitive complaining about chronic tinnitus as early symptoms of dementia due to Creutzfeldt–Jakob disease (Lopez et al., 1997). He also became "obsessed" with the details of his early life. The authors refer to these symptoms as obsessive–compulsive "features," but the resemblance is modest.

Pick's disease and other frontal lobe degenerative disorders

Ames et al. (1994) review the literature on degenerations that affect the frontal lobes, including Pick's disease and frontal lobe degeneration of the non-Alzheimer's type, both of which have been associated with repetitive and "compulsive" behavior in the context of dementia. They note that complex ritualistic behavior is usually limited to the early phase of the degeneration, while elementary stereotyped, repetitive behaviors occur later. They present the case of a 66-year-old man who developed obsessional slowness, rigid rituals, counting of environmental objects and intrusive, ego-alien thoughts about violence in the context of a progressive dementia associated with diminished blood flow in the frontal and temporal lobes and caudate nuclei.

Bilateral caudate nuclei atrophy was observed in a 36-year-old woman several months after she developed an agitated depression and began compulsive hand washing and rituals to avoid contamination of her hands (Tonkonogy and Barreira, 1989). Within two years she demonstrated a progressive dementia, bilateral Babinski signs and MRI evidence of bilateral frontal lobe atrophy of unknown etiology.

Neuroacanthocytosis

This rare, familial neurodegenerative disorder, which is associated with atrophy of the caudate nuclei, is characterized by motor and vocal tics, choreiform movements and lip and tongue biting that can be confused with compulsions (Wyszynski et al., 1989). The absence of typical symptoms of OCD and the presence of other signs, including generalized seizures, dysarthria, orofacial and orobuccal dyskinesia, areflexia or hyporeflexia, muscle atrophy and pes cavus deformity, should prevent misattribution of the neurological symptoms to OCD. Red blood cell acanthocytosis (greater than 2%), elevated serum creatine phosphokinase level and EMG signs of peripheral neuropathy are present.

Multiple sclerosis

George, Kellner and Fossey (1989) and Miguel et al. (1995) present four cases of OCD associated with multiple sclerosis. A causal connection is rendered unlikely in these cases by the periods of 3–20 years between the onset of the OCD and the first signs of multiple sclerosis.

Endocrine/metabolic disorder

Idiopathic hypoparathyroidism and OCD both began at about age 15 in a man found to have diffuse calcification of the basal ganglia, thalamic pulvinar, frontal lobes and other structures at age 36 (Kotrla et al., 1994). The authors note that a review of 62 cases with symmetrical striopallidodentate mineralizations due to various causes included only one patient with "compulsions," though 40% had other dramatic psychiatric symptoms. Nonetheless, given the involvement of the basal ganglia in idiopathic OCD and OCD patients' proclivity to hide their symptoms, the authors recommend careful evaluation of patients who are discovered to have basal ganglia mineralizations. Lopez-Villegas et al. (1996), for example, found that 6 of 18 patients with basal ganglia calcification without other radiological findings met criteria for OCD.

Acute intermittent porphyria

Hamner (1992) describes the case of a 50-year-old man whose chronic OCD was worsened during his attacks of acute intermittent porphyria, which were also accompanied by episodes of major depression that persisted for one to two months after each attack. During the attacks, the content of the patient's obsessions would change to thoughts of killing his wife, an obsession not present at any other time. The patient's OCD and depressions ultimately responded well to fluoxetine.

Diabetes insipidus, vasopressin and oxytocin

Barton (1965) attempted to establish a syndromal relationship between diabetes insipidus and OCD, presenting nine cases of diabetes insipidus in whom various obsessive or compulsive features were reported. Only four cases, however, appeared to have OCD; the others were marked only by "compulsive" water-drinking or meticulous behaviors. Of the four OCD patients, two had onset 10 or more years apart from the onset of diabetes insipidus. A third patient, with probable post-encephalitic Parkinsonism, appeared to have near concurrent onset of diabetes insipidus and OCD. The fourth patient had the onset of diabetes insipidus during her first pregnancy, followed a week later by the onset of drinking rituals; six years later typical OCD symptoms began. The absence of a close temporal relationship between diabetes insipidus and OCD in three of these four cases, argues strongly against a syndromal relationship.

Vasopressin (antidiuretic hormone), oxytocin and other central nervous system peptides that affect arousal and conditioned behaviors are being studied for potential roles in the pathophysiology of OCD (Altemus et al., 1994; Leckman, et al., 1994a). In an open-label trial in three patients, however, neither vasopressin nor oxytocin had any significant effect on obsessions or compulsions (Salzberg and Swedo, 1992). In a separate report, an OCD patient treated with intranasal oxytocin for two weeks experienced improvement, but simultaneously acquired gross memory impairment, hallucinations and delusions associated with hyponatremia (Ansseau et al., 1987). The authors note that rather than reflecting any beneficial biological effect of the oxytocin, the memory impairment or psychotic symptoms could have been responsible for the patient's lessened concern with his OCD symptoms.

Toxin or drug

Carbon monoxide poisoning with bilateral globus pallidus infarction produced typical OCD symptoms within a week of the insult (Escalona et al., 1997). The patient had the sudden onset of obsessions concerning harming others, sexual obsessions, fears of contamination, irresistible urges to spit, even indoors, and checking, counting and hand washing rituals. He was started on fluoxetine but failed to return for follow-up. Laplane et al. (1989) report two cases in which carbon monoxide poisoning produced obsessive–compulsive symptoms. In the first case, bilateral lesions of the globus pallidus were associated with compulsive mental counting. In the second case, bilateral lesions of the lentiform nuclei (globus pallidus and putamen) were associated with compulsively repeating the time, counting others' spoken words and repeating a mandatory sentence before certain actions. The patient was aware of the absurdity of the compulsions, but could not resist. In another case, carbon monoxide poisoning with basal ganglia lesions produced tic-like movements of the head and neck, forced grabbing and grasping behaviors, palilalia, echolalia, fits of shouting (klazomania) and involuntary, repetitive utterance of obscenities, so that the clinical picture was reminiscent of Tourette's syndrome (Pulst, Walshe and Romero, 1983).

Laplane et al. (1989) also describe a case in which hypoxia-induced, bilateral damage to the lentiform nuclei was associated with compulsive checking, turning light switches on and off and reciting of the alphabet. The patient was not disturbed by these behaviors and became angry if anyone interfered. Another of their patients with bilateral lentiform lesions, secondary to an allergic reaction to wasp venom, engaged in long periods of switching lights on and off and counting, and became angry when interrupted. The patient also exhibited choreiform movements, a parkinsonian gait and apathy. Weilburg et al. (1989a) report the case of a man who suffered probable anoxic brain injury at birth and developed OCD in his late teens. When examined at age 24, he had a decrease in the volume of the left caudate nucleus and putamen. The long delay between the brain insult and the onset of OCD, however, raises a question about the linkage.

Manganese poisoning

Compulsive behaviors, with retained insight, are an early sign of chronic manganese poisoning. Studying Chilean manganese miners, Mena et al. (1967) observed compulsive running, singing, dancing or chasing passing cars until exhausted as early symptoms of poisoning, often accompanied by irritability and depression. About a month after the onset of compulsive behaviors, the miners developed irreversible neurological signs, including muscular weakness, abnormal gait, increased motor tone, impaired speech and expressionless facies.

Drugs

Nefazadone was implicated in the case of a 40-year-old woman who developed obsessive ruminations about whether she had taken her medication and about the possible recurrence of breast cancer within a week of starting the drug (Sofuoglu and DeBattista, 1996). The obsessions worsened when the dose was increased to 400 mg/day and disappeared one day after nefazodone was discontinued.

Drug-induced OCD associated with clozapine or risperidone is described in Chapter 5.

Abuse of stimulant drugs can produce stereotyped, repetitive behaviors (Rylander, 1969), and therapeutic use of these drugs in children with attention deficit disorder has been associated with choreiform movements and tics (Denckla, Bemporad and MacKay, 1976) and rare instances of Tourette's syndrome (Lowe et al., 1982). Only a few cases of children with typical obsessions and compulsions apparently induced by stimulants have been reported. The OCD symptoms began six days (Frye and Arnold, 1981) to six months (Koizumi, 1985) after initiation of stimulant treatment, and persisted for one to three months after stimulants were discontinued. One patient (Frye and Arnold, 1981) remitted while taking 5 mg/kg of pyridoxine, a cofactor in the synthesis of serotonin and other catecholamines, one while taking pyridoxine and tryptophan, and one spontaneously (Koizumi, 1985). The absence of subsequent similar reports in more than a decade greatly weakens the presumption of a causal link between the OCD symptoms and the stimulant treatment.

Part III

Obsessive–compulsive spectrum disorders

7

Tourette's disorder

This is a tic disorder. When one develops this disorder, a series of problems occur, behavioral and physical in various combinations.

Charcot, *Nine Case Presentations on General Neurology Delivered at the Salpêtrière Hospital in 1887–88*

After more than a century, medical investigators are reexamining the nineteenth-century separation of Tourette's Disorder (formerly Tourette's Syndrome) from Sydenham's chorea and other childhood movement disorders. Kushner and Kiessling (1996) provide a lively summary of the decades of medical discourse during which the separation came into existence. In 1885, Jean-Martin Charcot, renowned neurologist of Paris' Salpêtrière hospital, created the eponym, *La Maladie des Tics de Gilles de la Tourette*, in honor of his 28-year-old assistant. At Charcot's direction, Tourette described and published nine cases of "variable choreas" or "convulsive tics," distinguishing their symptom picture from Sydenham's chorea. Tourette emphasized the triad of multiple motor tics, copro-lalia (uttering obscenities) and echolalia (repeating someone else's words), the latter two symptoms representing forms of vocal tics. Charcot's aim, in opposition to 80 years of medical opinion, was to dissociate the choreas from rheumatic fever, creating another of his distinct neurological syndromes. One of Tourette's cases was that of Madame (later Marquise) de Dampiere, who suffered from persistent motor tics, barking sounds and coprolalia. Her case was first published by Jean Itard in 1825 and was appropriated 60 years later by Tourette. Ironically, hers was the only case in Tourette's series that exhibited the full syndrome bearing his name, and neither Tourette nor Charcot ever personally examined her (Kushner and Kiessling, 1996). Itard, along with many physicians before and after his time, had argued that all choreas were linked to rheumatic fever. Charcot disagreed.

Today, we know that Charcot, at least in part, was wrong. Group A β-hemolytic streptococcal infection triggers rheumatic fever not only in the forms of acute rheumatic arthritis and endocarditis, but also as Sydenham's chorea. In the past decade, it has been discovered that streptococcal infection can also trigger OCD, which appears concurrently with the symptoms of Sydenham's chorea (Swedo, 1994). Because OCD commonly occurs in Tourette's Disorder (TD), this discovery has renewed interest in potential connections between the events producing

Table 7.1. DSM-IV diagnostic criteria for Tourette's disorder (307.23)

A. Both multiple motor and one or more vocal tics have been present at some time during the illness, although not necessarily concurrently. (A *tic* is a sudden, rapid, recurrent, nonrhythmic, stereotyped motor movement or vocalization.)

B. The tics occur many times a day (usually in bouts) nearly every day or intermittently throughout a period of more than one year, and during this period there was never a tic-free period of more than three consecutive months.

C. The disturbance causes marked distress or significant impairment in social, occupational, or other important areas of functioning.

D. The onset is before age 18 years.

E. The disturbance is not due to the direct physiological effects of a substance (e.g., stimulants) or a general medical condition (e.g., Huntington's disease or postviral encephalitis).

Source: Reprinted with permission from the *Diagnostic and Statistical Manual of Mental Disorders, Fourth Edition.* Copyright 1994, American Psychiatric Association, p. 103.

rheumatic fever and the unknown etiology of TD (Kushner and Kiessling, 1996). For example, a study of immune markers in a small group of children with TD revealed that all were positive for a B lymphocyte antigen identified by monoclonal antibody D8/17. This antigen is notable as a trait marker for rheumatic fever susceptibility and is also prevalent in children with streptococcal-induced (auto-immune) OCD (Murphy et al., 1997). Does an autoimmune diathesis link rheumatic fever to the new syndrome that Charcot named in honor of Tourette?

Although this book is intended to aid clinicians in their treatment of adult patients, the vast majority of the literature concerning TD is concerned with children. As a result, the descriptive and outcome data summarized in this chapter are largely derived from child and adolescent studies. Nonetheless, these data can inform the clinician's exploration of an adult patient's symptoms and the formulation of an effective treatment plan.

Having long suffered from impaired self-control and an often embarrassing and stigmatizing illness, an adult TD patient may have a negative self-concept, disturbed family and peer relationships and limited educational attainment. The adult patient's life history in these domains must be carefully, though gently, probed.

Diagnosis

The DSM-IV (American Psychiatric Association, 1994) diagnostic criteria for Tourette's Disorder are shown in Table 7.1 The essential feature is the daily occurrence of multiple motor tics and vocal tics, although not necessarily concurrently.

DSM-IV lowered the diagnostically permissible age of onset from the 21 years allowed in DSM-III-R to 18 years, perhaps because onset after age 18 is rare (Robertson, 1989). The ICD-10 Diagnostic guidelines for TD, termed "combined vocal and multiple motor tic disorder [de la Tourette's syndrome]" (code F95.2) (World Health Organization, 1992), are consistent with the DSM-IV criteria. ICD-10, however, does not mention that tics should be present daily nor specifically limit the age at onset. ICD-10 also implies greater disability, describing TD as a "chronic, incapacitating disorder," whereas DSM-IV merely requires that the symptoms cause significant impairment.

Differential diagnosis

Tics, described in DSM-IV as "sudden, rapid, recurrent, nonrhythmic, [and] stereotyped" (American Psychiatric Association, 1994, p. 103) are distinguished from other involuntary movements, although not always easily. *Choreiform movements* are not individually repetitive, they wander through the limbs, are irregular, and may have a "dancing" quality. ("Chorea" is derived from the Greek, *choreia*, a choral dance). Like tics, choreiform movements most often affect the face, hands and arms, but the individual may also be generally fidgety. Additional signs of Sydenham's chorea include weakness, diffuse hypotonia, inability to maintain a continuous muscular contraction (e.g., inconstant grip, termed "milkmaid's grip") and dysrhythmic speech. *Dystonic movements* are slow, twisting movements that grow out of and often return to a state of increased motor tone. *Athetoid movements* (from the Greek, *athetos*, without position) are slow, writhing movements of alternating flexion and extension or pronation and supination, usually of the fingers and hands, less often of the toes and feet. Muscles of the face or neck may also be affected. *Myoclonic jerks* (from the Greek, *mys*, muscle, and *klonos*, a tumult) are very brief, rapid, variable intensity contractions of a muscle fascicle, whole muscle or muscle group. Unlike tics, they do not migrate from body part to body part and cannot be suppressed by voluntary effort. *Hemiballismic movements* are intermittent, unilateral, large-amplitude, violent limb movements. *Synkinesias* are involuntary movements that accompany a voluntary movement.

TD is differentiated in both DSM-IV and ICD-10 from *chronic motor* or *vocal tic disorder*, which is the presence, for 12 months or more, of either motor or vocal tics, but not both. *Transient tic disorder* is characterized by motor or vocal tics that are present for at least four weeks, but less than 12 months. *Tic disorder not otherwise specified* is diagnosed when tics last less than four weeks or have their onset after age 18 years.

Tics and syndromes resembling TD have also been reported in *Huntington's disease, neuroacanthocytosis* and *Asperger's syndrome* (Jankovic, 1993). Sacks coined the term "acquired Tourettism" for cases of TD caused by cerebral insult, e.g., following *encephalitis, head trauma, stroke* or *carbon monoxide poisoning* (Robertson, 1989). The medical history and the additional neurological (or ancillary) findings lead to the appropriate diagnosis. Tics are associated rarely with neuroleptic-induced *tardive dyskinesia* (Jankovic, 1993). *Stimulant drugs* can exacerbate existing tics or precipitate tics in individuals with attention deficit disorder (Sandor, 1993); these drugs can often be utilized successfully, however, in a coordinated treatment plan for individuals with comorbid attention deficit disorder and TD (Singer and Walkup, 1991) (see pp. 146–9 for discussion).

Complex motor tics can be quite difficult to distinguish from *compulsions* such as touching, tapping, rubbing, blinking or staring, particularly in individuals who suffer from both TD and OCD (Holzer et al., 1994). Typically, compulsions are voluntary, purposeful acts that must be performed properly in order to ward off or undo some negative event. They are preceded by related thoughts or images and by autonomic anxiety symptoms (Miguel et al., 1997). Tics are purposeless, and unlike compulsions, are frequently preceded by premonitory sensory experiences such as an increasingly uncomfortable muscular sensation of tightness, tension or "itching," or of dry throat before a grunt or cough; performance of the tic produces relief, which may be short-lived. Complex motor tics are involuntary or only partially voluntary (i.e., temporarily suppressible) and, although they are coordinated movements, have no purpose other than to relieve uncomfortable premonitory feelings (Jankovic, 1992; Leckman et al., 1997b). Tics may persist during sleep, although they are almost always less frequent and less intense.

Clinical picture

The modal age of onset of motor tics in TD is between five and seven years (Leckman et al., 1997b), but onset between ages 1 and 21 years has been reported (Sandor, 1993). Simple vocal tics usually begin one to two years after motor tics (Robertson, 1989), but are the presenting symptom in 12–37% of children (Bruun and Budman, 1993). Onset of the syndrome is usually gradual, with one or more episodes of transient tic disorder preceding persistent symptoms (Leckman et al., 1997b). Individual tics, however, may begin suddenly. Common first signs are excessive eye blinking, facial grimacing, head jerking and lip licking or biting (Peterson, 1996). New tics usually appear in a rostral to caudal order, but the march of symptoms may be irregular in the individual patient.

Motor tics gradually evolve into complex behaviors characteristic of the patient. These may take the form of grooming, facial expressions, spitting, touching oneself or others, gesturing, stretching, neck-cracking, trunk-bending, slapping the face or body, squatting, hopping, stamping, jumping or other complex motor acts. Self-injurious behavior, e.g., head banging, pressing the eyes, biting the lips, cheeks or fingernails, and occasionally, scratching, picking scabs or sticking sharp objects into the skin, may affect up to one-third of patients (Robertson and Yakely, 1993). Obscene gestures (copropraxia) and forced sexual touching are uncommon, but quite troubling.

Simple vocal tics include sniffing, grunting, throat clearing, snorting, sucking, coughing, squeaking, barking and other meaningless sounds. Complex vocal tics may present as stereotyped words or phrases, palilalia (repeating one's own words), echolalia or coprolalia. Coprolalia occurs in only a minority of patients (Robertson, 1989), and is reported in non-Western as well as Western cultures (Staley, Wand and Shady, 1997). It disappears in up to one-third of patients (Robertson, 1989).

In children, tics typically occur in bouts, which wax and wane over weeks or months, exacerbated by stress, emotional upset and fatigue (Leckman et al., 1997b). In adults, symptom severity, although potentially exacerbated by the same factors, is more stable over long periods. Perhaps three-quarters of patients experience a gradual decrease in tic symptom severity during adolescence, but an unfortunate few suffer increased symptoms, or emergent or aggravated obsessions, compulsions, depression or anxiety (Peterson, 1996). During adolescence, temper tantrums, aggressiveness and behavioral problems often worsen, and coprolalia may first appear. These developments and the increased social demands of adolescence can contribute to an increased need for professional attention (Bruun and Budman, 1993). Reviewing retrospective and follow-up studies, Bruun and Budman (1993) concluded that about one-third of patients remit during late adolescence or early adulthood; one-third experience substantial lessening of tic frequency and severity; and, the final third remain significantly affected. These statistical averages hide the variability of individual experience; some patients suffer a worsening of symptoms in adulthood. In one follow-up study, more than half of TD patients continued to require medications for tics into adulthood (Goetz et al., 1992).

The clinical picture appears to be quite similar across cultures, although coprolalia is reported in a larger proportion of case reports from outside the United States and Europe, probably as a result of ascertainment or reporting bias (Staley et al., 1997).

Assessment instruments

The available assessment instruments vary in their ease of administration and in the clinical domains measured, but all provide reliable measures of tic severity (Leckman et al., 1989; Walkup et al., 1992). The Shapiro Tourette Syndrome Severity Scale contains five ordinal scales that focus on whether tics are noticeable to others, elicit comments and impair functioning. The Tourette Syndrome Global

Scale allows the clinician to rate the frequency and impact of tics and the intensity of behavioral problems, motor restlessness and school/work impairment. The Tourette's Syndrome–Clinical Global Impression Scale is a seven-point ordinal scale for rating symptom severity derived directly from the Global Impression Scale (Guy, 1976) provided in Appendix 2. The Hopkins Motor–Vocal Tic Scale provides linear analog scales on which parents and the physician can rate the severity of each tic, taking into account its frequency, intensity, interference and impairment. Finally, the Yale Global Tic Severity Scale (YGTSS) provides ordinal scales for separately rating motor and phonic tics with regard to number, frequency, intensity, complexity, interference with behavior or speech and impairment of self-esteem and functioning (Leckman et al., 1989). Because the anchor points of the YGTSS are well defined, this scale is provided in Appendix 2.

Prevalence

No studies have generated prevalence statistics by examining all members of a geographically defined population. Apter et al. (1993) examined a cohort of more than 28,000 sixteen- and seventeen-year-olds entering the Israel Self-Defense Force. After completing a self-report form inquiring about lifetime history of tics, all individuals were examined by physicians trained to recognize tics and TD. Those manifesting tics underwent a structured, confirmatory assessment. The prevalence of TD was 4.9 per 10,000 males (1 in 2,041 males) and 3.1 per 10,000 females (1 in 3,226 females).

A few studies have attempted to determine prevalence by contacting treatment sources and soliciting affected individuals through media outreach. Using these methods in Monroe County (New York, USA) Caine et al. (1988) reported a prevalence in children of 7.1 per 10,000 for males (1 in 1,400) and 0.8 per 10,000 (1 in 11,900) for females. On the basis of responses to questionnaires mailed to physicians and others in North Dakota, USA, Burd and colleagues (1986) estimated the prevalence of treated TD cases aged 18 years and younger at 9.9 per 10,000 males and 1.0 per 10,000 females. These authors' estimates for adults were 0.77 per 10,000 for males and 0.22 per 10,000 females. The majority of studies suggest that the prevalence of TD is three to four times higher in males than in females (Robertson, 1989).

Undoubtedly, the community prevalence of TD is several times the treated prevalence rate, since many affected individuals go uncounted: the ascertainment of treated cases is admittedly incomplete; and, many individuals do not seek care because they have symptoms too mild to motivate help-seeking, experience barriers to care or do not know their tics are treatable (Robertson and Gourdie, 1990).

Genetics

Family linkage and twin studies in the 1970s and 1980s suggested that most cases of TD represented autosomal dominant inheritance with greater penetrance in males than females (Robertson, 1989). Recent studies suggest that there may be several different modes of inheritance, including mutations at varying genetic loci and multifactorial inheritance (Sadovnick and Kurlan, 1997). To date, the genetic roots of TD have escaped detection.

Family and twin studies indicate that in TD pedigrees, chronic motor tics and obsessions and compulsions without tics are all phenotypes of the TD vulnerability gene or genes (Pauls, 1992). By examining TD patients' first-degree relatives instead of relying on family history data, Pauls and colleagues (1991) were able to describe more accurately the genetic relationship between TD and these phenotypes. TD and chronic motor tics were more likely to occur in male relatives, whereas OCD without tics was more likely to occur in female relatives. The relatives' age-adjusted rate of TD was 9%, of chronic motor tics, 17% and of OCD, 11.5%. The risk for OCD was the same in the relatives of TD patients with and without comorbid OCD.

A study utilizing mailed questionnaires to assess 43 twin pairs in which at least one twin had TD, found that 16 of 30 monozygotic pairs (53%) were concordant for TD compared to only 1 of 13 dizygotic pairs (8%) (Price et al., 1985). When two-thirds of the monozygotic pairs were examined by direct interview, 89% were found to be concordant for TD and 100% for either TD or chronic motor tics (Singer and Walkup, 1991). Since the severity of TD symptoms can vary in monozygotic cotwins concordant for the disorder, nongenetic factors, not clearly established at present, must somehow influence TD severity (Peterson, 1996).

Concordance for OCD appears to be high in monozygotic twin pairs in which at least one twin is affected by TD and at least one by OCD. Among nine such pairs examined by direct interview, 7 (78%) were concordant for OCD (Singer and Walkup, 1991).

Comorbidity

Since Gilles de la Tourette remarked upon obsessions and compulsions in patients with the syndrome bearing his name, numerous studies have confirmed his observation. The precise degree of association, however, has not been established. Three modern studies using structured interviews to evaluate OCD in TD patients report comorbidity figures ranging from 28% to 62% (Frankel et al., 1986; Pauls et al., 1986; Pitman et al., 1987).

Certain kinds of obsessions and compulsions appear to be more common in TD patients with comorbid OCD than in patients with OCD alone. Studies suggest that comorbid patients are more likely to have obsessions involving sexual content, violent thoughts or images, symmetry and exactness (Leckman et al., 1995, 1997b). Compulsions involving counting, hoarding, ordering, touching, tapping, rubbing, blinking or staring are more common, and those involving cleaning are less common (Holzer et al., 1994; Leckman et al., 1995; Petter, Richter and Sandor, 1998). As noted earlier, determining whether many of these behaviors represent compulsions or complex motor tics can be difficult. TD patients with OCD often report a need to experience "just right" perceptions before they can stop performing a compulsion (Leckman et al., 1994b).

Tic onset usually precedes the onset of OCD, e.g., by an average of three years in one study (Holzer et al., 1994) and by nine years in another (Pitman et al., 1987). As a result, children with TD should be evaluated periodically for the appearance of obsessive–compulsive symptoms (Peterson, 1996).

Attention deficit hyperactivity disorder (ADHD) is common in children with TD who come to clinical attention (Singer and Walkup, 1991; Sverd et al., 1992). In addition, individual elements of the syndrome – inattention, distractibility, impulsivity or hyperactivity – frequently appear in isolation. The association between TD and ADHD is believed to reflect in large measure an ascertainment bias (individuals with both conditions are more likely to be referred for treatment), as well as difficulty in segregating TD and ADHD symptoms (Robertson, 1989; Towbin and Riddle, 1993). In most cases, ADHD manifests itself before TD (Singer and Walkup, 1991). The effects of ADHD on the child's self-concept, school performance, peer relationships and family relationships may outweigh the effects of TD and require more vigorous intervention. In any case, the burden of having two chronic, disruptive illnesses can be heavy indeed. Fortunately, ADHD often remits in adulthood (Towbin and Riddle, 1993) and TD often improves. TD with comorbid ADHD has not been well studied in adults.

Treatment

In creating a treatment plan for an adult with TD, the clinician should assess the severity of motor and vocal tics, the presence of comorbid conditions such as OCD and ADHD, and the effects of TD and these comorbidities on the patient's self-concept, relationships and social functioning, both during maturation and currently. When mood or anxiety disorders are present, their treatment may indirectly alleviate tic symptoms by reducing stress. An approach to planning integrated treatment for TD is shown in Table 7.2 (p. 150).

Medications will ameliorate tics, often markedly, but usually do not abolish them. Behavior therapy aimed at tics is no longer thought to be effective.

Psychotherapy may be needed to relieve and redress the psychological or social aftermath of the disorder. A first step in treatment is educating the patient and his concerned others regarding the nature of TD. In the United States, the Tourette Syndrome Association offers educational materials and scientific reprints for this purpose (See Appendix 1). Kindred organizations have been established in other countries, including Australia, France, Germany, Holland, New Zealand, Norway and the United Kingdom. Patients who present with mild to moderate symptoms may need only education and the reassurance that treatment is available if symptoms worsen.

Pharmacotherapy

When TD symptom severity and related impairments justify medication, the clinician has several drug classes from which to chose. The choice involves balancing symptom severity, comorbid conditions, drug side-effects and the likelihood of effectiveness.

Drug therapy of TD is thought to work by decreasing neuronal activity in the basal ganglia, thereby quieting a cortico–striato–thalamo–cortical circuit (Leckman et al., 1997b). The basal ganglia in each hemisphere consist of the globus pallidus and the striatum (caudate nucleus and putamen). Recent pathophysiological models of TD link therapeutic drug action to effects on the neurotransmitters utilized by and impinging upon this brain region (Singer and Walkup, 1991; Leckman et al., 1997b).

Possible neurotransmitter dysfunctions are being actively investigated. Leckman et al. (1997b) summarize neurobiological evidence suggesting that TD is related to abnormally increased dopaminergic innervation of the striatum or to supersensitivity of striatal dopaminergic D2 receptors; they note, however, that not all evidence supports this hypothesis. These authors describe how the hypothesized dopaminergic abnormality may, in turn, reflect abnormalities in GABAergic striatal neurons, and be influenced by opioid, noradrenergic and other systems. Most drugs now used to treat TD target dopaminergic or noradrenergic neurotransmission.

In patients with isolated TD, first-line drugs include clonidine and certain neuroleptics. Clonidine is an α_2 adrenergic agonist that inhibits presynaptic norepinephrine release. It is primarily marketed for the treatment of hypertension. By decreasing activity of locus coeruleus projections to the substantia nigra and ventral tegmentum, clonidine indirectly decreases their dopaminergic stimulation of the basal ganglia (Peterson, 1996). Unlike the neuroleptics, clonidine never gives rise to tardive dyskinesia. The drug's primary disadvantage is its lower likelihood of effectiveness. Although more than half of patients treated in open-label studies reportedly improved, the results of double-blind trials are highly variable

(Goetz, 1993). One trial found no advantage of clonidine over placebo (Goetz et al., 1987). A second study, involving 12 subjects, reported that 7 (58%) improved (Borison et al., 1992). A 12-week, randomized, double-blind study compared 21 subjects (children and adults) given clonidine (mean dose 4.4 ± 0.7 µg/kg per day) with 19 subjects given placebo. The active drug group exhibited significantly greater, though not impressive, improvement on most measures of motor and phonic tics (Leckman et al., 1991). For example, clonidine-treated patients improved a mean of 26% on a global scale compared to a mean of 11% in the placebo group.

Clonidine has a half-life of 12.7 ± 7 hours in adults, necessitating twice or three times daily dosing (Medical Economics Company, 1998). The starting dose in adults is 0.025 to 0.050 mg twice or three times daily, with increases of 0.025 to 0.050 mg every three to four days, and a target dose of 0.2 to 0.5 mg/day (Peterson, 1996). The smallest tablet marketed in the United States is a 0.1 mg dose. Transdermal patches designed to deliver clonidine doses of 0.1, 0.2 or 0.3 mg/day for a week are also available. Benefit may not be apparent for three to four weeks (in part because of the necessity of titrating the dose), and some investigators recommend a trial of 8–12 weeks before reaching a conclusion (Robertson, 1989). Common side effects are drowsiness, dry mouth, irritability, headache and insomnia; symptomatic postural hypotension can occur at higher doses. Because abrupt discontinuation of clonidine can provoke hypertension, agitation or exacerbation of tics, the dose should be tapered over two to four days (Goetz, 1993; Medical Economics Company, 1998).

The efficacy of haloperidol and pimozide have been established in double-blind trials, and both are approved by the federal Food and Drug Administration for the treatment of TD. Both drugs block dopamine D2 receptors and are thought to act by reducing dopaminergic input from the substantia nigra and ventral tegmentum to the basal ganglia (Peterson, 1996). Although more effective than clonidine, both drugs, with prolonged use, carry the disadvantage of tardive dyskinesia risk. About 70–80% of patients treated with either drug experience substantial benefit (Kurlan and Trinidad, 1995).

The starting dose of haloperidol in adults is 0.5 mg/day, with dose increases no more often than every five to seven days to a maximum dose of 8 mg/day (Peterson, 1996). A slow upward titration allows time to evaluate tic response and avoid unnecessarily high doses, which increase tardive dyskinesia risk. Haloperidol tablets are available in the United States in 0.5, 1, 2 and 5 mg doses, among others. Patients frequently discontinue treatment because of sedation, cognitive dulling, fatigue, dysphoria or extrapyramidal side effects such as tremor, akathisia or acute dystonia. A small minority experience a loss of therapeutic effect (Silva et al., 1996).

The starting dose of pimozide in adults is also 0.5 mg/day, one-quarter of the smallest dose tablet available in the United States. As with haloperidol, a slow upward titration is recommended to a maximum dose of 8 mg/day (Peterson, 1996). In equivalent doses, pimozide appears to be less likely than haloperidol to cause sedation and extrapyramidal side effects (Shapiro et al., 1989) and may have lower discontinuation rates (Sandor et al., 1990). Pimozide can prolong the QT_c interval, and in rare instances has induced arrhythmias, but this is unlikely at the doses used to treat TD (Kurlan and Trinidad, 1995). The manufacturer recommends obtaining an electrocardiogram at baseline and considering a lower dose if the QT_c interval becomes greater than 0.52 seconds or increases by more than 25% (Medical Economics Company, 1998). Macrolide antibiotics (e.g., erythromycin, clarithromycin) are contraindicated in patients taking pimozide since rare instances of fatal ventricular arrhythmias have been associated with this combination (Medical Economics Company, 1998). Patients who respond poorly to or cannot tolerate haloperidol may have a good response to pimozide, and vice versa (Kurlan and Trinidad, 1995).

Smaller bodies of evidence support the effectiveness of other neuroleptics including fluphenazine, trifluoperazine and sulpiride (a selective D2 receptor antagonist available in Europe) (George, Trimble and Robertson, 1993b; Kurlan and Trinidad, 1995).

A few open-label studies suggest that the novel neuroleptic risperidone is effective in doses of 0.5 to 6 mg/day, but the magnitude of its therapeutic effect may be somewhat smaller than that of haloperidol or pimozide (Lombroso et al., 1995; Bruun and Budman, 1996). At the time of writing, a double-blind trial is underway. Risperidone is a weaker D2 receptor antagonist than haloperidol or pimozide and a strong 5-HT$_2$ receptor antagonist. Sedation and weight gain are common complaints, but because of its receptor blockade profile, risperidone may carry a lower tardive dyskinesia risk than standard neuroleptics and, at doses up to 6 mg/day, may cause fewer extrapyramidal side effects. Patients who have not responded to haloperidol, pimozide or clonidine may respond to risperidone (Bruun and Budman, 1996).

Ziprasidone, another novel neuroleptic that blocks both 5-HT$_2$ and D2 receptors, moderately inhibits serotonin and norepinephrine reuptake and acts as a 5-HT$_{1A}$ agonist, has been found effective in children and adolescents with TD (Sallee et al., 1998. The tolerability and efficacy of ziprasidone in the treatment of children and adolescents with Tourette's syndrome, unpublished data). In a multicenter, double-blind, placebo-controlled, eight-week trial, ziprasidone 20–40 mg/day decreased tic severity scores by a mean of 54% ($n = 15$), compared to a mean of 1% in the placebo group ($n = 11$). Ziprasidone seems less likely than risperidone to cause weight gain, but may be associated with somnolence, postural hypotension, nausea, vomiting, constipation and akisthisia. At the time of writing, ziprasidone is being evaluated in the United States for the treatment of schizophrenia. Additional studies will be needed to define its place in the TD armamentarium.

The literature concerning drugs of which the use in TD is supported only by occasional case reports or small case series is reviewed by Kurlan and Trinidad (1995); a few newer series are described by Peterson and Cohen (1998). These drugs include botulinum toxin (for painful dystonic tics or blepharospasm), calcium channel blockers, clonazepam, lithium, naltrexone and nicotine.

Treating comorbid ADHD

In planning treatment for an adult patient with comorbid TD and ADHD, the clinician must carefully delineate all of the disorders present and determine their impact on past and current psychological and social functioning. It may be necessary to interview (with the patient's permission) those living with the patient in order to uncover the entire clinical picture. Adults with ADHD often have comorbid antisocial personality disorder, substance abuse, mood, anxiety or learning disorders (Biederman et al., 1993). They frequently exhibit stubbornness, low frustration tolerance, anger outbursts and chronic interpersonal conflicts. Deciding when and how to treat each of the patient's problems is a challenging exercise in the art of medicine. Active substance abuse, however, is a contraindication to the prescription of stimulants and seriously compromises the use of tricyclic antidepressants because of potential noncompliance, medication abuse and dangerous interactions between abused substances and prescribed drugs.

As with uncomplicated TD, psychotherapy may be indicated to relieve and repair the psychological and social consequences of a life experience marred by ADHD. Educating the patient and his significant others regarding the nature of ADHD can relieve guilt and facilitate cooperation with the treatment plan. The nonprofit organizations, Children and Adults with Attention Deficit Disorders and the National Attention-Deficit Disorder Association, offer educational materials and sponsor local chapters and support groups (see Appendix 1).

Well-controlled studies suggest that cognitive–behavioral therapy can help patients learn techniques for managing and diminishing impulsivity, inattention and affective instability (Barkley, 1990), but their exposition is beyond the scope of this book.

Pharmacotherapy

Stimulant drugs and tricyclic antidepressants have established efficacy in treating ADHD in children with TD (Peterson and Cohen, 1998). I could find no controlled trials centered on adults with both conditions. Moreover, few controlled trials of pharmacotherapy for adults with ADHD have been published. Attempts to reach firm conclusions by comparing the available ADHD treatment studies are confounded by methodological differences in sampling, diagnostic criteria, drug dosing and outcome measures (Spencer et al., 1995).

A few well-controlled trials support the use of the tricyclic antidepressant, desipramine, in treating patients with comorbid TD and ADHD. Desipramine was more effective than clonidine or placebo in a double-blind crossover trial in 37 children with comorbid ADHD and TD (Singer et al., 1995). In this trial and in a chart review study of 30 similarly diagnosed children, desipramine also tended to improve tic severity (Spencer et al., 1993a). A chart review study of 12 children with comorbid ADHD and TD treated with nortriptyline suggests that it may be as effective as desipramine for both ADHD and tics (Spencer et al., 1993c).

In adults with ADHD, desipramine in doses of 100–200 mg/day is effective in about two-thirds of patients; the therapeutic effect is noticeable within two weeks or less (Wilens et al., 1996). Whether tricyclics ameliorate ADHD symptoms in adults to the same degree as do stimulants is controversial. However, in a well designed, six-week, double-blind, placebo-controlled study of 41 adults with DSM-III-R ADHD, desipramine, but not placebo, produced clinically and statistically significant improvement over baseline in 12 of 14 ADHD symptoms (Wilens et al., 1996). The side effects of desipramine and nortriptyline include anticholinergic effects, symptomatic postural hypotension (in 5–10% of patients), tremor, jitteriness and either sedation or insomnia. In healthy adults, cardiac side effects other than tachycardia are rare.

Well-controlled trials have demonstrated the efficacy of bupropion in treating ADHD in children, and open-label trials suggest it may be as effective as the stimulants in adults (Popper, 1997). Bupropion, however, appears to share a disadvantage of the stimulants – it can exacerbate tics (Spencer et al., 1993b). Bupropion may be preferable to the stimulants in treating patients with a history of substance abuse.

Because stimulants exacerbate tics in some individuals, their use in children (and adults) with comorbid ADHD and TD is controversial (Sverd et al., 1992; Golden, 1993). Still, they are often well tolerated, sometimes ameliorate tics and are not contraindicated (Castellanos et al., 1997). In ADHD adults without TD, d-amphetamine, methylphenidate and pemoline are each effective in about 75% of patients, although individuals may respond to one drug and not another (Popper, 1997). The effectiveness of methylphenidate and pemoline in adults has been established in controlled trials. Clinical experience indicates that the longer acting stimulant methamphetamine is also effective, but it is far more expensive (Bhandary et al., 1997). D-amphetamine and methylphenidate have a clinical duration of action of three to six hours, whereas pemoline acts for 4–10 hours, allowing twice daily instead of three or four times daily dosing and producing a somewhat smoother clinical response (Popper, 1997). Patients taking stimulants with shorter durations of action may experience rebound symptoms before the next dose, including anxiety, irritability, confusion and verbosity (Bhandary et al., 1997). Although sustained release preparations of d-amphetamine and methylphenidate are marketed, they have not been studied in adults.

A double-blind, controlled study of methylphenidate in adults with ADHD, but without TD, demonstrated that a dose of 1.0 mg/kg per day was more effective than lower doses and was well tolerated (Spencer et al., 1995). The usual starting dose is 5 mg three times daily with weekly increments of 5–10 mg/day and a usual dose range of 10–90 mg/day (maximum 140 mg/day) (Bhandary et al., 1997). The usual starting dose of d-amphetamine is 2.5 mg twice daily with weekly increments of 5–10 mg/day and a usual dose range of 5–45 mg/day in two or three divided doses (maximum 70 mg/day) (Bhandary et al., 1997). Individuals vary widely in their dose requirements. Therapeutic effects are usually apparent within a week.

In their review of the pharmacotherapy of adult ADHD, Wilens and colleagues (1995) note that stimulant side-effects in ADHD adults are usually mild. The most common are insomnia, nervousness, decreased appetite, weight loss, dysphoria and headaches. Increases in heart rate and blood pressure are generally minimal and benign. Pemoline, however, has been associated with life-threatening hepatic failure and 11 deaths in children and adolescents over a 20-year period and is not a first line choice (Popper, 1997). If pemoline is prescribed, liver function must be evaluated at baseline and at least every six months thereafter. Long-term safety and efficacy of the stimulants in adult ADHD have not been established.

The α_2-adrenergic agonist clonidine helped 95% of children with comorbid ADHD and TD in one chart review study (Steingard et al., 1993); however, a double-blind crossover trial in a similar comorbid group found that clonidine was no better than placebo and that desipramine was better than clonidine (Singer et al., 1995). In an open-label study of 10 children with comorbid ADHD and TD, the more selective α_2-adrenergic agonist guanfacine was associated with modest improvement in ADHD in four children and moderate decrease in phonic, but not motor, tics in five (Chappell et al., 1995). Both drugs are thought to ameliorate ADHD by blocking α_2-adrenergic receptors in the prefrontal cortex, thereby enhancing working memory and attention (Chappell et al., 1995). Guanfacine tends to be less sedating than clonidine. The dosing of clonidine is the same as was described earlier for use in treating TD. Guanfacine can be started at 0.5 mg once daily and increased by 0.5 mg every three to four days to 1–3 mg/day as tolerated (Chappell et al., 1995). The therapeutic value of these drugs in adults with ADHD has not been established.

Open-label trials suggest very modest efficacy for L-deprenyl (selegilene) in comorbid ADHD and TD (Feigin et al., 1996); additional trials are needed to determine its utility.

This literature leads me to recommend desipramine or nortriptyline as first-line treatments in adult patients with comorbid ADHD and TD. These drugs appear to be nearly as effective as the stimulants and may modestly improve tics. If the patient is receiving a neuroleptic for TD, a tricyclic or a stimulant can be cautiously added, with attention to additive anticholinergic, cardiovascular and cognitive side effects (Golden, 1993). While clonidine and guanfacine may also relieve TD, they appear to be less effective for ADHD than the tricyclics and stimulants. If a tricyclic drug fails to relieve a patient's comorbid ADHD, the clinician must weigh the greater effectiveness and risks of the stimulants (and possibly bupropion) against the lesser effectiveness and risks of clonidine and guanfacine. Alternately, the clinician might consider combined treatment with methylphenidate and clonidine, although this combination has not been investigated in comorbid ADHD and TD. Since these drugs affect the noradrenergic system by different mechanisms, and since clonidine is often beneficial in TD, their use in combination might relieve both ADHD and TD symptoms (personal communication, F.R. Sallee, M.D., April, 1998).

Treating comorbid OCD

Open-label studies (Riddle et al., 1990; Como and Kurlan, 1991; Eapen, Trimble and Robertson, 1996) and two controlled trials (Kurlan et al., 1993; Scahill et al., 1997) indicate that fluoxetine is effective in treating OCD in TD patients. In a double-blind, placebo-controlled crossover trial involving 14 TD patients (eight with OCD or obsessive–compulsive symptoms), fluoxetine 20 mg/day had no significant effect on tic severity (Scahill et al., 1997). A small ($n = 11$), double-blind crossover trial, marred by its short, six-week treatment period, found that OCD symptom severity decreased 25% after fluvoxamine treatment, but this change was not statistically significant (George et al., 1993b). Case reports support the use of clomipramine (Ratzoni et al., 1990), which may also reduce tic severity (Iancu et al., 1995), perhaps because it blocks norepinephrine as well as serotonin reuptake.

I have had success in a few cases with each of the selective serotonin reuptake inhibitors (SSRIs) in treating OCD in adult patients with mild to moderate TD symptoms. Most patients were not receiving concomitant TD medications, and some experienced a lessening of tic severity during SSRI treatment. The drug doses were those ordinarily used to treat OCD alone (See Chapter 3).

When comorbid OCD fails to respond to the first adequate SSRI trial, adding haloperidol or pimozide in gradually escalated doses up to 2–10 mg/day, or risperidone up to 6 mg/day, is a reasonable next step. In a double-blind, placebo-controlled trial, eight of eight patients with chronic tics and fluvoxamine-refractory OCD responded during a four-week trial of added haloperidol (mean dose, 6.3 ± 3.0 mg/day) compared to none of seven given added placebo (McDougle et al., 1994a). The tic severity ratings of the eight patients decreased by a mean of 50%.

Table 7.2. Tourette's disorder (TD): treatment planning guidelines

- Assess the severity of motor and vocal tics.
- Assess psychological, interpersonal and occupational problems related to TD and consider psychotherapeutic intervention.
- Identify and treat comorbid mood disorder.
- Assess for comorbid ADHD and OCD.
- Educate the patient and concerned others about TD.
- Consider an 8–12 week trial of clonidine for tics, and continue it long-term if effective.
- If clonidine fails, consider a trial of haloperidol or pimozide.
- If clonidine and haloperidol or pimozide fail, consider a trial of risperidone.
- If necessary, consider trials of less well established drugs.

When comorbid ADHD is present:
- Assess psychological, interpersonal and occupational problems related to ADHD and consider psychotherapeutic intervention.
- Assess for comorbid antisocial personality disorder, substance abuse and learning disorder.
- Treat active substance abuse before treating ADHD.
- Educate the patient and significant others about ADHD.
- Consider referral for expert cognitive–behavioral treatment of ADHD symptoms.
- Consider a four to six week trial of desipramine or nortriptyline and continue long-term if effective.
- If a tricyclic fails, weigh the risks and benefits of a stimulant (or bupropion) versus clonidine or guanfacine. Alternatively, consider a combination of methylphenidate and clonidine.

When comorbid OCD is present:
- Treat with an SRI, as in isolated OCD; (clomipramine may ameliorate both conditions).
- If the SRI fails, consider adding haloperidol, risperidone or pimozide.

Notes:
ADHD: attention deficit hyperactivity disorder; OCD: obsessive–compulsive disorder; SRI: serotonin reuptake inhibitor.

The 100% OCD responder rate in this small trial far exceeds the rate one would expect from a trial of a second SSRI. This lends support to the strategy of neuroleptic addition for TD patients whose OCD has failed to respond to an SSRI trial, although additional studies of this strategy should be undertaken.

Isolated cases of onset or exacerbation of tics during SSRI treatment exist (Fennig et al., 1994; Kotler et al., 1994), but these do not constitute a reason to withhold SSRI treatment of comorbid OCD. Such events are rare and can be managed by trials of alternate SSRIs or by the addition or dose adjustment of clonidine, guanfacine or a neuroleptic.

8

Body dysmorphic disorder

But I, that am not shaped for sportive tricks
Nor made to court an amorous looking glass

Shakespeare, *Richard III*

The term, "body dysmorphic disorder," was introduced in DSM-III-R to describe a disorder first reported by Morelli in 1891 as dysmorfophobia (Phillips et al., 1993). The term is derived from the Greek word, *dysmorfia*, first used by Herodotus in the *Histories*. He was referring to the "ill looks" of the "ugliest girl in Sparta," who miraculously married the king of Sparta after a goddess transformed her into a beauty (Philippopoulos, 1979). Janet termed the condition, *obsession de la honte du corps* (obsession with shame of the body), and considered it similar to OCD (Phillips et al., 1995). The term most often used in the earlier scientific literature was dysmorphophobia, but European psychiatrists also utilized the terms, "beauty hypochondria" and "dermatological hypochondriasis." When the belief in being egregiously unattractive reached delusional intensity, cases were often grouped together with cases of monosymptomatic hypochondriacal psychosis, which includes delusions of parasitosis and the olfactory reference syndrome (the delusion that one gives off a noticeable, objectionable odor) (Munro and Chmara, 1982).

Diagnosis and differential diagnosis

DSM-IV diagnostic criteria (300.7)

Body dysmorphic disorder entered the American Psychiatric Association's diagnostic classification system with the 1987 publication of DSM-III-R (Phillips, 1991). DSM-III included it only as a form of atypical somatoform disorder described in an appendix, and did not assign the delusional variety a specific classification. The DSM-IV criteria (American Psychiatric Association, 1994) are given in Table 8.1.

ICD-10 diagnostic criteria (F45.2)

ICD-10 (World Health Organization, 1992) is the first edition of the international coding system to include body dysmorphic disorder, but it does not provide

Table 8.1. DSM-IV diagnostic criteria for body dysmorphic disorder (300.7)

A. Preoccupation with an imagined defect in appearance. If a slight physical anomaly is present, the person's concern is markedly excessive.
B. The preoccupation causes clinically significant distress or impairment in social, occupational, or other important areas of functioning.
C. The preoccupation is not better accounted for by another mental disorder (e.g., dissatisfaction with body shape and size in Anorexia Nervosa).

Source: Reprinted with permission from the *Diagnostic and Statistical Manual of Mental Disorders,* Fourth Edition. Copyright 1994 American Psychiatric Association, p. 468.

diagnostic criteria and includes this condition within the category, hypochondriacal disorders.

Differential diagnosis

When the preoccupation with imagined ugliness is delusional, DSM-IV allows the patient to be given two diagnoses – body dysmorphic disorder and *delusional disorder, somatic type.* DSM-III-R criteria had called for patients to be placed in one diagnostic group or the other. The expert panel revising the criteria noted that the two diagnoses may not represent separate disorders, since the intensity of belief can fluctuate during the disorder's course.

Whether body dysmorphic disorder is a form of *OCD* or a separate disorder is not clear (Phillips et al., 1995). Both disorders are characterized by ideas that are repetitive, persistent and difficult to resist, and by repetitive behaviors that the patient has difficulty controlling. However, the preoccupations of body dysmorphic disorder are more likely to be accepted as natural (ego–syntonic), to be dwelt upon without resistance, and to take the form of overvalued ideas or delusions accompanied by ideas of reference. Obsessions, by contrast, are usually experienced as irrational (ego–dystonic) and are resisted. The preoccupations of body dysmorphic disorder appear to be more often linked to shame, low self-esteem and rejection sensitivity. Moreover, the compulsive behaviors in body dysmorphic disorder less often relieve anxiety and may increase it if they subjectively confirm the patient's fears of ugliness as, for example, mirror-checking may. OCD is diagnosed in patients with body dysmorphic disorder if obsessions and compulsions are not limited to concerns about appearance.

Body dysmorphic disorder can be distinguished from *anorexia nervosa* by the focus on body weight and "fatness" in the latter condition, and from *gender identity disorder* by the patient's discomfort with or rejection of primary and secondary sex characteristics in this disorder. The degree of concern with unattractive features in *social phobia* and *avoidant personality disorder* is distinguished by the fact that the patients' appearance to some extent justifies their concern and by the concern's more limited intrusiveness, frequency, persistence, associated distress and resultant impairment. In the Japanese and Korean literature, however, body dysmorphic disorder is grouped within a class termed "Taijin-phobia," which bears resemblances to social phobia and avoidant personality disorder (Phillips, 1991). The high rate of co-occurrence of body dysmorphic disorder and social phobia suggests that they may be related (Phillips et al., 1994). The low self-esteem and shame of *major depression* are not focussed on the patient's appearance, but instead involve self-denigration of abilities, accomplishments, actions and personality traits. Moreover, the somatic symptoms of major depression will be present.

Clinical picture

Patients are consumed with the belief that they are ugly and suffer intensely. They feel that because they are truly ugly, deformed, grotesque or repulsive, others dislike, ridicule or scorn them. Referring to the suffering of these patients, Phillips (1991) coined the phrase, "the distress of imagined ugliness." The body area that most commonly troubles these patients is the face or head, with a focus on skin flaws, defects, blemishes, wrinkles, spots, scars, facial hair, supposed acne, thinning hair, or a nose the patient considers misshapen or too large. One patient, for example, complained of "dead skin" on his face "with small holes and imperfections all over it" especially on the eyelids and eyebrows (Koran and Pallanti, 1996). The eyes, ears, mouth, lips, teeth, jaw, chin, cheeks, head, breasts, buttocks or genitals can also be areas of focus. Both men and women may focus on signs of gender identity. Men become preoccupied with their genitals, loss of scalp hair and height. Women become preoccupied with breasts, hips and legs (Perugi et al., 1997a; Phillips and Diaz, 1997). Men will occasionally present with the complaint that their body is too small and not muscular enough and will be spending countless hours in body-building exercises. This condition has recently been termed, "muscle dysmorphia" (Phillips, O'Sullivan and Pope, 1997b). Many patients have several concomitant foci or develop new foci over the course of their illness.

Typically patients are preoccupied with their appearance for many hours per day, although some manage to function reasonably well. The preoccupations are either overvalued ideas or reach delusional intensity. The majority of patients have ideas of reference, thinking that others notice their imagined defect and react to it with derision or dislike. As a result, they limit their social exposure and may refrain from dating, shopping, attending school or working (Phillips, 1991).

Rituals accompany the preoccupations (Phillips, 1991). Patients spend hours each day examining the "ugly" feature in a mirror or other reflective surfaces, comparing themselves to others, engaging in camouflaging behaviors such as applying unneeded makeup, combing or arranging their hair, or adopting postures that hide the offending body part. They may grow a beard or wear hats or special clothes to hide the "defect." Picking at minor flaws in the skin or at mild acneiform lesions is not unusual and can produce serious damage and scarring. In three large series, 26% (Veale et al., 1996a,b), 30% (Phillips et al., 1994) and 40% (Hollander, Cohen and Simeon, 1993) of patients had obtained cosmetic surgery, but good results should not be expected, since these patients' expectations are unrealistic and magical (Andreasen and Bardach, 1977; Veale et al., 1996a,b). Other patients pursue fruitless consultations and treatments with various medical specialists, asking dermatologists about skin flaws, endocrinologists about body hair, urologists about "small" genitals (Phillips et al., 1995) or, in one of my cases, ophthalmologists about "uneven" eyelids.

In one series of 48 nondelusional patients (Phillips et al., 1994), males comprised 58%, three-quarters were single, and half were unemployed. The mean age at onset was 17 years, but the disorder made its appearance from childhood to the twenties. The course was continuous in more than 90% of cases. Excessive mirror checking and camouflaging behaviors each affected 81%. Nearly one-third made excessive requests for reassurance about their appearance. Almost every patient exhibited impairment in school, social or work relationships. Approximately one-fourth had been housebound for a week or more because of anguish over ugliness; a similar proportion had been hospitalized because of their disorder. One fourth had made suicide attempts, 10% because of the suffering induced by their disorder. (Suicide attempts were equally common in a British series of 50 patients – Veale et al., 1996a.) A comparison group of 52 patients with body dysmorphic disorder of delusional intensity contained a smaller percentage of men (42%), but otherwise exhibited clinical features that were quite similar, suggesting that this is merely a more severe form of the disorder.

In the case report and case series literature of the past 100 years reviewed by Phillips (1991), the disorder usually ran an unremitting course, lasting for years or decades, although a few cases with a waxing and waning course or a remission were described.

Assessment instruments

Although somewhat time-consuming, the use of an assessment instrument can help facilitate rapport and convey the interviewer's familiarity with the many manifestations of body dysmorphic disorder. In addition, an assessment instrument permits a quantitative comparison of the results of sequential treatment trials. If several trials each result in only partial response, quantitative outcome measures help the clinician judge the trade-offs between benefits and side effects.

A quantitative measure of illness severity should be obtained at the first or second interview. Two assessment instruments are available.

Phillips et al. (1997a) modified the Yale–Brown Obsessive Compulsive Scale (Y–BOCS) to assess severity of body dysmorphic disorder (BDD–YBOCS). The Y–BOCS items concerning time occupied, interference, distress, resistance and control were focussed on the perceived defect in appearance. In addition, these authors modified and included the Y–BOCS items for insight and avoidance, which are not included in standard scoring; thus, the total possible score on the BDD–YBOCS is 48, compared to 40 for the standard Y–BOCS. The BDD–YBOCS can be found in Phillips' book for patients (1996d). Alternatively, the clinician can modify the Y–BOCS given in Appendix 2 by simply focussing each question, as did Phillips (1996d), on the patient's thoughts and activities related to the perceived body defect. The BDD–YBOCS demonstrates excellent inter-rater reliability, internal consistency and concurrent validity when compared to scores on the Global Assessment of Functioning (GAF) scale (DSM-IV 1994, p. 32) and the Clinical Global Impressions scale (Guy, 1976). Change in the BDD–YBOCS is a valid measure of treatment response.

Rosen and Reiter (1996) developed a semi-structured interview, the Body Dysmorphic Disorder Examination, which can be used to measure baseline and treatment effects on preoccupation with appearance, negative evaluation of appearance, weighting of appearance in self-evaluation, body checking and camouflaging behaviors and avoidance of activities. The interview has good internal consistency and test–retest and inter-rater reliability.

Prevalence and comorbidity

The prevalence in the general population is unknown. One plastic surgeon estimated that such patients comprised 2% of his practice (Andreasen and Bardach, 1977).

Patients with body dysmorphic disorder seem to be more likely than control groups to have comorbid depression, OCD or social phobia (Phillips et al., 1993, 1994; Veale et al., 1996b). The lifetime prevalence of comorbid disorders in one study of 48 patients with nondelusional body dysmorphic disorder was: major depression (84%); social phobia (40%); OCD (33%); alcohol abuse or dependence (29%); and dysthymia (13%) (Phillips et al., 1994). The lifetime prevalence of these disorders did not differ significantly in 52 companion cases of delusional body dysmorphic disorder, again supporting the view that this is merely a more severe form. Comorbid depression usually begins within the same year or after, rather than before, body dysmorphic disorder and is often chronic (Phillips et al., 1993). Social phobia precedes body dysmorphic disorder in most comorbid cases (Phillips et al.,

1993). In a UK series of 50 patients evaluated with a structured clinical interview, the prevalence of comorbid conditions at the time of interview was: dysthymia (18%); major depression (8%); social phobia (16%); OCD (6%); other anxiety disorders (16%); and substance abuse/dependence (2%) (Veale et al., 1996a). Comorbid personality disorders were common, particularly avoidant (38%), paranoid (38%) and obsessive–compulsive (28%). Confusion of state with trait variables may have affected these diagnoses.

Patients with atypical depression, OCD or social phobia should be asked about concerns with appearance. In one study of atypical depression, which is marked by abnormal sensitivity to social rejection, 14% of patients had comorbid body dysmorphic disorder (Phillips, 1995). Reports of the lifetime rate of body dysmorphic disorder in OCD patients range from 8% (Brawman-Mintzer et al., 1995) to 37% (Phillips et al., 1995), which suggests that an accurate figure has yet to be established.

Body dysmorphic patients may be so ashamed or humiliated by their concerns that they hide them for decades, not only from family and friends, but also from their therapists (Phillips, 1991). To screen for body dysmorphic disorder, the clinician can ask patients with depression, social phobia or OCD, "Have you been very worried about how you look?" Or, "Do you feel especially unattractive?" A positive response is grounds for inquiry about preoccupations, compulsive behaviors, distress and avoidance behaviors related to bodily appearance.

Treatment

Pharmacotherapy

Although there are no controlled trials yet published, the available literature indicates that serotonin reuptake inhibitors (SRIs – clomipramine, fluoxetine, fluvoxamine, sertraline and paroxetine) are the treatment of choice. All of these SRIs have been used successfully, but improvement is more likely than cure. Given their greater propensity to cause anticholinergic side effects and weight gain, clomipramine and paroxetine should be saved for later trials. Studies cited subsequently indicate that the dose of the chosen drug should be increased over several weeks to the maximum tolerated dose. One should wait at least 12 weeks after reaching this dose before making a judgment about efficacy. A successful pharmacotherapy should be continued. In my experience and in published cases, discontinuation of medication is followed within a few weeks by a return of symptoms. Until research makes clear how and when to discontinue pharmacotherapy, continuous treatment remains the conservative approach. If the patient wishes a trial off medication, the dose should be tapered over three to four months with careful monitoring for symptom return. Slow tapering has proven more successful than tapering over one month in preventing relapse or recurrence of major depression (Kupfer, 1991).

In some patients, body dysmorphic disorder responds to an SRI, but a comorbid major depression or social phobia does not. There are no studies to guide the clinician. In instances of comorbid major depression, I have instituted combined therapies with good results, often adding bupropion in doses of 150 mg/day to 300 mg/day (See Chapter 2). If a tricyclic antidepressant is added, one must keep in mind that SSRIs can inhibit tricyclic metabolism, producing higher plasma levels and more side effects (See Chapter 2). Desipramine in doses of 25 mg/day to 75 mg/day, or equivalent doses of nortriptyline (10 mg/day to 50 mg/day), will often produce adequate serum levels, which should be checked. When comorbid social phobia fails to respond, a reasonable strategy is to add a drug with demonstrated efficacy in this disorder, such as clonazepam, 1 to 6 mg/day (Jefferson, 1995) or buspirone 45 to 60 mg/day (Schneier et al., 1993). Because all of the selective serotonin reuptake inhibitors (SSRIs) are effective in social phobia (Marshall et al., 1994; Katzelnick et al., 1995), the clinician can consider switching to another SSRI. This strategy carries some risk, since the new drug may fail to benefit both conditions. Alternately, cognitive–behavioral therapies for social phobia, including social skills training, graduated exposure, cognitive restructuring or combinations of these can be utilized (Heimberg, 1993). (See Chapter 2.)

For nondelusional patients, cognitive–behavioral therapy, described subsequently, should be provided with all medication trials. Clinical experience with OCD patients suggests that patients who engage in behavioral treatment while taking medications may be less likely to relapse once medication is stopped, but this impression awaits firm research confirmation. Cognitive–behavioral therapy is not recommended for delusional patients; they are unlikely to be dissuaded by logical argument or to comply with exposure and response prevention.

Summarizing the literature on pharmacotherapy for body dysmorphic disorder, Phillips (1995) reports that 54% of 113 trials of various SRIs produced clinically significant improvement (Clinical Global Impression scale, CGI, rating of much or very much improved), compared to 30% of 23 trials with an monoamine oxidase inhibitor (MAOI), 15% of 56 trials with tricyclic or other antidepressants, 6% of trials with other drugs such as benzodiazepines and mood stabilizers, and 2% of 83 trials with antipsychotics.

Phillips, Dwight and McElroy (1998) reports an open-label 16-week trial in 30 subjects given fluvoxamine, mean daily dose 238 mg/day (range, 50–300 mg/day), in which 9 (30%) achieved CGI ratings of much improved and 10 (33.3%) of very much improved. Delusional and nondelusional patients were equally likely to respond and delusional belief significantly diminished (5 of 7 delusional patients were responders). Six of the 19 responders were not rated as much improved until week 10 or later, indicating the need for lengthy therapeutic trials in this disorder. In 6 of 19 patients with comorbid major depression, the body dysmorphic disorder responded while the depression did not; in one patient, depression improved without a response of body dysmorphic disorder. Body dysmorphic disorder symptoms were just as likely to respond in patients without as in those with comorbid depression. Patients who discontinued fluvoxamine relapsed within four days to two months, but responded again when an SRI was restarted.

The use of SRIs is also supported by an observation in one patient with comorbid body dysmorphic disorder and OCD and a history of major depression; experimentally induced, acute tryptophan depletion caused an immediate worsening of her body dysmorphic disorder and a deterioration of mood, without any effect on OCD (Barr, Goodman and Price, 1992).

If the patient has failed to respond to one SRI, the most reasonable medication strategy is to try another. Phillips (1996c), who has extensive clinical experience, expects about one-third of nonresponders to one SRI to respond to another, but well-designed studies are needed to establish an accurate figure. Since response is unpredictable and the side effects of these drugs are usually tolerable, serial three-month trials of several should be conducted when necessary. As in OCD, the available data suggest that higher doses are often needed to treat body dysmorphic disorder than to treat major depression. After several failures, switching to an MAOI seems as reasonable as trying the remaining SRIs. Note that a 'washout' period of at least two weeks is required before switching from an SRI to an MAOI, except in the case of fluoxetine, which requires a washout period of at least five weeks.

Trials of augmenting medications should be pursued in both partial responders and nonresponders. In a study of 13 nonresponders or minimal responders to fluoxetine or clomipramine (Phillips, 1996a), six benefitted from the addition of buspirone 30–90 mg/day (mean dose 48±15 mg/day). The mean time to response was a little more than six weeks (range 5–9 weeks). Delusional and nondelusional patients were equally likely to respond, but partial responders to an SRI were more likely to respond (56%) than were nonresponders (25%). Given the small number of patients, the distinction between partial responders and nonresponders must be regarded as quite tentative. Phillips (1996c) reports that decreasing or discontinuing buspirone led to relapse. Because of the danger of precipitating the serotonin syndrome, buspirone cannot be added to an MAOI.

Patients with delusional body dysmorphic disorder who do not respond sufficiently to an SRI may benefit from the addition of a neuroleptic. Nine of 15 such patients experienced either increased insight or decreased ideas of reference with neuroleptic augmentation (Phillips, 1996b). Pimozide should not be combined with clomipramine (CMI), however, because of additive cardiac toxicity.

Adding CMI to an SSRI has also been reported helpful (Phillips, 1995), but plasma CMI and desmethylclomipramine (DCMI) levels should be monitored. Combined levels of somewhat greater than 1000 ng/ml have been tolerated without serious subjective side effects, albeit with intracardiac conduction changes (Szegedi et al., 1996). My work with intravenous CMI in OCD (Koran, Sallee and Pallanti, 1997), leads me to believe that plasma levels of 250–350 ng/ml of CMI alone should be sufficient, and that combined levels under 450 ng/ml, with a CMI/DCMI ratio of at least 2.2/1, are well tolerated. These levels are achievable in most patients by combining oral doses of 75–150 mg/day of fluvoxamine with 100–150 mg/day of CMI (Szegedi et al., 1996). The combination is started at low doses (25–50 mg/day of each drug), with weekly increases of 50 mg/day of one or both drugs and careful monitoring of plasma levels. Steady state levels of CMI are reached after two weeks of a constant dose, while steady state for DCMI requires three weeks (Medical Economics Company, 1998).

Very rapid, favorable results were observed in two patients with delusional body dysmorphic disorder who were treated with pulse-loaded, intravenous CMI (Koran and Pallanti, 1996). The patients received 150 mg over 90 minutes on the first day and 200 mg over 90 minutes on the second day, followed by a five-day drug holiday. At that point their Y–BOCS scores had decreased by about one-third and they began oral CMI 200 mg/day. Within two weeks both patients had markedly increased their socialization and returned to work or school. After eight weeks of oral CMI treatment, their Y–BOCS scores had decreased by about 55%. Given the apparent rapidity of response to pulse-loaded, intravenous CMI, this treatment deserves evaluation in a randomized, double-blind study. In the United States, intravenous CMI is available only on a research basis.

The literature gives little reason to treat body dysmorphic disorder with neuroleptics alone, and electroconvulsive therapy is not helpful (Phillips, 1995; 1996c).

If the patient is suffering from delusions of parasitosis or the olfactory reference syndrome rather than body dysmorphic disorder, pimozide in doses of 2–12 mg/day, reached over one to three weeks, can be expected to produce excellent results in about two-thirds of patients within 2–12 weeks (Munro, 1988). Other neuroleptics, such as haloperidol, risperidone and olanzapine, should be effective, although no large case series have been published. The clinician must be careful not to challenge the patient's delusional beliefs. In my experience, offering the medication with the explanation that it is being given to reduce the patient's anguish, anxiety or distress while a definitive plan is developed to deal with the parasites or the odor will facilitate compliance.

In patients with delusions of parasitosis, the clinician should consider organic etiologies, including stimulant abuse, tuberculosis, syphilis, hematological disorders such as polycythemia vera and chronic lymphocytic leukemia, B-vitamin deficiencies, renal failure, occult neoplasm and dementia (May and Terpenning, 1991).

Combining psychotherapy with medication

Because body dysmorphic disorder markedly impairs self-esteem and social functioning, psychotherapy is a necessary part of treatment. As noted earlier, cognitive-behavioral treatment should be aimed at the symptomatic beliefs and behaviors, but other forms of therapy, such as psychodynamic or interpersonal therapy or assertiveness training, may be needed to deal with life issues and social deficits. With delusional patients, the clinician should await the beneficial effects of medication before attempting to add cognitive–behavioral or other intensive therapies. Supportive and psychoanalytic psychotherapy, without concomitant SRI drug therapy, have produced mixed findings in case reports. They may help with life issues, but they rarely decrease substantially patients' preoccupations or rituals.

As mentioned earlier, an empathetic interview guided by an assessment instrument can help in establishing rapport. This careful review of the symptoms and their effects also helps the patient to recognize how time consuming the preoccupations are and how dramatically they impair school, work or social life. The review can help strengthen the patient's motivation to confront his or her fears and engage in planned attempts to reduce suffering.

Body dysmorphic patients are often reluctant to seek psychiatric treatment. Psychiatrists can attract patients by making their interest known to plastic surgeons and dermatologists, to whom these patients often turn, and by educating these colleagues about likely presenting complaints.

Cognitive–behavioral therapy

A few studies, which suffer from the absence of blinded outcome ratings, suggest that cognitive–behavioral therapy can benefit motivated patients (Veale et al., 1996b). Although the data are sparse, I recommend that the clinician attempt to implement these techniques as part of a comprehensive treatment plan that encompasses medications and problem-focussed psychotherapy. Whether cognitive techniques add to behavioral interventions remains to be determined, but for the present I recommend that both be utilized.

Once a thorough case history and understanding of the patient as a person have been obtained, the clinician asks the patient to make a written list of behaviors related to checking defects, camouflaging or otherwise responding to them and avoiding social exposure. The Liebowitz Social Anxiety Scale (Liebowitz, 1987; see Appendix 2) is a useful tool for cataloging avoided social situations and the degree of attendant anxiety. Together, the patient and clinician choose one behavior, the change of which would cause only modest anxiety. The patient is told to give up this behavior, or to pursue a specific social exposure daily, allowing a week or more for the resultant anxiety to abate. When this change has been completed, another behavior is chosen for modification or resistance. The patient and clinician arrange a gradual but steady abandonment of the patient's symptomatic rituals. Asking the patient to abandon all of the rituals simultaneously is too anxiety-provoking a demand.

On the cognitive front, the clinician repeatedly points out that beauty is subjective and that the value of a human being is not solely determined by his or her appearance. He challenges the patient's belief that one's appearance must be "perfect" and that if one is ugly one is worthless or unlovable. When no real defect is apparent to the therapist, he encourages the patient to accept uncertainty about the presence of a defect.

Veale et al. (1996b) report that after 12 weekly sessions utilizing these techniques, seven of nine nondelusional patients, an unspecified number of whom had comorbid OCD, social phobia or depressive disorder, were either free of body dysmorphic symptoms or very much improved, compared to none of 10 similar patients placed on a waiting list. The treated patients' mean score on the BDD–YBOCS fell by 50% while their mean scores on the Montgomery–Åsberg Depression Rating Scale (Appendix 2) fell nearly 60%, from mild depression to subclinical levels. No long-term follow-up is provided.

McKay et al. (1997) report that 10 nondelusional patients improved statistically significantly, as measured by the BDD–YBOCS, after being treated five days per week for six weeks with 90–minute sessions of exposure and response prevention, plus imaginal exposure (30 sessions in all). The baseline and endpoint BDD–YBOCS scores are not provided. Exposure and response prevention consisted of having the patient sit in crowded waiting rooms, go to supermarkets, department stores and restaurants, talk to others at varying distances, all without camouflage of the "ugly body parts." Imaginal exposure involved having the patient imagine that the perceived defect was even uglier and more noticeable and that the response of others to attempted social encounters was intensely negative as a result of the perceived defect. Those randomly assigned to a relapse prevention program improved more after six months on self-rated measures of anxiety (Beck Anxiety Inventory) and depression (Beck Depression Inventory), but not on the BDD–YBOCS, than those assigned to simple follow-up. The relapse prevention program included education about how to manage lapses (temporary recurrence of symptoms at lesser intensity), continued self-imposed exposure and response prevention, and freedom to contact the therapist if symptoms began to return or worsen.

In addition to Phillips' (1996d) helpful book for patients, *The Broken Mirror: Understanding and Treating Body Dysmorphic Disorder*, the OC Foundation has

Table 8.2. Body dysmorphic disorder: treatment planning guidelines

---

- Identify all body parts involved.
- Identify maladaptive coping behaviors.
- Assess whether the patient is delusional.
- Explore impairments in social functioning.
- Assess depression and suicide risk and intervene.
- Measure baseline severity (Y–BOCS or other instrument).
- Treat comorbid mood, anxiety or substance use disorders.
- Institute a 12-week trial of an SRI (clomipramine, fluoxetine, fluvoxamine, paroxetine, sertraline, or perhaps, citalopram).
- If the response is inadequate, try sequentially:
  - a second SRI;
  - buspirone augmentation;
  - an SSRI plus clomipramine, or an MAOI alone.
- In nondelusional patients, institute cognitive–behavioral therapy (cognitive restructuring and exposure and response prevention) along with pharmacotherapy.
- In delusional patients, add a neuroleptic to the SRI.
- Consider a trial of intravenous clomipramine (available in the United States only as an experimental treatment).
- Utilize bibliotherapy.
- As symptoms improve, institute psychotherapy for functional deficits and life problems.

Notes:
SRI: serotonin reuptake inhibitor; MAOI: monoamine oxidase inhibitor; Y–BOCS: Yale–Brown Obsessive–Compulsive Scale.

published a thoughtful educational pamphlet, *Learning to Live with Body Dysmorphic Disorder*, (Phillips, Van Noppen and Shapiro, 1997c) designed to aid both patients and families. Patients should be encouraged to read these materials, and to return with questions.

After a century of descriptive case reports and largely ineffective treatments, body dysmorphic disorder is now quite treatable. Gentle inquiry should be directed to patients at high risk of suffering from this disorder, particularly those with atypical depression, OCD or social phobia. An approach to planning integrated treatment for body dysmorphic disorder is shown in Table 8.2.

9

Hypochondriasis

They importune their doctors, beg for cures, try various remedies, and unless they are soon relieved, they change their doctors and their drugs.

Felix Platter (1536–1614), *Praxeos Medicae Tomi Tres*

The term "hypochondria" originated in the medical theories of ancient Greece and Rome: Claudius Galen of Pergamon (130–200 AD), whose works were the sacred texts of Western medicine for more than 1200 years, used the term, *melancholia hypochondriaca* to refer to one of three forms of melancholia – illnesses characterized by a mixture of fears and despondency (depression) (Jackson, 1986). Galen elaborated on Hippocratic theories of the humoral origins of health and disease. He asserted that when the liver, spleen and stomach malfunctioned and allowed an excess of black bile to appear in the blood, smoky vapors of black bile ascended to the brain, giving rise to hypochondriacal melancholia and its symptoms (Jackson, 1986). Galen's appellation embodied both anatomical and physiological concepts – hypochondria, referring to the area located below the xiphoid cartilage and ribs (from *hypo*, beneath, and *chondria*, cartilage), and melancholia, from the Greek for black bile. Fifteen hundred years later, the English physicians, Thomas Willis and Thomas Sydenham, separated hypochondriasis from other forms of melancholia, but only recently did the term come to mean specifically a morbid preoccupation with one's bodily health (Barsky, Wyshak and Klerman, 1986). The idea that hypochondriasis (morbid preoccupation with health) could exist separately from melancholia, i.e., from depressive disorders as now conceived, was not widely accepted until well into the twentieth century.

Diagnosis and differential diagnosis

DSM-IV criteria (300.7)

Two modern studies confirm that the signs and symptoms constituting the DSM-IV diagnostic criteria for hypochondriasis represent a syndrome (Barsky et al., 1986; Noyes et al., 1993). These diagnostic criteria are set out in Table 9.1. Note that although hypochondriasis and body dysmorphic disorder share the same DSM-IV code number (300.7), their diagnostic criteria are distinct.

Table 9.1. DSM-IV criteria for hypochondriasis (300.7)

A. Preoccupation with fear of having, or the idea that one has, a serious disease based on the person's misinterpretation of bodily symptoms.

B. The preoccupation persists despite appropriate medical evaluation and reassurance.

C. The belief in criterion A is not of delusional intensity (as in Delusional Disorder, Somatic Type) and is not restricted to a circumscribed concern about appearance (as in Body Dysmorphic Disorder).

D. The preoccupation causes clinically significant distress or impairment in social, occupational, or other important areas of functioning.

E. The duration of the disturbance is at least six months.

F. The preoccupation is not better accounted for by Generalized Anxiety Disorder, Obsessive–Compulsive Disorder, Panic Disorder, a Major Depressive Episode, Separation Anxiety, or other Somatoform Disorder.

Specify "poor insight" if, for most of the time during the current episode, the person does not recognize that the concern about having a serious illness is excessive or unreasonable.

Source: Reprinted with permission from the *Diagnostic and Statistical Manual of Mental Disorders*, Fourth Edition. Copyright 1994 American Psychiatric Association, p. 465.

ICD-10 criteria (F45.2)

Unlike DSM-IV, ICD-10 does not require the signs and symptoms of hypochondriasis to have been present for at least six months. In addition, ICD-10 does not allow for poor insight; such cases are classified as delusional disorders (F22.0). Finally, ICD-10 considers body dysmorphic disorder a form of hypochondriacal disorder and intermingles the descriptions of the two disorders. The diagnostic guidelines speak of a persistent belief in having either a physical illness or a presumed abnormality of appearance, and of refusing to accept reassurance from several physicians that the illness or the abnormal appearance is not present.

Differential diagnosis

The early stages of *multisystem diseases*, such as hyperparathyroidism or other endocrine disorders, the onset of some neurological disorders, such as multiple sclerosis or myasthenia gravis, and the beginnings of certain pain syndromes can present puzzling diagnostic challenges. The physician confronted with a possible case of hypochondriasis must consider whether a reasonable search for credible organic etiologies has been conducted. Records of earlier medical encounters should be sought; conversing with the patient's previous physicians is often helpful. The physician should independently think through the differential diagnosis of the patient's complaints and if not satisfied with the investigation of organic possibilities, arrange for appropriate evaluations. Just as "even paranoids have enemies," even hypochondriacs get sick and eventually die of something.

A *transient form of hypochondriasis*, by definition lasting less than six months, can be induced by a major life stress, a life-threatening medical disorder or the death of a loved one, in which case the survivor may develop some of the symptoms of the deceased (Barsky, Wyshak and Klerman, 1990). Compared to patients with the chronic form, patients with transient hypochondriasis, matched for the level of medical morbidity, are less disabled and perceive themselves as less ill (Barsky et al., 1990). Supportive psychotherapy should be provided as a means to reduce such patients' suffering and perhaps speed recovery.

Secondary hypochondriasis may be caused by major depression, panic disorder, generalized anxiety disorder or schizophrenia, in which case the underlying disorder is the focus of treatment. In these situations, the signs and symptoms of the primary, underlying psychiatric disorder will be visible, but it may take several visits to disentangle the symptomatology.

In *somatization disorder*, the patient is preoccupied with the symptoms and their effects on functioning rather than with the possibility or belief that they signify the presence of serious disease.

A form of illness variously labelled "*environmental illness*," "*multiple chemical sensitivity*" and "*total allergy syndrome*" inhabits the borderlands between hypochondriasis and somatization disorder. These patients are convinced that they have become ill as a result of exposure to certain foods or common environmental chemicals (paints, pesticides, perfumes, plastics, tobacco smoke, new or poorly ventilated buildings, work place fumes or inhalants) (California Medical Association Scientific Board Task Force on Clinical Ecology, 1986). They radically alter their lives in attempts to avoid further exposure (Brodsky, 1983). Their symptoms range from fatigue, difficulty concentrating, impaired memory and irritability to headache, gastrointestinal complaints, urinary complaints, muscle and joint pains, paresthesias and skin rashes. Unlike patients with hypochondriasis, these patients do not believe their disorder is life-threatening. In both groups of patients, however, life and thought revolve around symptoms, their management and the seeking of medical attention. Although multiple chemical sensitivity patients usually reject conventional medical and psychiatric explanations for their symptoms (Simon, Katon and Sparks, 1990), their suffering and disability may be reduced by supportive care and structured desensitization programs (Staudenmayer, 1996; Weaver, 1996).

Unlike the obsessions of *OCD*, hypochondriacal preoccupations are experienced as sensible or rational, are not resisted, and concern the interpretation of physical signs and symptoms (Barsky, 1992). Some patients with OCD, however, obsess about whether they may have or will contract a serious disease, typically acquired immunodeficiency syndrome (AIDS) or cancer, from exposure to objects, activities or events that bear no medically recognized causal connection to the feared disease. Other OCD patients, like patients with hypochondriasis, insist on repeated, medically unnecessary diagnostic testing long after the risk period following truly hazardous exposure has ended. The distinction lies in the source of the patient's concerns: in hypochondriasis the source lies in somatic signs and symptoms; in OCD the source lies in exposure to external risk factors, either realistic or irrational.

Delusions of parasitosis and the *olfactory reference syndrome* (the delusion that one's body is emitting an unpleasant odor noted by others) are forms of delusional disorder, somatic type, and are considered along with body dysmorphic disorder in Chapter 8. These patients are certain they are ill, whereas the hypochondriacal patient is able to entertain the possibility that the feared disease is not present.

Irritable bowel syndrome (Dalton and Drossman, 1997), *fibromyalgia* (Wallace, 1997; McCain, 1996) and *chronic fatigue syndrome* (Abbey and Garfinkel, 1991) are recognizable syndromes for which medical treatment is often helpful. Afflicted patients are not preoccupied with the fear or belief that they have serious physical disease.

Irritable bowel syndrome is defined as the presence of recurrent or continuous abdominal pain relieved by defecation, which is often associated with changes in stool frequency or consistency, or the presence of disturbed defecation, usually associated with complaints of bloating (Walker, Roy-Burne and Katon, 1990). The psychiatrist can be helpful in several ways: by framing the condition as a biological vulnerability that results in symptoms under conditions of stress; by providing appropriate treatment for comorbid psychiatric conditions; and, by developing a management plan for maladaptive illness behaviors (Walker et al., 1990). Modest doses of tricyclic antidepressants (e.g., 50 mg/day of trimipramine, 150 mg/day of desipramine) have proven helpful in four of six double-blind, placebo-controlled trials of four to eight weeks duration (Gruber, Hudson and Pope, 1996). No clear relationship was seen between treatment outcome and the baseline severity of psychiatric symptoms. Emmanuel, Lydiard and Crawford (1997) report a single case in which fluvoxamine, begun at 50 mg/day and increased slowly to 150 mg/day, markedly reduced bowel symptoms after two months of treatment in a women who had no psychiatric comorbidity; symptoms returned when she discontinued fluvoxamine after an unspecified interval.

Fibromyalgia is defined by the American College of Rheumatology as widespread musculoskeletal aching associated with the presence of 11 of 18 specific, reproducible tender points (Wolfe et al., 1990). Morning stiffness, fatigue and poor sleep are common concomitant complaints. Persistent fear of underlying serious disease is absent. Amitriptyline, 25–50 mg at bedtime, and a structured program of physical exercise have been shown to be helpful in controlled trials (Powers, 1993).

Patients with fibromyalgia have no greater lifetime prevalence of psychiatric disorder than patients with rheumatoid arthritis, suggesting that fibromyalgia is not of psychopathological origin (Ahles et al., 1991).

Chronic fatigue syndrome (Sharpe, 1996) is marked by the new onset of medically unexplained, incapacitating fatigue, tiring with even mild exertion and the failure of rest to alleviate the fatigue. A widely accepted case definition for this condition also requires the presence of at least four of the following: muscle pain; joint pain; headache; tender lymph nodes; sore throat; unrefreshing sleep; malaise for more than 24 hours after exertion; and subjective memory impairment. Many patients meet DSM criteria for concurrent major depression and the majority have met criteria for major depression at some point in their lifetime. A minority meet criteria for concurrent anxiety disorders. Although patients with this syndrome usually insist, like patients with hypochondriasis, that they are suffering from an organic disease, chronic fatigue patients are more focussed on their symptoms and impaired functioning than on fears about a life-threatening disease. Hypothyroidism, anemia, Addison's disease and a sleep disorder need to be ruled out as occult causes. Sharpe (1996) describes a comprehensive approach to the evaluation and treatment of these patients, including both pharmacological and nonpharmacological treatments. A randomized, controlled trial of carefully graded structured exercise in patients free of comorbid psychiatric disorders demonstrated marked benefit in most patients (Fulcher and White, 1997). In studies that included patients with comorbid depression, graded structured exercise combined with cognitive therapy and treatment of the depression helped the majority (Sharpe et al., 1996; Deale et al., 1997).

Clinical picture and assessment instruments

The patients suffering from hypochondriasis pays exquisite attention to bodily sensations and physical signs. They attribute these to serious disease, whereas normal individuals attribute them to stress, overwork or aging. The most common complaints are pain, cardiac symptoms, respiratory symptoms, bowel complaints, nausea, weakness and fatigue (Kenyon, 1976). Headaches are the commonest form of pain complaint, followed by chest pain, abdominal pain and diffuse muscular pains, which may suggest or merit a diagnosis of fibromyalgia. Cardiac complaints include palpitations, missed beats, fears of a heart attack and nonexertional chest pain, which is often left-sided (Mayou et al., 1994). The patient may attribute easy tiring or inspirational dyspnea to feared heart disease. Nineteenth-century cases of neurasthenia, soldier's heart and effort (or Da Costa's) syndrome probably included many patients fitting modern criteria for hypochondriasis. Gastrointestinal complaints range from indigestion, regurgitation, dysphagia and bad taste in the mouth to lower abdominal cramping pain, flatulence and constipation.

Patients present their medical history and complaints in great detail and are difficult to interrupt. The clinician will soon recognize, however, that the description of the symptoms, their groupings, temporal patterns, and the exacerbating and relieving factors do not fit classical patterns of serious disease. Most patients will have visited many physicians seeking confirmation of their fears, demanding numerous, repeated diagnostic tests, becoming frustrated or angry with the physician's failure to find the cause of their symptoms and terminating the relationship only to begin the fruitless search anew. Unfortunately, some treating physicians convey subtle or overt criticism, rejection or dislike, producing legitimate angry feelings. Noyes et al. (1993) report that patients with hypochondriasis had at least 50% more physician visits, number of physicians seen, hospitalizations and medications taken in the previous six months than age- and gender-matched controls selected from the same medical clinic.

Hypochondriacal patients feel unsatisfied or angry with their physicians and dismiss any reassurance as lack of understanding and sometimes, as evidence of incompetence. In the doctor's office and every other venue, the patient's conversation focuses on bodily complaints and disease fears; little is said about human relations, life activities or feelings. The patient often uses the symptoms to control family and friends; special foods are required, the house must be kept quiet, "stressful" responsibilities are avoided. The secondary gains of the sick role, i.e., sympathy, attention, support and release from responsibilities, may be clearly visible as perpetuating factors (Barsky and Klerman, 1983).

Assessment instruments

The Whitely Index, a 14-item self-report questionnaire (Appendix 2), provides a reliable and reasonably valid screening instrument for use in medical populations (Pilowsky, 1967; Barsky et al., 1986). Each item can be scored "yes" or "no," as in the original study (Pilowsky, 1967) or on an ordinal 5–point scale (Barsky et al., 1992a; personal communication, A. J. Barsky, M.D., January, 1998). Factor analysis of the Index, using principal components analysis, yields three scales: disease conviction; disease fear; and bodily preoccupation (Pilowsky, 1967). The items contributing most heavily to each scale are shown in Appendix 2. No measure for following the change in severity of hypochondriasis has been developed, but the clinician can use the patient's scores on the three Whitely scales individually or as a sum.

Barsky et al. (1992a) developed and validated a structured diagnostic interview for DSM-III-R hypochondriasis that is useful for research purposes. Modified versions of the interview's questions have been incorporated into the Structured Clinical Interview for DSM-III-R (Spitzer et al., 1990) and the Structured Clinical

Interview for DSM-IV Axis I Disorders (First et al., 1995). The questions provided by Barsky et al. (1992a) are the most detailed.

Prevalence and course

The prevalence of hypochondriasis in the general population is unknown. Patients in medical and surgical practices very often present with somatic complaints that have no organic basis, and in one family practice study, about 9% of patients disbelieved the physician's reassurances (Kellner, 1985). The gender ratio in hypochondriasis appears to be nearly 1:1. No information is available on familial patterns, but a familial focus on symptoms in childhood may predispose to hypochondriasis (Kellner, 1985). Although cultures strongly influence the meaning of symptoms and the propensity to seek medical care (Barsky and Klerman, 1983; Kellner, 1985; Abbey and Garfinkel, 1991), the relative prevalence of hypochondriasis across cultures is unknown.

Hypochondriasis usually begins in adolescence, but patients may present to the clinician with symptoms that began after age 30. Several studies report that about half of adult patients recover or improve substantially after one to three years; they no longer believe that they have a physical disease and improve their social and occupational functioning (Kellner, 1985). In a follow-up study, Noyes et al. (1994) found that two-thirds of medical clinic patients with hypochondriasis still met criteria after a year; one-fifth were markedly improved; and, only 1 in 12 had recovered from their baseline problem or concerns. Those who will spontaneously recover cannot be distinguished at the time of presentation from those who will develop a chronic condition. Thus, treatment should be offered to all. Apparently favorable prognostic factors include: acute onset; short duration; the presence of anxiety or depression (in contrast to a lack of emotional reaction to symptoms); fewer physicians consulted; younger age; higher socioeconomic status; and the absence of personality disorder, comorbid organic disease, histrionic traits in women and prominent resentment in men (Kellner, 1985). Because of grave methodological limitations affecting studies that have reported on prognosis, firm conclusions about the validity of these prognostic factors cannot be drawn.

Comorbidity

Since antiquity, physicians describing hypochondriacal patients have commented on the presence of depressive and anxiety symptoms. A modern study utilizing structured interviews with 42 general medical clinic patients meeting criteria for DSM-III-R hypochondriasis found high prevalence rates for concurrent dysthymia (45%), major depression (33%), generalized anxiety disorder (24%) and somatization disorder (21%), all statistically significantly higher than in a comparison group of medical patients (Barsky, Wyshak and Klerman, 1992b). The lifetime prevalence rate for OCD (9.5%) was also elevated compared to the control group. Substance abuse was not more prevalent. A one-year follow-up of 48 general medicine clinic patients with DSM-III-R hypochondriasis reported lower, but still substantial, rates of comorbid psychiatric conditions, including 15% with panic disorder (Noyes et al., 1994). In a general medicine clinic sample, Barsky, Barnett and Cleary (1994) found that one-quarter of panic disorder patients had concurrent hypochondriasis. These high rates of comorbid mood and anxiety disorders help explain the millennial slowness in recognizing hypochondriasis as a separate disorder.

Treatment

The goals of treatment are to decrease disability, complaint behavior, the inappropriate use of medical care and the stress that provokes symptoms. Cure of chronic hypochondriacal attitudes and the disappearance of chronic, functional somatic symptoms are, in most cases, unrealistic expectations. No standard treatment exists, but a cognitive–behavioral treatment has been evaluated in a controlled trial of modest size (Warwick et al., 1996) and experienced clinicians have described a similar seemingly successful approach (Sharpe et al., 1996). Until additional evidence from controlled trials is available, these methods should constitute the core of the clinician's psychotherapeutic approach.

The start of any treatment is a careful assessment of the patient and the illness that has changed him. The psychiatrist should begin by reviewing the medical evaluations already performed to assure himself that no reasonable organic possibility has been overlooked. Once assured, he can embark on what will probably be a prolonged course of cognitive–behavioral and interpersonal psychotherapy, which can be augmented with pharmacotherapeutic trials. Treatment of comorbid mood and anxiety disorders may indirectly lessen the severity of primary hypochondriasis.

Psychotherapeutic approaches

The available data regarding the outcome of psychotherapeutic treatments are few. In the only published controlled trial, Warwick et al. (1996) randomly assigned 32 patients meeting DSM-III-R criteria for hypochondriasis, without a primary affective or psychotic disorder, to either cognitive–behavioral therapy, 16 sessions over four months, or a waiting list control. The mean duration of the patients' hypochondriasis was 86 months (range = 6–396 months).

Treatment consisted of multiple elements refined from an earlier successful, but uncontrolled trial (Warwick and Marks, 1988). The elements included: educating the patient about the nature of hypochondriasis and cognitive–behavioral treatment; teaching the patient to recognize how his negative thoughts about symptoms produced anxiety and how his behaviors maintained it; identifying and challenging misinterpretations of signs and symptoms; teaching more rational interpretations; modifying frightening mental images; and, changing dysfunctional assumptions. Patients were asked to listen to tape recordings of each session before the next one occurred. Graded exposure to feared illness-related situations was arranged and patients were instructed to refrain from anxiety-relieving rituals such as bodily checking and seeking reassurance. Patients were instructed to focus on a bodily area in order to discover that such focussing gave rise to "symptoms." Patients kept a daily log of negative thoughts and the new, rational responses to these thoughts.

At the end of treatment, the active treatment group had achieved significantly greater improvement than the waiting list control group on almost all outcome measures, whether self-rated, therapist-rated or rated by an assessor blind to the treatment condition. These measures included disease conviction, health anxiety, need for reassurance, time spent worrying about health and frequency of checking. Gains were maintained at a three-month follow-up evaluation. Additional research is needed to identify which of these many treatment elements is essential and the duration of the therapeutic effect.

A similar approach is described by Sharpe, Peveler and Mayou (1992), who derived their methods from their clinical experience, uncontrolled case series and a few small controlled trials involving patients with noncardiac chest pain, irritable bowel syndrome, chronic headaches or chronic pain syndromes.

In the assessment phase, Sharpe et al. (1992) advise the clinician to seek out the predisposing, precipitating and perpetuating factors for the patient's illness behaviors. The patient is asked to describe in detail his symptoms, his beliefs about their causes and implications, their effects on his life (including activities or situations that are avoided), and the reactions of concerned others. The patient's motivations for change and his attitudes toward other physicians and the clinician are elicited, along with any family history of similar symptoms or serious illness. The clinician evaluates the contribution of comorbid conditions such as generalized anxiety disorder, major depression, dysthymia or panic disorder and institutes appropriate pharmacotherapy.

The clinician must then negotiate the patient's agreement to the aims, methods and duration of treatment. The patient is asked to refrain from further diagnostic testing and evaluation and other forms of treatment, including prescribed and over-the-counter medications. Drug doses can be slowly tapered when necessary, and innocuous medications can be continued if they bring symptom relief or improved functioning, although this is rarely the case.

Cognitive–behavioral sessions, usually an hour in length, are scheduled weekly or bi-weekly. The patient keeps a daily diary that documents symptom intensity (0–10 scale), related activities or thoughts, the degree of anxiety, apprehension or depression accompanying the symptom (0–10 scale) and the degree of belief in symptom-related thoughts (0–10 scale).

Each session begins with setting the agenda; the focus is limited to a few complaints so that the patient's commitment to implementing the interventions can be obtained. The diary is reviewed with an aim of decreasing dysfunctional behaviors such as taking medication, seeking reassurance and avoiding activities. The clinician also attempts to unearth the illogical assumptions behind symptom-related beliefs. He educates the patient about comorbid conditions, about the effects of selective attention and about how stress causes the sensations which the patient is erroneously attributing to serious disease. Suggesting that the symptoms are due to psychological factors is not helpful. The patient is likely to resist such attributions and to hear them as accusations that "it's all in your head."

At each session, the clinician helps the patient choose a few new behaviors to implement in the coming week. These should be behaviors that the patient has desired but avoided because of symptoms. The behavioral changes should be small and realistically attainable within the time frame between visits. Exposure and response prevention are key treatment elements. Patients are instructed to expose themselves sequentially to feared situations and not to perform the reassuring rituals, just as one treats compulsions in OCD. Since the new behaviors are likely to elicit either anxiety or sensations related to unaccustomed physical exertion, the patient should be told to expect a temporary increase in the bodily sensations that have been frightening or depressing him. He is instructed to keep in mind the new, non-pathological explanations provided by the clinician.

Since social reactions to hypochondriacal complaining can reinforce this behavior, the clinician should strongly consider inviting one or more of the patient's concerned others to treatment planning sessions. These individuals should be asked to refrain from providing reassurance or sympathy for symptoms and complaints, and should attribute this refusal to "what we all agreed at the doctor's office." They should also reinforce the patient's improved familial, social or vocational functioning with praise and appreciation.

Patients should be educated about their illnesses whenever possible. In cases of hypochondriasis, Cantor and Fallon's (1996) book, *Phantom Illness: Shattering the Myth of Hypochondria*, is quite useful. The book describes the many symptoms of the disorder, theories about its origins and treatment approaches, and includes the case histories of many individuals who were helped. Patients should be encouraged to read this book and return with questions.

In some cases, the clinician can combine the cognitive–behavioral methods just described with attention to the conflicts, feelings and life problems that the patient is avoiding through his focus on somatic symptoms. Usually, this attention will be strenuously resisted until a solid therapeutic alliance has been established. The alliance will grow as the clinician pursues a detailed history of the illness and of the patient's life course and current circumstances, allows ventilation, educates the patient about his symptoms, engages in active problem solving, communicates empathy and caring and instills hope for improved functioning despite continued symptoms.

Pharmacotherapy

Some evidence exists that selective serotonin reuptake inhibitors (SSRIs) or imipramine may be helpful, but any trial should be combined with elements of cognitive–behavioral therapy. Fallon et al. (1993) gave fluoxetine, starting at 20 mg/day and increased every two weeks by 20 mg/day, to 16 patients with DSM-III-R hypochondriasis, unaccompanied by concomitant major depression. The patients had been ill a mean of 11 years. Most patients had concomitant panic disorder, generalized anxiety disorder or OCD. Statistically significant improvement in disease phobia and disease conviction (measured by the Whitely Index) and in anxiety (measured by the Hamilton Anxiety Rating Scale) were achieved, even though bodily preoccupation (Whitely Index) did not diminish. Two patients responded to 20 mg/day of fluoxetine, but five needed 60–80 mg/day to achieve a good response, suggesting that as in OCD, SSRI doses should be pushed to the maximum tolerated level. Five patients had responded by the fifth week and 10 by the end of the study. Only fixed dose, comparative trials, however, will establish whether dose or length of treatment is the critical factor. Only one of three patients with comorbid OCD responded, indicating that comorbid OCD is not necessary for therapeutic response. After 12 weeks of treatment, four patients were rated very much improved and six much improved on the Clinical Global Impression Scale (Guy, 1976; Appendix 2).

Viswanathan and Paradis (1991) report a case of cancer phobia that responded in week 6 to fluoxetine, (four weeks at 20 mg/day and two at 40 mg/day); the patient was unresponsive to seven weeks of treatment with buspirone 30 mg/day, three months of desipramine 150 mg/day and to 20 months of behaviorally oriented psychotherapy.

Wesner and Noyes (1991) report marked benefit in an open trial of imipramine begun at 25 mg/day and increased every three days by 25 mg to 150 mg/day. Of 10 patients meeting DSM-III-R criteria for hypochondriasis without comorbid depression, eight completed four weeks of treatment. Six were markedly improved and one was "back to normal." All aspects of the illness improved, including worry about health, anxious response to cues suggesting disease, avoidance behaviors and

Table 9.2. Hypochondriasis: treatment planning guidelines

- Rule out an organic cause for the symptoms.
- Rule out transient (stress-induced) hypochondriasis.
- Rule out secondary hypochondriasis (related to major depression, panic disorder, generalized anxiety disorder, schizophrenia).
- Assess the symptoms, the patient's beliefs, and his or her motives for treatment.
- Negotiate the patient's agreement to the aims, methods and duration of treatment.
- Measure baseline severity with the Whitely Index.
- Treat comorbid mood and anxiety disorders.
- Assess predisposing, precipitating, perpetuating factors.
- Institute cognitive–behavioral therapy (symptom diary, cognitive restructuring, exposure and response prevention).
- Consider a 12–week trial of an SSRI or imipramine.
- Reduce complicity by concerned others by means of joint treatment sessions.
- Utilize bibliotherapy.
- As preoccupation with bodily symptoms diminishes, institute psychotherapy for life problems.

Note:
SSRI: selective serotonin reuptake inhibitor.

the seeking of reassurance. Two patients discontinued treatment because of over-stimulation (jitteriness, insomnia or irritability) and one because of concern over tachycardia. The authors note that their patients were especially sensitive to side effects, indicating that the clinician, therefore, should be prepared to provide a good deal of reassurance and support. Starting at an even lower dose and increasing it more slowly may facilitate compliance.

The hypochondriacal patient's progress is slow, occurring over months rather than weeks. The clinician will, therefore, benefit from discharging in leisure pursuits the irritation and frustration these patients can engender. He can take pleasure in knowing that he is struggling intelligently with a difficult disorder, which in most cases will already have defeated many others. Treatment planning guidelines derived from the literature are shown in Table 9.2.

Treatment of hypochondriasis in primary care

Many hypochondriacal patients will refuse to see a psychiatrist. When a colleague in primary care asks for consultation about managing a patient with this disorder, the psychiatrist can communicate the management suggestions offered by experienced clinicians (Drossman, 1978; Kellner, 1985). The psychiatrist should explain that while these suggestions are derived from clinicians' experience, they have not been validated in research studies.

The primary care physician should be advised to avoid saying that he expects the patient to improve. The physician should not expect the patient to express appreciation for his efforts. These changes in expectations will reduce his frustration. The physician should schedule regular, time-limited appointments, not "as needed" visits. The visits, described subsequently, will combine symptom evaluation, education and, after some weeks, the planning of small changes in behavior. The frequency and duration of the visits should not change based on the patient's symptoms. A decreased frequency of office visits encourages the patient to have more symptoms to gain access to the doctor and punishes wellness by providing him with less physician time. If improvement occurs, appointments should not be diminished until the patient insists on this.

Managed care plans may resist approving these regularly scheduled visits. Reviewers can be informed that this treatment plan represents expert opinion and that the physician believes it will prove less costly than scheduling appointments, tests and investigations in response to the patient's symptoms. The physician should appeal to the highest level of the managed care plan adverse decisions regarding care that he believes is indicated and should document each step of the appeal. Hall (1994) notes that documentation should include:

- The clinical information provided to the reviewer.
- Reasons for the appeal.
- The reviewer's name.
- Time and date of the appeal.
- Notation that the reviewer was informed that the appeal is requested under the rules established by the Wilson and Wickline court decisions (although they are legally binding only in California).
- Notation that the clinician informed the reviewer of the risk to the patient if the treatment plan is not followed.

The risks include the morbidity associated with unnecessary diagnostic tests and the despair and depression, with adverse consequences, that can accompany inappropriately treated hypochondriasis (Barsky et al., 1992a).

Hall (1994) also reviews the legal doctrines evolving in the United States under which the patient can file suit against the managed care plan for unreasonably denying medical care.

After the initial evaluation is complete, the physician should tell the patient that it has helped him to understand the patient's concern and discomfort, and that he respects how well he has managed or how much he has done despite the symptoms. This intervention is aimed at improving the patient's often perilously low self-esteem. When presenting the results of a negative workup, the physician should state clearly that "no serious disease has been found." The physician adds that he nonetheless accepts the reality of the symptoms and of the patient's suffering. The physician should stress that the negative findings do not mean an end to the doctor–patient relationship; the physician intends to continue working with the patient to help improve his quality of life despite persistent symptoms. The physician should not promise relief or symptom removal because initially, at least, the patient needs the symptoms in order to relate to others and the world or to solve a conflict that generates anxiety. The symptoms elicit caring from others and provide an identity (one who is afflicted, who suffers, whose life accomplishment is to endure misery). Neither should the physician reassure the patient that "everything will be alright." This reassurance undercuts the legitimacy of the patient's need to complain and is rarely believed. Attempts to point to the psychological sources of the patient's symptoms are counterproductive.

A focal physical examination should be performed when new symptoms are presented, but should not be repeated for old, unchanged symptoms. Over time, the physician should attempt to teach the patient that his somatic symptoms do not signify serious disease, that he has learned to focus on his body and that he must unlearn the selective attention to symptoms that magnifies their intensity. It may be helpful to ask the patient to pay close attention for a week to a nonsymptomatic portion of the body, such as the nose or the toes of the right foot, to appreciate how selective attention creates symptoms. The physician should teach the patient to change his internal monologue about fears of serious disease to a self-statement such as: "My symptoms are a nuisance, but they don't mean serious disease." The patient must be given information repeatedly and in small doses; he is too frightened to learn well and will distort and forget.

The physician must clarify the diagnostic terms used by previous physicians, e.g., chondritis, irritable heart or rheumatism, explaining that they were unsuccessful attempts to give reassurance about the absence of serious disease or to provide a convenient label for the symptoms. Explanations for the presence of any symptom should be simple; medical jargon and pathophysiological explanations should be avoided.

The hypochondriacal patient usually requests medications despite repeated failures to benefit from them. The physician is subsequently blamed for the medication's failure to help. To avoid this trap, medications can be given with a statement like: "I'm not sure this will help, but we can try it if you would like." When the medication fails to help and the patient complains, the physician can respond, "Remember, we tried this because you wished to, not because I thought it was likely to help." This places responsibility for medication trials on the patient. When the patient complains that nothing works, the physician can respond, "Nonetheless, I'd like to continue to see and work with you. Our goals are to reduce your fears about serious disease and to increase your functioning, despite the symptoms." The physician understands that the relationship, not a medical intervention, is the therapeutic agent.

Like the psychiatrist, the primary care physician can encourage the patient to decrease the use of ineffective coping mechanisms, such as avoiding activity, seeking reassurance from family members and taking medications for symptoms. The patient should be told to expect that symptoms will temporarily increase as these behaviors are abandoned, but that adhering to changed behaviors will diminish the symptoms' stultifying effect on his life.

The physician must be willing to tolerate the patient's anger when symptoms and fears persist. Taking care of oneself, pursuing leisure activities and reflecting on a difficult job well done can help the physician cope.

10

Pathological jealousy

Dost think I am so muddy, so unsettled, to appoint myself in this vexation? sully the purity and whiteness of my sheets, – which to preserve is sleep; which being spotted, is goads, thorns, nettles, tails of wasps?

Shakespeare, *Winter's Tale*

Just as jealousy in fiction can be comical or tragic, a patient's jealousy can be normal or pathological. The distinction is not always easily made, since threats to love and fidelity may be real, valid but exaggerated, or wholly imagined. Jealousy occupies a divided place in our culture, valued on the one hand as a reasonable response to loss of love, and disdained on the other as a sign of inappropriate possessiveness and a source of violent crime (Tarrier et al., 1990; Mullen, 1991). A reading of classic literary portrayals of jealousy such as Shakespeare's *Winter's Tale* and *Othello*, or Tolstoy's *The Kreutzer Sonata* (1985) can enrich the clinician's grasp of the pathological distortions of this normal human experience (Seeman, 1979).

Clinicians confronted with a patient's jealous passion must uncover the facts that have been colored by the patient's perceptions. They must investigate how the patient's cultural background may be shaping these perceptions and legitimizing the patient's current and planned responses (Mullen's, 1991, review is a valuable resource). Finally, they must always evaluate the potential for violence. Often it will be necessary to interview the individual who is the object of jealousy. This chapter describes the varieties of pathological jealousy and reviews the limited data available regarding treatment.

Diagnosis

DSM-IV diagnostic criteria (297.1)

Pathological jealousy occurs in nondelusional and delusional forms. The delusional form, occasionally called the "Othello syndrome," is grouped in DSM-IV with other focal delusional disorders and termed, Delusional Disorder, Jealous Type (American Psychiatric Association, 1994), as shown in Table 10.1. The nondelusional form has been called "pathological jealousy," (Byrne and Yatham, 1989), "obsessional jealousy" (Stein, Hollander and Josephson, 1994a) and "morbid jeal-

Table 10.1. DSM-IV diagnostic criteria for delusional disorder, jealous type (297.1)

A. Delusional belief of at least one month's duration that the individual's sexual partner is unfaithful.
B. Criterion A for schizophrenia has never been met, i.e., the patient has not exhibited two or more of: delusions; hallucinations; disorganized speech; disorganized behavior and negative symptoms (e.g., avolition, flattened affect).
C. Apart from the impact of the delusion(s) or its ramifications, functioning is not markedly impaired and behavior is not obviously odd or bizarre.
D. If mood episodes have occurred concurrently with delusions, their total duration has been brief relative to the duration of the delusional periods.
E. The disturbance is not due to the direct physiological effects of a substance (e.g., a drug of abuse, a medication) or a general medical condition.

Source: Reprinted with permission from the *Diagnostic and Statistical Manual of Mental Disorders,* Fourth Edition. Copyright 1994 American Psychiatric Association, p. 301.

ousy," (Michael et al., 1995), and has no separate place in diagnostic systems.

Tarrier et al. (1990) have suggested criteria for distinguishing normal from non-delusional pathological jealousy: pathological jealousy is characterized by a pre-occupation with unfounded, irrational ideas about the partner's infidelity that are not supported by evidence, disrupt the person's functioning and are culturally aberrant. The jealous thoughts are persistent and intrusive, elicit intense feelings and motivate related behaviors. In contrast to obsessions, which are usually ego-dystonic, the fears or suspicions of infidelity are frequently ego-syntonic, although the individual will allow that they may be untrue; in this case, they can be considered over-valued ideas (Lane, 1990).

ICD-10 diagnostic criteria (F22.0)

ICD-10 includes delusional jealousy within the category, Delusional Disorder (World Health Organization, 1992). The ICD-10 Diagnostic Guidelines are consistent with the DSM-IV diagnostic criteria for Delusional Disorder, Jealous Type, but specify that the delusion must have been present for at least three months, whereas DSM-IV requires only one month. ICD-10 notes that the delusion must be out of keeping with the individual's cultural background.

Differential diagnosis

Delusional jealousy should be distinguished from jealousy of delusional intensity secondary to *dementia, schizophrenia, affective disorder, general medical conditions* and *substance-induced psychotic disorder.* In the first three disorders, additional signs and symptoms are present. In the latter two, the history, physical examination and laboratory studies should be revealing. When *alcohol* (the most common organic cause) is the etiological agent, DSM-IV assigns the diagnosis, Alcohol-Induced Psychotic Disorder, With Delusions (291.5); ICD-10 assigns the diagnosis, Psychotic Disorder, Predominantly Delusional, Due to Use of Alcohol (F10.51). Organic conditions that have been associated rarely with delusional jealousy include *hyperthyroidism* (resolving four weeks after successful treatment of the hyperthyroidism) (Hodgson, Murray and Woods, 1992); *epilepsy* (Enoch and Trethowan, 1979); *adrenocortical insufficiency*, with concomitant depression and reversible dementia (all reversed after 10 days of prednisolone therapy) (Hassanyeh, Murray and Rodgers, 1991); and, *amantadine* treatment of Parkinson's disease (onset after 200 mg/day for four and a half years, resolving within five days of stopping the drug) (McNamara and Durso, 1991). In the last instance, the fallacy of *post hoc, ergo propter hoc* seems particularly likely to be at work.

Prevalence

The prevalence of the two forms of pathological jealousy is unknown, but they appear only rarely in clinical practice. In a retrospective chart review in a Munich psychiatric hospital, Soyka, Naber and Völcker (1991) found the prevalence of jealousy of delusional intensity to be 1.1%, primarily in patients with organic psychoses, paranoid disorders (mostly delusional disorder), alcohol psychoses or schizophrenia. Chiu (1995) reported a prevalence of 0.9% for DSM-III-R delusional disorder, jealous type in 349 elderly Chinese inpatients and outpatients treated at a Hong Kong psychiatric unit, along with one case of delusional jealousy due to schizophrenia and one due to dementia.

Jealousy appears to be a common experience in nonclinical populations. A mailed questionnaire study of 351 subjects in a New Zealand university city found 40% reporting jealousy without good cause on at least one occasion and 10% indicating that their jealousy caused substantial problems in a relationship (Mullen and Martin, 1994). Since only 75% of those contacted by mail returned the questionnaire and respondents may have under-reported episodes, jealousy may be even more prevalent. How much of this is "pathological" is unknown. Mullen's (1991) review of the history of jealousy from the Renaissance to the Present makes clear how time and culture influence the dividing line between a socially engrained reaction to infidelity and a pathological state.

Clinical picture

In both the delusional and nondelusional forms of pathological jealousy, the morbid preoccupation with unfaithfulness is accompanied by endless inquiring. The jealous individual may repeatedly and vociferously ask the sexual partner about suspected liaisons or his or her whereabouts, check the partner's mail or pockets, call the partner's work place to ascertain if he or she is truly there, or check clothes for signs of sexual activity. The sufferer repeatedly accuses the partner of having affairs, and may follow the partner or insist that the partner provide a detailed account of daily activities. In delusional disorder, jealous type, ideas of reference are common, i.e., random events are interpreted as offering evidence of the suspected infidelity. The partner may be threatened with violence, and physical attack may occur (Enoch and Trethowan, 1979; Freeman, 1990; Michael et al., 1995).

The characteristics of jealousy reported in the New Zealand community study (Mullen and Martin, 1994) bear exploration in patients presenting for treatment. The most common fear was of losing the partner, followed by fearing loss of attention. Fears of losing psychological intimacy, sexual exclusivity or financial security and fears of being shamed or humiliated were less common. Both jealous men and jealous women reported feeling angry, sad, agitated and restless; women more often felt insecure.

Comorbidity

Nondelusional jealousy is often associated with alcohol abuse (Michael et al., 1995; Mullen and Martin, 1994), and occasionally occurs in conjunction with OCD (Stein et al., 1994a). In a study of 207 male inpatients with alcohol dependence in Kerala, India (a city "largely comparable to Western settings"), Michael et al. (1995) found a prevalence of morbid jealousy of 34%, including 62 nondelusional cases (30%), 7 delusional cases with delusional jealousy predating the alcohol dependence, and 2 delusional cases developing after alcohol dependence. About one-quarter of the individuals expressed their morbid jealousy only when intoxicated. Interviewing the spouses was important in recognizing the diagnosis, since only one-third of the morbidly jealous men volunteered the presence of jealousy.

Treatment

Psychotherapy

No controlled trials are available to guide the choice or implementation of psychotherapy. After determining that the pathological jealousy is not secondary to one of the disorders mentioned earlier, the clinician should evaluate the precipitating factors, projected sexual guilt, defensive maneuvers, the possibility that jealousy serves to increase sexual arousal in the couple (Seeman, 1979) and the potential for violence. In five female cases reported by Seeman (1979), events that lowered the jealous partner's self-esteem were common precipitants of jealousy. In fits of remorse, the patients berated themselves for their behavior, or tormented themselves with feelings of inferiority compared to the suspected rival. Some partners contributed to the jealousy by engaging in provocative behavior and teasing allusions, and several jealous spouses had themselves secretly been unfaithful in the past. The sexual excitement of one or both spouses was often increased by the presence of jealousy. Psychotherapeutic treatment conducted over one or more years utilized techniques of clarifying perceptual distortions, attending to the patient's self-esteem, allowing ventilation and providing couple therapy, but was not markedly effective in this small series.

A small study that included a waiting list control group utilized from one to six 50-minute sessions of cognitive–behavioral therapy in patients with chronic, nondelusional morbid jealousy, most of whom were women who sought help following a partner's threat to terminate the relationship (Dolan and Bishay, 1996). The sessions focussed on faulty assumptions and their origins, feelings of inferiority, guilt related to the patient's previous unfaithfulness or maltreatment of their partner, and strategies to help the patient control emotions and behaviors. Patients were instructed to counteract jealous self-statements with more logical self-statements and were given taped therapy sessions or written summaries of rational self-statements. More than half of the 30 patients who completed the study (8 additional patients dropped out) and their partners reported marked improvements, including disappearance of the belief that the spouse would leave or become involved with someone else, and cessation of interrogation and seeking clues. Improvement was maintained during a follow-up period of three to six months.

Pharmacotherapy

No controlled trials have been reported. Delusional disorder, jealous type, has responded well to pimozide in a few cases. Dorian (1979) and Munro (1984) report remissions beginning within one to three weeks of treatment with 4 mg/day and sustained over many months of continued treatment. Pollock (1982) reports marked improvement beginning within a few days of starting 4 mg/day and sustained over 6–12 months at reduced doses. Iruela et al. (1990) report marked improvement in two cases beginning after two months of treatment with 8 mg/day and persisting during 6–18 months of continued treatment with 2 mg/day. These two patients continued to believe that infidelity had occurred, but agreed that it had ceased, and no longer dwelt on it.

Selective serotonin reuptake inhibitors (SSRIs) have been helpful or curative in a number of cases. In one case, nondelusional pathological jealousy remitted after eight weeks of fluoxetine 60 mg/day and continued in remission during four months of treatment followed by four months without medication (Lane, 1990). In another case, remission occurred after four weeks of fluoxetine 20 mg/day and persisted during six months of continued treatment (Gross, 1991). In patients with

Table 10.2. Pathological jealousy: treatment planning guidelines

- Determine whether the patient is delusional.

For delusional disorder, jealous type:
- Rule out other psychoses (paranoid, affective, alcoholic, schizophrenic), dementia and rare medical etiologies.
- Interview the partner to assess the relationship and the partner's possible contributions to jealousy.
- Evaluate the risk of violence and intervene.
- Institute neuroleptic treatment (consider pimozide).
- For nonresponders, consider haloperidol, a novel neuroleptic such as risperidone or olanzapine, or adding an SSRI.

For non-delusional pathological jealousy:
- Assess for alcohol abuse/dependence and treat.
- Interview the partner to assess the relationship and the partner's possible contributions to jealousy.
- Evaluate risk of violence and intervene.
- Initiate an eight-week trial of an SSRI and continue an effective drug long-term.
- Institute cognitive-behavioral therapy.
- Consider couple therapy.
- For an SSRI nonresponder, try a second SSRI or clomipramine.

Note:
SSRI: selective serotonin reuptake inhibitor.

comorbid OCD, cases of nondelusional pathological jealousy and cases with partial insight improved moderately to markedly after treatment with various SSRIs: fluoxetine 40 mg/day for six weeks, with sustained improvement during nine months of continued treatment (Wright, 1994); fluoxetine 80 mg/day for 12 weeks (two cases); fluoxetine 80 mg/day plus pimozide 1 mg/day (one case); 30 mg/day (one case); clomipramine 50–75 mg/day plus pimozide 1 mg/day (one case); and, sertraline 200 mg/day (one case) (Stein et al., 1994a). The case reported by Wright (1994) was remarkable in that three family members (grandmother, mother and maternal uncle) also suffered from pathological jealousy and two children had OCD, suggesting the possibility of a biological relationship between these disorders in this pedigree.

For delusional disorder, jealous type, controlled trials are needed to investigate the utility of pimozide and other neuroleptics, including the new dopamine/serotonin blockers such as risperidone and olanzapine. The available case literature suggests that a trial of combined neuroleptic and selective serotonin reuptake inhibitor (SSRI) treatment is reasonable in poorly responsive cases.

In nondelusional pathological jealousy, studies of SSRIs alone and SSRIs plus augmenting drugs, as well as studies of cognitive–behavioral approaches alone and combined with SSRIs are indicated. The necessary duration of drug treatment requires study. Cognitive–behavioral techniques should be described in detail and measures of specific therapeutic elements should be provided. Long-term follow-up will be required to validate short-term results.

Table 10.2 translates the available data and case reports into suggested treatment planning guidelines.

11

Trichotillomania

Even a single hair casts its shadow.

Publius Syrus (ca. 42 BC), *Maxims*

In 1889 Hallopeau, a French dermatologist, described a case of self-inflicted depilation of the scalp and coined the term, *trichotillomania* (from the Greek, *thrix*, hair; *tillein*, pulling out; and, *mania*, madness) (Hallopeau, 1889). More than a century later, the incidence, prevalence, etiology, natural history and appropriate treatment of trichotillomania are still unclear. This chapter considers trichotillomania in adults aged 18 years and older. The literature concerning trichotillomania in children and adolescents is reviewed by Adam and Kashani (1990) and by Reeve, Bernstein and Christenson (1992).

Diagnosis

DSM-IV diagnostic criteria (312.39)

Trichotillomania entered the American Psychiatric Association's diagnostic classification system with the 1987 publication of DSM-III-R, where it was grouped with the Impulse-Control Disorders Not Elsewhere Classified. DSM-IV (American Psychiatric Association, 1994) added the criterion, "causes clinically significant distress or impairment," to the four criteria contained in DSM-III-R (Table 11.1). Approximately 20% of individuals who chronically pull out their hair do not meet DSM-IV criteria for trichotillomania in that they deny the presence of either tension (criterion B) or gratification (criterion C) (Christenson, Mackenzie and Mitchell, 1991a; Christenson, Chernoff-Clementz and Clementz, 1992a). Whether they differ in important clinical respects from those meeting full criteria is unknown.

ICD-10 diagnostic criteria (F63.3)

ICD-10 (World Health Organization, 1992) places trichotillomania in the analogous category, Habit and impulse disorders. This category is characterized by impulses "that cannot be controlled." Because the suggestion that an impulse is irresistible carries implications of diminished responsibility under the law,

Table 11.1. DSM-IV diagnostic criteria for trichotillomania (312.39)

A. Recurrent pulling out of one's hair resulting in noticeable hair loss.

B. An increasing sense of tension immediately before pulling out the hair or when attempting to resist the behavior.

C. Pleasure, gratification, or relief when pulling out the hair.

D. The disturbance is not better accounted for by another mental disorder and is not due to a general medical condition (e.g., a dermatological condition).

E. The disturbance causes clinically significant distress or impairment in social, occupational, or other areas of functioning.

Source: Reprinted with permission from American Psychiatric Association. (1994). *Diagnostic and Statistical Manual of Mental Disorders,* Fourth Edition. Copyright 1994 American Psychiatric Association, p. 621.

DSM-IV avoided ascribing irresistibility to the Impulse-Control Disorders. Although the ICD-10 description of trichotillomania is generally consistent with the DSM-IV diagnostic criteria, ICD-10 does not mention associated distress or impairment of functioning.

Differential diagnosis

Trichotillomania must be distinguished from other causes of patchy hair loss including *alopecia areata* (a patchy loss of unknown etiology); *tinea capitis* (ringworm); alopecia caused by *medications* or by *poisons* such as thallium; *alopecia toxica* (loss from a febrile illness); *alopecia traumatica* (loss from excessive use of hair "softeners" or hot combs); *alopecia syphilitica* (seen in secondary syphilis); alopecia secondary to *irradiation*; *myxedematous alopecia*; and, *alopecia mucinosa* and other rare dermatological conditions. In adults, these diagnoses need be considered only in patients who deny or rationalize the signs; denial is more common in children and adolescents (Greenberg and Sarner, 1965). If necessary, the diagnosis can be established or confirmed by a punch biopsy of the affected area, which will usually reveal multiple catagen hairs (follicles in regression), melanin casts and dilated follicular ostia with keratin plugs (Muller, 1990). The presence of traumatized hair bulbs without inflammation, found in 21% of a series of 66 patients, is diagnostic (Muller, 1990). The presence of both normal and damaged follicles in the same area is typical. Inflammation suggests alopecia areata.

Not all chronic hair pulling is trichotillomania, and the DSM-IV diagnostic criteria probably identify individuals suffering from differing psychopathological or pathophysiological conditions. For example, Christenson and Crow (1996) have drawn attention to the distinction between patients who experience mounting tension and center their attention on pulling and those who pull while distracted by other activities. These authors suggest a closer relationship to OCD in the former group. Whether the degree to which trichotillomanic behavior is associated with tension, impulsivity, pleasure and awareness has important treatment implications deserves investigation.

Chronic hair pulling has been reported in association with *severe anxiety* (Krishnan, Davidson and Miller, 1984), *major depression* (Sachdeva and Sidhu, 1987), *dysthymia* (Sunkureddi and Markovitz, 1993) and *psychosis* (Childers, 1958). Hair pulling that occurs in *infancy* and *early childhood* appears to be a different syndrome; males predominate in treated preschool children and the behavior appears to be more likely to remit spontaneously or with minimal treatment (Swedo and Leonard, 1992). One childhood case of hair pulling concomitant with Sydenham's chorea has been reported (Stein et al., 1997c).

Clinical picture

In the majority of cases, trichotillomania results in patchy or full alopecia of the scalp (Muller, 1987; Christenson et al., 1991a). Many individuals also pull out eyelashes, eyebrows or facial hair, and some extract pubic, axillary or chest, abdominal or extremity hair. Hair pulling usually occurs daily, or nearly daily, and can occupy several hours or more (Soriano, et al., 1996).

Feelings of shame and humiliation lead patients to avoid exposing the damaged areas. They commonly attempt to conceal the alopecia with creative hair styling, wigs, hair pieces, constant use of hats or bandannas, makeup or false eyelashes. Patients have presented to me for treatment after long evading dating, intimate relationships, sports such as swimming, and outdoor exposure to windy places. More frequent hair pulling, greater body dissatisfaction, and greater anxiety and depression are associated with lower self-esteem (Soriano, et al., 1996).

A study of 60 adult chronic hair pullers helps delineate the clinical picture (Christenson et al., 1991a). The mean age of onset was 13 ± 8 years (median $=12$). The majority of subjects pulled from more than one site, with an average of eight years elapsing between the start of hair pulling and the involvement of the second site. Some patients used the dominant hand, others the non-dominant or both hands in pulling. Somewhat less than half the patients had used tweezers to pull out hair. The median number of pulling episodes per week was 16 for those primarily plucking scalp hair and seven for those primarily plucking eyelashes. A little more than half the patients sought out hairs with special tactile qualities, whether coarse, thick, curly or short. Hair pulling was not motivated by pruritus. Oral behaviors were associated with hair pulling in 48%: chewing hair or biting off the hair bulbs, rubbing hair around the mouth, licking the hair or ingesting it. No patient had a history of a trichobezoar (gastric or intestinal hairball). The vast majority reported some pulling episodes that began or remained out of complete awareness. High risk situations for hair pulling included watching television, reading, talking on the telephone, lying in bed, driving and writing. Hair pulling was worse in the evening for 95% of patients.

In a study of the effects of the menstrual cycle on pulling, slightly more than half of 45 women providing data reported that in the week prior to menses, pulling urges were more frequent and intense, pulling more frequent and the ability to resist weaker, with a return to baseline during menses or soon thereafter (Kethuen et al., 1997). With the exception of this gender-specific finding, men and women hair pullers exhibit no clinically important differences (Christenson, MacKenzie and Mitchell, 1994b).

Trichotillomania appears to be commonly associated with other problematic behaviors such as nail biting, skin picking, picking at acne, nose picking, lip biting and cheek chewing (Christenson et al., 1991a; Simeon, et al., 1997a).

Medical complications of trichotillomania are uncommon but may be serious. Trichobezoar is rare, but potentially life-threatening, and may cause intestinal obstruction, gastric or intestinal bleeding or perforation, acute pancreatitis, or obstructive jaundice, as well as discomfiting symptoms such as abdominal pain, nausea, vomiting, constipation, diarrhea, flatulence, anorexia and foul breath (Muller, 1987). A recent study of 24 primarily lower class children and adolescents in India suggests that trichobezoar may be more common in poor children: 9 of the 24 patients had trichobezoars or trichophytobezoars (hairball with vegetable matter) (Bhatia et al., 1991). Since trichophagia in children is associated with iron deficiency anemia (Sullivan, 1989), this symptom should trigger a complete blood count and serum iron estimation, even in adults. Other unusual medical complications include: skin infection at the site of pulling; blepharitis; chronic neck, shoulder or back pain from prolonged abnormal pulling postures; carpal tunnel syndrome; and, avoiding health care to escape shame, e.g., avoiding treatment for basal cell carcinoma of the scalp (O'Sullivan et al., 1996).

Christenson and Crow (1996) discuss the hypothesis put forward by researchers at the National Institute of Mental Health (NIMH) that trichotillomania may represent a pathological release of innate, fixed action patterns of grooming behavior. These investigators suggest that certain animal models, including canine acral lick dermatitis, feather picking in birds and psychogenic alopecia in cats, each of which is responsive to treatment with selective serotonin reuptake inhibitors (SSRIs), may illuminate the neurobiological basis of trichotillomania.

Assessment instruments

The relative merits and disadvantages of many assessment methods and instruments have been reviewed by Winchel et al. (1992a). For clinical purposes, one can ask the patient to count daily and collect in envelopes the pulled hairs. However, patients who swallow their plucked hairs must first give this up. Patients can also be asked to keep a diary that records each pulling episode (duration, situation, precipitants and response), but some find this too time consuming. The NIMH Trichotillomania Questionnaire (Swedo et al., 1989b), a modified form of the Yale–Brown Obsessive–Compulsive Scale (Y–BOCS), rates pulling behavior, but not related thoughts. The Psychiatric Institute Trichotillomania Scale allows the clinician to record the sites of pulling and to rate on a 0–7 scale the quantity of observable hair loss, time spent pulling and thinking about pulling, success in resisting the impulse to pull, distress related to trichotillomania and the degree to which hair pulling interferes with activities. Definitions and examples are provided for each scale point (Winchel et al., 1992b).

The only validated self-rating scale is the Massachusetts General Hairpulling Scale (Ketheun et al., 1995; O'Sullivan, et al., 1995). The patient rates seven items weekly on a 0–4 scale: the frequency of urges to pull, their intensity, ability to control the urges, frequency of hairpulling, attempts to resist, control over hair-pulling and associated distress.

In my clinical practice, I record the sites of pulling and rate symptom severity using the first 10 items of the Y–BOCS (provided in Appendix 2). I reword the questions to focus on trichotillomania-related thoughts and behaviors (Koran, Ringold and Hewlett, 1992; Stanley et al., 1993). For research purposes, the other rating scales offer advantages (Winchel et al., 1992a).

In my experience, engaging the patient in any assessment method that enhances awareness of pulling behavior and increases accountability for the amount of hair pulled aids in treatment.

Prevalence

Until the 1990s, trichotillomania was thought to be quite rare. For example, case frequency was reported as 2 per 1200 patients treated for psychiatric disorders in a university outpatient clinic (Fabbri and Dy, 1974), and 5 per 10,000 children treated for psychiatric disorders (Schacter, 1961). The disorder was thought to be more common, though still infrequent, in dermatological practice (Mehregan, 1970; Muller, 1987). Now that media attention is increasing awareness of treatments for trichotillomania, affected individuals are increasingly seeking care.

The prevalence of trichotillomania in the general population has not been studied. A 1989 questionnaire survey of approximately 2500 college freshman in the United States at two state universities and a liberal arts college, with a 97.9% response rate, indicated a lifetime prevalence of DSM-III-R trichotillomania of 0.6% for both male and female students (Christenson, Pyle and Mitchell, 1991d). When the investigators ignored the diagnostic criteria referring to tension, pleasure and gratification, the prevalence increased to 3.4% of females and 1.5% of males. A similar survey of about 700 college freshman found that 11% pulled their hair on a regular basis for other than cosmetic reasons, and that 1% met DSM-IV criteria for trichotillomania by self-report (Rothbaum et al., 1993).

In treated case series, women outnumber men by a ratio that approximates 3.5:1 (Muller, 1990; Azrin, Nunn and Frantz, 1980). In modern pharmacological trials, the female-to-male ratio has been 7:1 or higher (Christenson et al., 1991c; Streichenwein and Thornby, 1995; Stanley et al., 1997). The female preponderance may be due in part to women's greater willingness to seek medical care.

About 5–8% of the first-degree relatives of probands with trichotillomania also have the condition, but whether this reflects nature or nurture is unknown (Christenson, Mackenzie and Reeve, 1992b; Lenane, et al., 1992; Schlosser et al., 1994a).

Comorbidity

The available data concerning the prevalence of comorbid conditions are tainted by serious methodological shortcomings such as ascertainment bias and limited geographical representation. These problems preclude generalizing the reported figures. Still, the data begin to suggest that the prevalence of comorbid mood and anxiety disorders is higher than in the general population. In the largest methodologically strong study, Christenson et al., (1991a) evaluated 60 patients aged 18–61 years (mean$\pm$SD$=34\pm8$) with a semi-structured interview utilizing DSM-III-R criteria (Table 11.2). Another set of estimates is provided by a study of 43 older children, adolescents and adults (mean age$=30\pm11$) who responded to advertisements for drug studies at the NIMH and were evaluated with a semi-structured interview (Table 11.2) (Swedo and Leonard, 1992). This study utilized modified diagnostic criteria for trichotillomania: neither gratification nor tension relief was required.

In a study severely limited by its methods, respondents to print media materials seeking individuals with trichotillomania or self-injury were mailed a survey package (Cohen et al., 1995). Only 16% of 772 individuals surveyed returned usable questionnaires and recorded their "formally diagnosed" disorders on a self-report form. In addition to trichotillomania, reported by 40% of these 123 respondents, 13% reported a formal diagnosis of OCD; 14%, depressive disorder; 3%, bipolar disorder; 15%, anxiety disorder; and, 7%, substance abuse.

Case reports and small case series link trichotillomania to a variety of other disorders, but the diagnostic criteria vary widely. Most cases in the literature reporting behavioral and hypnotic treatments do not carry additional diagnoses, although patients are frequently described as guilty, ashamed, anxious, depressed

Table 11.2. Lifetime prevalence of selected psychiatric disorders in two convenience samples of trichotillomania patients

Disorder	Study A[a] (%)	Study B[b] (%)
Major depression	55	39
Dysthymia	8	
Panic disorder	19	5
Obsessive–compulsive disorder	15	16
Generalized anxiety disorder	27	32
Social phobia	8	2 (Phobic disorder)
Simple phobia	32	
Bulimia	8	
Anorexia nervosa	0	5 (Anorexia/bulimia)
Eating disorder NOS	12	
Alcohol abuse	18	15 (Substance abuse)
Other substance abuse	17	

Notes:
[a] Christenson et al., 1991b: $n = 50$.
[b] Swedo and Leonard, 1992; $n = 43$.
NOS: not otherwise specified.

or suffering low self-esteem. Because of ascertainment and reporting bias, conclusions about comorbid risk cannot be drawn from these sources.

The prevalence of DSM Axis II personality disorders has been examined in three convenience samples, but again, these figures cannot be generalized (Table 11.3). The limited diagnostic validity of all structured instruments used to evaluate personality disorders (Perry, 1992) further complicates the interpretation of these data.

The only study to examine the prevalence of personality disorders in trichotillomania patients and gender-matched patients seeking psychiatric treatment at the same center found no difference between the two groups (Christenson et al., 1992a).

Relationship to obsessive compulsive disorder

A number of similarities suggest a relationship between trichotillomania and OCD. Patients often describe their pulling as "compulsive." Available data suggest, but do not prove, that the rate of OCD in probands (as noted earlier) and in their first degree relatives (Lenane et al., 1992; Schlosser et al., 1994a) is increased over the rate in the general population. Like OCD, trichotillomania has been thought to have origins in psychosexual development and traumas (Galski, 1981; Singh and

Table 11.3. DSM-III-R personality disorders in convenience
samples of trichotillomania patients

Personality disorder	Study A[a] (%)	Study B[b] (%)	Study C[c] (%)
Paranoid	4	0	5
Schizoid	2	0	14
Schizotypal	0	0	5
Obsessive–compulsive	8	0	27
Histrionic	15	30	0
Dependent	8	7	9
Antisocial	0	0	5
Narcissistic	0	3	9
Avoidant	10	3	14
Borderline	2	23	14
Passive–Aggressive	6	17	14

Notes:
[a] Christenson et al., 1992b; $n = 48$ female trichotillomanics.
[b] Swedo and Leonard, 1992; $n = 30$ female trichotillomanics.
[c] Schlosser et al., 1994a; $n = 20$ female and 2 male trichotillomanics.

Maguire, 1989). The case-report literature suggests that like OCD, hair pulling is poorly responsive to psychoanalytic psychotherapy (Greenberg and Sarner, 1965; Monroe and Abse, 1963; Saper, 1971; Galski, 1981; Barabasz, 1987) and often responds to serotonin reuptake inhibitors (SRIs) (discussed subsequently). Response to similar treatments, however, is a weak argument for a relationship between disorders, e.g., many unrelated conditions respond to propranolol.

On the other hand, important differences separate trichotillomania and OCD. OCD compulsions are ego-dystonic, never pleasurable, are performed in full awareness, and aim at avoiding increased anxiety. Although hair pulling is ego-dystonic insofar as patients feel ashamed and dislike the physical stigmata, they often report that hair pulling itself is pleasurable (Stanley et al., 1992), engaged in with minimal awareness, and carried out in response to, rather than to avoid, increased anxiety. In addition, hair pulling is not elicited by an obsession and is less strenuously resisted than are compulsions (Stanley et al., 1992). Hair pulling appears to be much more common in females than in males, whereas the female-to-male ratio for OCD in epidemiological studies rarely exceeds 1.5:1 (Karno et al., 1988; Weissman et al., 1994). Finally, hair pulling has been successfully treated (at least in the short-term) with brief courses of hypnosis and many behavioral therapy techniques to which OCD is resistant.

Neurobiological studies, reviewed by Christenson and Crow (1996), provide the strongest evidence that the relationship between trichotillomania and OCD is at most, limited. For example, unlike patients with OCD, those with trichotillomania do *not* exhibit an increased number of neurological soft signs, abnormalities of serotonin's cerebral spinal fluid metabolite (5–HIAA), blunted neuroendocrine response to *meta*-chlorophenylpiperazine (*m*-CPP), or elevated resting glucose metabolism in the orbital frontal, anterior cingulate and caudate regions. (Compared to gender- and age-matched controls, female trichotillomania patients exhibit increased resting glucose metabolism in the cerebrum globally, in the cerebellum and in the right superior parietal region – Swedo et al., 1991.)

Treatment

Treatment begins with taking a careful history of the disorder and its effects and inquiring after possible comorbid conditions. The data reviewed earlier suggest that mood and anxiety disorders will be commonly found. No treatment approach has been established as effective in a large controlled trial. Case reports, small series, and a few uncontrolled and controlled trials present a variety of treatment methods that merit exploration. Patients are often quite relieved to find that others pull out hair and should be guided to organizations offering educational material and contact with kindred sufferers (See Appendix 1).

Behavior therapy

The behavior therapy literature shares the shortcomings of the pharmacotherapy literature: mostly uncontrolled observations, short follow-up periods, and a publication bias toward favorable outcomes. Much of this literature is presented in detail elsewhere (Friman, Finney and Christophersen, 1984). All reports include at least two treatment elements and most include at least four, making it difficult to identify the essential factors. Placebo effects and the nonspecific elements of supportive psychotherapy may have contributed to the reported results.

The largest published experience concerns habit reversal treatment, which includes 13 components. Azrin et al. (1980) randomly assigned 34 subjects to one 2-hour session of instruction in either habit reversal or negative practice. The results were remarkable: 14 of 19 habit reversal subjects (74%) reported no hair-pulling at the four-week follow-up, starting with the first post-treatment day, compared to only 5 of 15 negative practice subjects (33%). At the four-month evaluation, 11 of 18 habit reversal subjects were still refraining from hair pulling. At 22 months, 9 of 12 habit reversal subjects reached were in remission, compared to 2 of 8 negative practice subjects. The four-month and 22-month follow-ups appear to have been conducted largely by telephone, but reports from family and friends "were generally in agreement." Similarly positive results were reported in four patients who had mild hair pulling (Rosenbaum and Ayllon, 1981) and in one severely affected patient (Tarnowski et al., 1987).

In patients with trichotillomania uncomplicated by serious comorbidity, I have had good results with a modified form of habit reversal derived from the behavioral literature. The seven treatment elements I utilize are: hair collection; identifying preventive strategies for high-risk situations; motivation enhancement; changing the internal monologue; awareness training; competing response training; and, relaxation training.

• *Self-monitoring.* Ask the patient to collect all the hairs pulled each day in an envelope, count them, write the number and the date on each envelope, and bring the envelopes to the next treatment session. Explain that this will provide the patient and the clinician with a daily measure of progress, and will help the patient be accountable to herself, since she will know exactly how much she is pulling. This task seems to reduce hair pulling by increasing the behavioral cost of pulling, and by drawing on patients' reluctance to share this embarrassing information. Azrin et al. (1980) used a daily diary, and some patients find this method more practical and acceptable.

• *Coping strategies.* After identifying the situations in which pulling occurs, help the patient develop coping strategies. For example, ask the patient to commit to keeping both hands on the steering wheel unless shifting or turning a radio dial. Or, ask the patient to commit to keeping both hands on the book while reading. If pulling occurs during long stays in the bathroom, ask the patient to set a timer to 1–2 minutes and leave when it goes off. Making these commitments to the clinician seems to be an important motivator.

• *Motivation enhancement.* Give the patient a list of possible reasons for wanting to stop hair pulling (Table 11.4). Ask her to check off all that apply and write in any additional reasons she wishes. Explain that the motives driving the pulling behavior have overwhelmed the motives to stop. Ask the patient to strengthen the motives to stop by posting this list where she will review it at least once a day, e.g., on the refrigerator door or bathroom mirror. Keep a copy for review during therapy.

• *Changing the internal monologue.* Ask the patient to become aware of the internal monologue that gives her permission to pull, e.g., "I'll only pull a few," or, "I've already done so much damage, it doesn't matter," or, "It feels good." Ask her to change her "self-talk," and to substitute a more functional message for these rationalizations each time they occur. Offer a positive and a negative statement, since patients vary in the approach preferred: "I deserve to take better care of myself than to pull out my hair." Or, "Hair pulling is damaging, disfiguring and self-destructive, and I don't want to do that to myself."

Table 11.4. Reasons for stopping hair pulling

Patient's Name   *Date*

Please check off all of the reasons for stopping hair pulling that are true for you at this time:

I want to stop hair pulling because I want to:
___ like and respect myself more
___ be more attractive
___ look more normal
___ take better care of myself
___ be proud of myself
___ feel more comfortable with people I know
___ feel more comfortable with strangers
___ be able to participate in sports activities
___ please my significant other
___ provide a good example for my children (or others)
___ find healthier ways to express my feelings
___ put an end to an expensive habit
___ other (describe)

___ other (describe)

___ other (describe)

I want to stop hair pulling because I don't want to:
___ have to wonder what other people are thinking about me
___ have to explain anything to people
___ feel people are laughing at me
___ have people feel sorry for me
___ feel embarrassed when meeting strangers
___ have to tell lies about my condition
___ avoid certain social or athletic activities
___ express my tension, frustration, or boredom this way
___ feel out of control
___ have to avoid certain hair styles
___ have to avoid certain ways of dressing
___ have to conceal my habit
___ look funny or abnormal
___ other (describe)

___ other (describe)

___ other (describe)

- *Awareness training.* Ask the patient to slowly bring her hand(s) to the pulling area and while doing so, to become exquisitely aware of the sensations in every part of the arm, from the shoulder to the finger tips. Ask her also to pay attention to the hand as it enters the peripheral and central visual fields. Azrin et al. (1980) utilized practice in front of a mirror. Explain that you do not want her to be able to pull without being fully aware of it, and ask her to practice this awareness training 1–2 minutes twice a day.
- *Competing response.* Ask the patient to lightly clench her thumbs inside her fists for 3 minutes whenever she has the urge to pull, or to perform some other socially inconspicuous, incompatible response. Explain that this precludes pulling and that the urge will usually pass within this time. Some patients prefer to substitute a form of tactile stimulation, and you can suggest holding a soft eraser, stroking a soft makeup brush, squeezing a rubber isometric hand exerciser or fingering a string of beads.
- *Relaxation training.* Explain that tension and anxiety promote pulling. Ask the patient to choose a form of relaxation exercise (visualization of a pleasant scene, progressive muscle relaxation or diaphragmatic breathing) and to practice it for a few minutes one to several times a day "to lower your general level of tension."

Every element needs not be utilized with each patient. I tailor this package to the patient's presenting picture and motivations. After the treatment package is in place, I review at each session whether or not the patient has followed through with her commitments. When the patient fails to carry out a treatment task, I adopt a problem solving approach, e.g., "What prevented you from doing this?" I explore both motivational factors, such as ambivalence about stopping, and situational factors, including continued environmental stressors. This non-critical stance helps to maintain the therapeutic alliance, contradicts the expectations of reprimand, and counterbalances the internalized criticism that patients usually bring from parental responses to their hair pulling.

Once hair pulling has ceased, sustained improvement seems to require teaching the patient relapse prevention strategies and arranging three- to six-month follow-up visits. I ask patients to continue to rehearse the changed internal monologue, review the motivations for stopping and utilize the competing response as needed. In addition, I encourage patients to view lapses as signals to return to active treatment, rather than as occasions for self denigration or signs of an inescapable, prolonged relapse.

Pharmacotherapy

Many drugs appear promising, but the only one found effective to date in a controlled trial is clomipramine. Approaches to choosing medication are presented after a review of the available literature, which consists of uncontrolled observations. The published data are biased toward favorable outcomes, since these are more likely to find their way into print.

Pharmacotherapies supported by case series or uncontrolled trials are shown in Table 11.5. Instead of and in addition to drug effects, the improvements reported may reflect nonspecific therapeutic factors, e.g., the placebo effect, self-monitoring, or the benefits of supportive psychotherapy. Frequently, the duration of improvement is unspecified or the follow-up period is limited to a few weeks or months, too soon to evaluate outcome in this chronic condition. In many cases, improvement was transitory. Nevertheless, these uncontrolled observations represent hypotheses to be weighed critically and tested, both in the clinical situation and in carefully designed, controlled trials.

Case reports of response to isocarboxazid (Krishnan, Davidson and Miller, 1984), imipramine (Sachdeva and Sidhu, 1987), trazodone (Sunkureddi and Markovitz, 1993) and sertraline (Bradford and Gratzer, 1995; Rahman and Gregory, 1995) share a distinction. In these cases, trichotillomania improved concomitantly with comorbid major depression or dysthymia, suggesting that treatment of comorbid mood disorders may ameliorate trichotillomania. Isolated cases have responded to amitriptyline (Snyder, 1980) and the progestin levonorgestrol (Perciaccante and Perciaccante, 1993) in the absence of mood disorders, and to buspirone in the presence of generalized anxiety disorder (Reid, 1992). Two patients with a partial response to clomipramine had substantial further improvement when topical fluocinolone, 0.01%, was prescribed for pruritus in the areas subject to pulling (Black and Blum, 1992b; Gupta and Freimer, 1993).

Uncontrolled observations have also suggested efficacy for the combination of SRIs and neuroleptics. In a chart review study, two patients with a moderate response to adequate trials of clomipramine had marked improvement, sustained for six months, after the addition of 1–2 mg/day of pimozide; and, two of four patients with unsatisfactory or unsustained response during a fluoxetine trial, had a moderate to marked sustained response during a subsequent trial of clomipramine (50–200 mg/day) combined with pimozide (2–3 mg/day) (Stein and Hollander, 1992). All of the patients had comorbid conditions; in the four with OCD, the two disorders responded similarly to pimozide augmentation (two patients improved). Weight gain was problematic in this case series. In a second chart review study, three of four patients reported significant clinical improvement sustained for "some months" after risperidone 1 mg/day was added to clomipramine; a fifth patient, receiving citalopram, did not respond to added risperidone (Stein et al., 1997a). One patient discontinued risperidone because of worsening depression. A third chart review study, reported in abstract form, found that four of six patients (or five of six, the abstract is ambiguous) who were unresponsive to a SRI markedly improved after the addition of haloperidol 0.5–2.5 mg/day, experiencing "almost complete hair regrowth" (Van

Table 11.5. Drug treatments for trichotillomania supported by uncontrolled observations

Study	Drug	Dose	Treatment duration	Patients (N)	Outcome
Stein et al., 1997b	CIT	M = 36.2 mg	12 weeks	13	5 much or very much improved
Black et al., 1992	CMI	75–100 mg	9 months	1	improved, + topical steroid → remission
Iancu et al., 1996	CMI	75–200 mg	7–15 weeks	4	3 responded but relapsed on drug
Ninan et al., 1992	CMI	M = 125 mg	M = 11 weeks	2	"significant clinical improvement"
Pollard et al., 1991	CMI	50–150 mg	7–24 weeks	4	all responded; 3 relapsed on drug
Alexander 1991	FLU	40–60 mg	6 months	1	Relapsed when dose decreased
Iancu et al., 1996	FLU	20–60 mg	6–20 weeks	6	3 responded but relapsed on drug
Koran et al., 1992	FLU	20–80 mg M = 48 mg	7–12 weeks	17	5/13 completers markedly improved
Ninan et al., 1992	FLU	M = 45	M = 11 weeks	5	"significant clinical improvement"
Stanley et al., 1991	FLU	60–80 mg	12 weeks	5	4/5 markedly improved
Winchel et al., 1992c	FLU	M = 74 mg	12–16 weeks	16	8/12 completers improved
Iancu et al., 1996	FLV	200–300 mg	15–16 weeks	2	1 responded but relapsed on drug
Stanley et al., 1997	FLV	50–300 mg	12 weeks	21	no clear effect in 13 completers
Christenson et al., 1998	FLV	up to 300 mg	8 weeks	19	4 responded, but 3 relapsed on drug
Christenson et al., 1991c	LITH	900–1500 mg 0.5–1.2 mEq/L	3–12 months	10	8/10 responded, 5 within 1–3 weeks
Christenson et al., 1996	NLT	50 mg?	?	7	3 responded
O'Sullivan[a]	PAR	?	2–24 weeks	14	6 responded
Reid 1992	PAR	40 mg	4+ weeks	1	marked response, duration uncertain
O'Sullivan et al., 1998	VEN	M = 274 mg	8–28 weeks	10	5 responded, but inconsistently

Notes:

[a] Cited in Minichiello et al. (1994).

CIT: citalopram; CMI: clomipramine; FLU: fluoxetine; FLV: fluvoxamine; LITH: $LiCO_3$; NLT: naltrexone; PAR: paroxetine; VEN: venlafaxine; M: mean.

Ameringen and Mancini, 1996). Controlled trials are needed to evaluate these hopeful observations.

Controlled drug trials have been less encouraging. Two placebo-controlled, double-blind crossover trials have failed to corroborate the effectiveness of fluoxetine. In a study of 21 adults treated for five-week periods with up to 80 mg/day or placebo, fluoxetine had no greater effect than placebo on the number of hair pulling episodes per week, estimated amount of hair pulled per week, subjective severity of hair pulling or urge to pull hair (Christenson et al., 1991b). The second trial, involving 23 adult subjects, lengthened the active treatment period to 12 weeks (six weeks at 80 mg/day), but still found no significant drug effect (Streichenwein and Thornby, 1995). In a case report, a therapeutic response to fluoxetine stopped when isotretinoin was started for cystic acne and resumed when this medication was discontinued (Mahr, 1990).

In contrast, a 10-week, double-blind crossover trial comparing clomipramine (100–250 mg) to desipramine (100–200 mg) in 13 severely affected patients reported that clomipramine decreased hair pulling by 50% or more in nine subjects and induced complete remission in three (Swedo et al., 1989a). Only one patient responded more favorably to desipramine than clomipramine. A follow-up evaluation indicated that benefit was maintained for six months; after about four years, however, less than half the patients continued to be at least moderately improved, despite intervening treatments (Swedo, Lenane and Leonard, 1993).

An unpublished, double-blind, placebo-controlled trial of the opiate antagonist, naltrexone, reported benefit in three of seven naltrexone-treated patients, but evaluation of this claim awaits publication of the study (Christenson and Crow, 1996). In a single case report of comorbid trichotillomania and OCD, naltrexone 50 mg/day, added to fluoxetine 60 mg/day, decreased the duration and intensity of pulling episodes sufficiently to allow substantial hair regrowth (Carrion, 1995). The therapeutic benefit, which the patient attributed to diminished impulsivity and pleasure in pulling, was sustained during a four-month follow-up.

Choosing a medication

Since clomipramine is the only medication whose effectiveness has been demonstrated in a double-blind trial, it deserves primary consideration. Clomipramine's adverse effects, particularly sedation, weight gain and anticholinergic side effects, are often problematic, and relapse has been reported in a number of cases despite continued treatment (Table 11.5). Venlafaxine and mirtazapine, which like clomipramine, strongly enhance both serotonergic and noradrenergic functioning, may ultimately prove to be alternatives, but their use in trichotillomania has not been investigated. The addition of a low dose of pimozide, risperidone or haloperidol can be considered in patients with a partial or unsustained response to clomipramine. The small risk of tardive dyskinesia must be weighed and disclosed.

In the absence of better guides to treatment, the patient's subjective experience may provide clues. In those unusual cases where pruritus motivates pulling, a short trial of adding topical fluocinolone 0.01% to a partially effective regimen is indicated. The observation of long-term benefit from lithium, albeit uncontrolled, suggests that lithium and other drugs that diminish neuronal excitability, such as valproate or gabapentin, are worth investigating in patients who complain of overwhelming impulses to pull. Patients whose pulling is strongly motivated by pleasurable sensation may deserve a trial of the opiate antagonist, naltrexone.

Comorbid conditions will influence drug choice. From among all the drugs known to be effective for the comorbid condition, the clinician should select one that available data suggest is also beneficial in trichotillomania.

My clinical impression is that combining a drug trial with supportive psychotherapy and behavior therapy aimed at trichotillomania is more effective than medication alone. I utilize the modified version of habit reversal described earlier.

Hypnotic treatments

A variety of hypnotic techniques have been applied in case reports or small series of patients, usually as adjuncts to other behavioral or psychotherapeutic treatment elements. These elements have included awareness training (Galski, 1981; Barabasz, 1987), relaxation training (Fabbri and Dy, 1974; Galski, 1981; Hall and McGill, 1986; Barabasz, 1987), counseling (Fabri and Dy, 1974; Barabasz, 1987), competing response training (Hall and McGill, 1986) and changing self-statements about hair pulling (Rowen, 1981). Treatment outcome seems unrelated to the number of hypnotic sessions, but Hynes (1982) noted a correlation between outcome and his patients' hypnotizability, as reflected in their abilities to engage in age regression and to learn autohypnosis. Hypnotic suggestions have included pain on touching the scalp or pulling hair (in cases where pulling was pleasurable) (Galski, 1981; Rowen, 1981), increased awareness of hair pulling behavior through associated hand warming (Hall and McGill, 1986) and rituals other than hair pulling to decrease anxiety (Fabbri and Dy, 1974). Several authors emphasized the importance of shaping posthypnotic suggestions to enhance the patient's sense of self-control (Fabbri and Dy, 1974; Galski, 1981; Hynes, 1982; Barabasz, 1987).

In view of the heterogeneity of techniques employed and the absence of controlled studies, no conclusions can be drawn about the utility of hypnosis in treating trichotillomania.

An approach to planning integrated treatment for trichotillomania is displayed in Table 11.6.

Table 11.6. Trichotillomania: treatment planning guidelines

- Assess all sites of pulling and measure baseline rates.
- Assess motivation for treatment.
- Inquire about trichophagia; order serum iron and complete blood count if it is present.
- Assess and treat comorbid conditions, including skin picking, mood disorders, anxiety disorders and substance abuse. When choosing a drug, consider whether it may also benefit trichotillomania.
- Guide patient toward educational and support groups.
- Institute modified habit reversal.
- Consider pharmacotherapy:
    - clomipramine (plus a topical steroid if pruritus is present) – SSRIs are less well supported by the data;
    - add low dose haloperidol, pimozide or risperidone for partial or unsustained response to clomipramine (or an SSRI);
    - lithium carbonate;
    - naltrexone.
- Consider introducing post-hypnotic suggestions.
- Institute relapse prevention strategies.

Note:
SSRI: selective serotonin reuptake inhibitor.

12

Skin picking

Scratching is one of the sweetest gratifications of nature, and as ready at hand as any.

Michel de Montaigne, *Essays*

Skin picking was first described in the late 1800s by Brocq, who termed it "acné excoriée," or excoriated acne (Bach and Bach, 1993). Although others subsequently used the label, "neurotic excoriations," the etiology remains unknown. Since patients with skin picking are far more likely to present to dermatologists than psychiatrists and often refuse psychiatric referral, the psychiatrist should expect to be helpful more often as a knowledgeable consultant rather than as the primary treating physician.

Diagnosis

In that skin picking is not an official diagnosis, no accepted diagnostic criteria exist. It is not included in the DSM-IV diagnostic category of Impulse–Control Disorders or in the ICD-10 diagnostic category of Habit and impulse disorders. Skin picking behavior resembles the compulsive behavior of OCD in that it is repetitive, ritualistic, usually preceded by increasing tension, followed by tension relief and experienced as ego–dystonic and senseless. As a result, some authors have suggested that it be considered an OCD spectrum disorder (Stein et al., 1993).

Clinical picture

The lesions are usually found on the face, limbs or upper back – areas which the patient can easily reach – and may vary from a few to hundreds. They are produced by repetitive self-excoriation that begins in the absence of physical pathology, or in response to a benign skin abnormality, mild acne (Stout, 1990) or sensations of itching (Gupta, Gupta and Haberman, 1986), smarting, burning, stinging or prickling (Fruensgaard, 1991a). The lesions are usually a few millimeters in diameter, and depending on the recency of picking, may be open, scabbed or scarred; post inflammatory hypopigmentation or hyperpigmentation may be present (Gupta et al., 1986).

In one series of more than 60 patients referred to a university dermatology department, scratching and picking episodes usually occurred late in the day, when the patient was tired, or just before or after retiring to bed. Some patients experienced an altered state of consciousness while picking, resembling a dissociative state, and more than 90% did not experience significant pain while picking. Low self-esteem, lack of self-confidence and anticipation of criticism and hypersensitivity to it were common (Fruensgaard, 1991a).

Phillips and Taub (1995) describe the clinical features of skin picking behavior in 33 patients with body dsymorphic disorder (BDD). Nearly all of these patients were motivated to pick by a preoccupation with the appearance of their skin, and worried about nonexistent or minimal acne or various subjectively perceived imperfections. They compared their "defect" with the analogous region on others' bodies and engaged in mirror checking and in camouflaging behaviors (e.g., wearing makeup, covering the area with their hands, turning their "defect" away from the observer). Approximately half frequently sought reassurance, avoided mirrors and touched their "defect." Many picked for hours a day, usually while looking in a mirror. Some used tweezers, pins, needles or other sharp objects. Although picking usually reduced tension, the patients often felt depressed or anxious later, fearing they had further worsened their appearance. Like a larger comparison group of BDD patients, those with skin picking almost always experienced impaired social and occupational or academic functioning. One-third had been hospitalized because of BDD and one-quarter had made suicide attempts that were attributed to BDD.

Differential diagnosis

In *dermatitis artefacta* (manifest in burns, abrasions, scratches, ulcers or bullae), the patient consciously creates the lesions in order to gain the benefits of the sick role. Severe, comorbid personality disorder, e.g., borderline personality disorder, is frequently present (Van Moffaert, 1992). In *malingering*, the patient consciously produces lesions to obtain some material gain. Patients with *borderline personality disorder* may scratch or pick as one of several self-mutilating behaviors (including cutting and burning the skin) in response to anger, frustration or boredom. Patients with *delusions of parasitosis* (a form of delusional disorder, somatic type) may excoriate themselves attempting to remove the imagined parasites.

Skin picking can be a manifestation of the *Prader-Willi syndrome* (characterized by hypotonia at birth, childhood obesity, hypogonadism, and in most cases, mental deficiency) (Warnock and Kestenbaum, 1992), and, rarely, a symptom of Tourette's Disorder (American Psychiatric Association, 1994).

To uncover *BDD* motivating skin picking, patients should be asked why they pick (Phillips and Taub, 1995). The BDD patient is usually picking to reduce or remove an imagined defect or minimal imperfection (scar, pimples, "large" pores, "spots" or "bumps") and is preoccupied with it (see Chapter 8). Since picking can create lesions or defects, and since BDD patients may be unable to report accurately whether the defect was present before picking began, the clinician should attempt to examine pre-existing photographs or interview someone who knew the patient before picking began to determine whether the defect was minimal at the onset (Phillips and Taub, 1995).

Prevalence

The prevalence in the general population is unknown. In dermatology clinics, the prevalence may approach 2% (Stein et al., 1993). Skin picking is more common in women. The age of onset can range from the teens and 20s to the 60s (Gupta et al., 1986).

In a series of 33 patients with skin picking as a symptom of BDD, women constituted 58%, and the age of onset of BDD ranged from 9 to 36 years (Phillips and Taub, 1995).

Comorbidity

Since the early 1900s, skin picking has been reported in association with a variety of psychiatric conditions, but the absence of modern diagnostic criteria limits interpretation. In some modern cases, no other psychiatric condition has been found (Bach and Bach, 1993). The most commonly reported comorbid conditions have been anxiety and depressive symptoms, obsessive–compulsive traits or perfectionism, and conversion reaction; hypochondriasis and paranoid schizophrenia have also been mentioned (Fruensgaard 1991a; Bach and Bach, 1993; Simeon et al., 1997a). Skin picking may occur with other self-injurious behaviors such as trichotillomania (Christenson, Mackenzie and Mitchell, 1991a) and less often, with nail biting, skin cutting and skin burning (Simeon et al., 1997a). Skin picking appears to be common in patients with BDD (Phillips and Taub, 1995).

Anxiety and depression may be a cause of the picking behavior or a result of the embarrassment and social discomfort occasioned by visible skin lesions. This distress can be severe enough to precipitate suicide (Phillips and Taub, 1995). Less distressed patients may be concerned about being unattractive, without being desperate about it (Bach and Bach, 1993). Psychosocial stress has been considered a precipitating factor in many reported cases (Gupta et al., 1986; Fruensgaard, 1991a).

Treatment

Dermatologic treatment with antihistamines and topical steroids is generally ineffective (Gupta et al., 1986). In a series of 63 dermatology clinic patients followed-up one to five years after referral, only six had achieved stable healing, and seven intermittent healing (Fruensgaard, 1991a). The clinician, whether dermatologist or psychiatrist, should begin treatment by empathetically assessing in detail the patient's reasons for picking, mental state during picking and motivations for wishing to stop.

Pharmacotherapy

Case reports and small controlled trials suggest that serotonin reuptake inhibitors (SRIs) are often helpful. How long patients should be treated and the likelihood of response to a second selective serotonin reuptake inhibitor (SSRI) after the first has been ineffective remain to be determined.

Fluoxetine has been beneficial in a small, double-blind, placebo-controlled trial and several case reports. Simeon et al. (1997b) used newspaper advertisement to recruit subjects with skin picking of at least six months duration associated with noticeable lesions and significant distress or impaired functioning into a 10-week, double-blind trial of fluoxetine versus placebo. The subjects' mean duration of skin picking was nearly 18 years, and the mean age at onset was 16 years. Fluoxetine was begun at 20 mg/day and increased as tolerated weekly over three weeks to 80 mg/day. Of the 10 patients who received fluoxetine, four dropped out (two for side effects, two with improvement), four achieved a Clinical Global Improvement score (Guy, 1976) of much and two of very much improved. Three of 11 placebo patients were much improved, but none was very much improved. Change in skin picking was not related to change in measures of depression, anxiety or obsessive–compulsive symptoms.

Stout (1990) reports the case of a young woman who responded to fluoxetine begun at 20 mg/day and increased after two weeks to 40 mg/day. She noted a marked decrease in skin picking within one month, and after three months, her lesions had largely resolved. Stein et al. (1993) report two cases that responded to fluoxetine 20 mg/day with marked improvement within three weeks, which was sustained over six months in the case followed that long.

In a four-week, double-blind, placebo-controlled trial of fluvoxamine plus supportive psychotherapy in a group of patients with "psychocutaneous disorders" and "anxious and depressive features," five patients experienced marked reduction in skin picking (Hendrickx et al., 1991). The starting dose was 100 mg/day; no skin picking cases had been assigned to placebo.

Sertraline, begun at 25–50 mg/day and titrated to 100–200 mg/day, was beneficial in 19 of 28 (68%) evaluable patients with "neurotic excoriations" or "acne excoriée" treated in a dermatology clinic (Kalivas, Kalivas and Gilman, 1996). These 19 patients exhibited a 50% or greater decrease in open skin lesions within a month of starting treatment. The authors note the need for data on the length of treatment necessary to induce sustained response.

Gupta et al. (1986) administered clomipramine to an elderly woman with pruritus and skin picking unresponsive to 4½ years of dermatological treatment that included antihistamines and topical steroids. Three months of twice monthly supportive psychotherapy successfully encouraged the cultivation of new interests, but brought only modest improvement in skin picking, and then the patient developed major depression. She was started on clomipramine 25 mg/day, increased to 50 mg/day after one week. The patient noted benefit within the first week and marked improvement in pruritus and skin picking after three weeks, along with improvement in her depression. Discontinuation after six weeks resulted in recurrence of skin picking. After retreatment for six months, her pruritus, skin picking and depression remained in abeyance during a two-month follow-up. Gupta et al. (1986) note that their five elderly patients developed skin picking shortly after physical illness limited their physical activity, and recommend supportive therapy that includes efforts to facilitate physical activity.

In skin picking associated with BDD, Phillips and Taub (1995) report that dermatological treatment may alleviate the skin damage, but usually leaves the BDD preoccupations unchanged or worse. Their 33 patients reported that by history, about half the trials of SRIs had led to significant improvement, compared to only 10% for other psychotropic medications. Of nine patients unresponsive to dermatological treatment whom Phillips and Taub treated with an SRI, seven responded well; several apparently required trials of more than one such drug. In the one case described, fluoxetine 80 mg/day produced "near remission" during three years of treatment.

Because skin picking may be a form of self-injurious behavior, and the opiate antagonist, naltrexone, has been helpful in some such cases (Smith and Pittelkow, 1989; Roth, Ostroff and Hoffman, 1996), it can be considered in treatment-resistant skin picking. The absence of pain while picking (Fruensgaard, 1991a), also reported in cases of skin cutting responsive to naltrexone (Roth et al., 1996), also argues for a therapeutic trial of this drug (see Chapter 13 for a discussion of naltrexone's side effects). Naltrexone, 50 mg/day has resulted in cessation of self injurious behavior within a few days to two weeks. Patients often stopped the self-injurious behavior when naltrexone treatment restored the normal pain response. In a series of patients with borderline personality disorder, the self-injurious behavior returned when patients briefly discontinued naltrexone, but remained in abeyance during continuous trials lasting 4–16 weeks (Roth et al.,

Table 12.1. Skin picking: treatment planning guidelines

- Assess motivations for treatment.
- Assess motivations for skin picking.
- Assess subjective experience during picking.
- Evaluate for underlying body dysmorphic disorder and treat.
- Evaluate for other self-injurious behaviors and treat.
- Treat comorbid depressive and anxiety symptoms, low self-esteem, deficient self-assertion.
- Help the patient cope with or resolve social stressors.
- Initiate a 10-week trial of a serotonin reuptake inhibitor and continue an effective drug long term.
- Consider a four-week trial of naltrexone and continue if effective.
- Consider a trial of habit reversal.

1996). Bystritsky and Strausser (1996) report the cessation of cutting behavior during five weeks of treatment with naltrexone 50 mg/day in a patient with pre-existing epilepsy and OCD.

Psychotherapy

I am unaware of any controlled trials or studies in which outcome was evaluated by independent raters. Even the case report literature is sparse. Insight-oriented psychotherapy has been reported to exacerbate the symptoms (Seitz, 1953), but an eclectic psychotherapy incorporating psychodynamic elements has been reported helpful (Fruensgaard, 1991b). Fruensgaard (1991b) treated 22 patients referred from a dermatology clinic with a history, on average, of eight years of skin picking. The patients received psychotherapy at least once weekly for 3–55 months (mean = 14). The therapy included careful, but empathetic exploration of the patient's picking episodes, attention to developmental issues and current conflicts, cognitive restructuring with regard to picking, aggression management and self-assertion, and help in improving social relations. At follow-up three to nine years after starting psychotherapy, 7 (32%) had achieved stable healing and 10 (45%) had experienced intermittent healing. The variable lengths of treatment and follow-up, as well as the individualized application of therapeutic elements, make it difficult to evaluate this report.

Because the phenomenology of skin picking closely resembles that of trichotillomania, a form of therapy, termed habit reversal therapy, which is effective in trichotillomania, deserves investigation and exploratory clinical use. Habit reversal therapy is described in Chapter 11. Treatment planning guidelines are shown in Table 12.1.

13

Nail biting

Some devils ask but the paring of one's nail.

Shakespeare, Comedy of Errors

Adults do not come to psychiatrists seeking treatment for nail biting. Nonetheless, because unwanted, self-injurious nail biting is likely to be seen in patients presenting with other disorders, the psychiatrist should be familiar with treatment options. This behavior is not specifically mentioned in DSM-IV, but can reasonably be classified in the category, Impulse–Control Disorder, Not Otherwise Specified (code 312.30). Like the impulse-control disorders, self-injurious nail biting involves failure to resist an impulse or temptation to carry out an act harmful to the person, and is often followed by regret. In ICD-10 terminology, nail biting can be considered a habit control disorder within the category, Habit and impulse disorder, unspecified (code F63.9). Like these disorders, it is a persistent, maladaptive behavior characterized by a failure to resist impulses associated with anticipatory tension, and by subsequent tension relief. The initiating cause or causes of nail biting are unknown.

Prevalence

Habitual nail biting (onychophagia) is common in children and adults. In teenage, the prevalence begins to fall, dropping to approximately 20% at ages 16 to 17, then to about 10% in adults older than 35 (Leung and Robson, 1990). Although nail biting appears to run in families, the familial risk of OCD or other anxiety disorders does not appear to be increased (Leonard et al., 1991). Monozygotic twins are twice as likely to be concordant for nail biting as dizygotic twins (66% versus 34%) and four times as likely to be concordant for severe nail biting (75% versus 18%) (Leonard et al., 1991).

Clinical picture

Most nail biters bite only their fingernails and bite all the nails equally. Some also pick or clip the cuticles, and others clip their toenails excessively. Stress, tension and anxiety can precipitate biting episodes (Leung and Robson, 1990). The complications are not limited to social disapproval. Severe nail biting commonly brings on subungual infection and paronychia. Nail biting may also result in fungal infections, periungual warts and damage to the nail matrix or nail bed, with loss of the nail. Dental complications include spread of infection to the mouth, small fractures of the incisor edges, and apical root absorption (in severe nail biters) (Leung and Robson, 1990; Leonard et al., 1991).

Treatment

Psychological and behavioral treatments

Many psychological and behavioral treatments have been utilized for nail biting, but most reports are short-term, uncontrolled and do not distinguish among individuals with nail biting of varying degrees of severity. Two small controlled studies that utilized objective outcome measures begin to suggest that certain treatment elements may be helpful. Neither, however, describes the severity of the subjects' condition or provides long-term outcome data.

Silber and Haynes (1992) combined keeping a daily written log of biting episodes with executing a competing response when the urge to bite occurred (lightly clenching the hand for three minutes). This combination was more effective than either self-monitoring alone or self-monitoring combined with applying a bitter substance to the nails twice a day. Four of seven subjects in the competing response group stopped biting completely over the three-week study period compared with one of seven in each of the other two groups. Subjects in the bitter substance group reported getting used to the taste. Subjects in all three groups felt that the weekly contact with the therapist was the most important treatment element.

Wagstaff and Royce (1994), in a single session treatment intervention, found that adding a hypnotic induction procedure to four suggestions designed to discourage nail biting was more effective than giving the suggestions alone. The suggestions emphasized that nail biting was a habit that could be broken, and that success would enhance social attractiveness and self-esteem; encouraged subjects to repeat to themselves that they would not bite nails "today/tomorrow;" enhanced feelings of self-efficacy; and, predicted that within 10 days or so, the desire to bite would disappear and the idea of biting would be repulsive. At the five-week evaluation session, 7 of 11 hypnotic induction subjects reported that they had stopped nail biting completely, compared to one of six in the control group. Self-rated belief at baseline in the efficacy of the treatment was related to the degree of improvement, but the degree of motivation to improve was not. The authors note that the hypnotic induction subjects may have been more motivated to please the experimenter and thus may have put more effort into stopping nail biting. Like the study of Silber and Haynes (1992), this study suggests the importance of establishing a comfortable doctor–patient relationship.

In my experience, severe nail biting in patients with comorbid OCD can be successfully treated by combining elements from these studies with elements of habit reversal (see Chapter 11). My patients were also receiving a selective serotonin reuptake inhibitor (SSRI) for their OCD, but without significant effect on nail biting. In addition to suggesting that treatment "stands a good chance of being effective," the treatment elements are:

- Self-monitoring. Ask patients to monitor the frequency and conditions under which they engage in nail biting by keeping a daily log, divided into two-hour blocks, of biting episodes and their circumstances. If patients fail to perform self-monitoring, discuss their motivation for treatment.
- Competing response. Once self-monitoring is established, introduce a competing response, which can take many forms. Some patients prefer competing responses that provide tactile stimulation, such as fingering a string of beads or stroking a soft brush. Others find that lightly clenching their hands for three minutes, with the thumb inside the fist, or lightly clenching a soft eraser, works well.
- Relaxation exercises. Prescribe a relaxation exercise to be performed for a few minutes several times a day. The exercise can take the form of progressive muscle relaxation, visualization of a pleasant scene or diaphragmatic breathing.
- Motivation enhancement. Ask the patient review daily a written list of his or her motivations for stopping nail biting.

When patients fail to comply with a treatment element, I adopt a stance of mutual problem solving, e.g., "What prevented you from being able to do X?" We explore both motivational and situational factors. This non-critical stance helps to maintain the therapeutic alliance and counterbalances the internalized criticism that patients usually bring from parental responses to nail biting.

Pharmacotherapy

Only one controlled drug trial for severe nail biting has been published – a 10-week double-blind crossover study of clomipramine versus desipramine (Leonard et al., 1991). None of the 25 subjects had a concurrent anxiety or affective disorder; seven had no lifetime psychiatric diagnosis. Recruiting subjects for this study was difficult, suggesting that nail biters without comorbid psychiatric conditions are reluctant to take psychotropic medications for their disorder. Only 14 subjects completed the study and many dropouts were related to medication side effects or to withdrawal syndromes during crossover. Five subjects could not tolerate the side effects of the initial 25 mg dose of clomipramine or desipramine and several were unable to tolerate more than 50 mg of one drug or the other. Clomipramine was more effective than desipramine, but improvement was modest. Only 7 of 14 study completers experienced at least a 30% decrease in nail biting and only two stopped nail biting. Drug response was not related to baseline measures of anxiety or depression, drug dosage or steady state drug plasma levels. Nine study completers chose to continue taking a medication, but two of the three who continued on clomipramine discontinued within two months. Of the six who elected an open trial of fluoxetine, only two continued for six months or more; they reported an improvement of 50%.

Naltrexone has a beneficial effect on other self-injurious behaviors such as skin cutting (Roth et al., 1996). In two OCD patients whose severe nail biting did not respond to an SSRI or to behavioral approaches, I added naltrexone 50 mg/day with good results. The patients reported a markedly decreased urge to nail bite within the first week and have maintained an 80% or better improvement, as reflected in regrowth of most nails and reduced biting episodes, over five and nine months of continued treatment. The patients' self-esteem was enhanced by their control of a previously intractable and unsightly habit. Although these observations are clinical and uncontrolled, naltrexone merits study and exploratory use in clinical practice for patients with severe nail biting.

Naltrexone should not interact adversely with the SSRIs since it is metabolized by extrahepatic as well as hepatic sites. My patients had no side effects. Since naltrexone has been studied chiefly in patients undergoing treatment for narcotic addiction or alcoholism, identifying side effects likely to be common in other patient groups is difficult. In clinical trials, the common side effects have been gastrointestinal complaints (nausea, vomiting, abdominal pain and cramping), nervousness, low energy, muscle and joint pains and headache. Excessive doses, e.g., five times the recommended dose of 50 mg/day, can cause hepatocellular injury (Medical Economics Company, 1998).

The outcome of treatment for nail biting should be monitored both by self-report and by clinician rating. The patient's daily log of nail biting episodes provides a self-report index. In addition, the clinician can modify the compulsion subscale of the Yale–Brown Obsessive–Compulsive Scale (Appendix 2), as did Leonard et al. (1991), to rate: the time spent daily; interference in daily life (from time spent or embarrassment); intensity of the urge to nail bite; degree of resistance to the urge; and, success in resistance. If a 35 mm or Polaroid camera is easily available, the clinician can periodically take standardized photographs of each hand to quantify nail length and record skin damage (Silber and Haynes, 1992).

Research is needed to identify the effective and necessary elements of behavioral treatment and the efficacy of drug treatments for severe nail biting. The necessary duration of treatment requires study. Effective treatment for patients with and

Table 13.1. Severe nail biting: treatment planning guidelines

---

- Assess the medical complications of nail biting
- Treat comorbid mood and anxiety disorders
- Institute modified habit reversal treatment:
  - suggestion of treatment efficacy
  - self-monitoring of nail biting
  - competing response
  - relaxation exercise
  - enhancing motivation for stopping
- Consider sequential, 10-week trials of serotonin reuptake inhibitors
- Consider using hypnotic suggestion
- Consider a trial of naltrexone with or without a serotonin reuptake inhibitor

---

without comorbid psychiatric conditions may differ. The roles of SSRIs and nal-trexone, alone and in combination with behavioral treatment, should be evaluated. Meanwhile, in cases of severe nail biting, clinicians can utilize these treatments knowing that the risk of important adverse reactions is small. Treatment planning guidelines are shown in Table 13.1.

14

Compulsive buying

See how possession always cheapens the thing that was precious.

William Dean Howells, *Pordenone*

Compulsive buying (also called compulsive shopping, addictive or impulsive buying) is not officially recognized as a mental disorder. Kraepelin (1915) and Bleuler (1924) both briefly referred to compulsive buying in their early twentieth-century textbooks, calling it "oniomania," (urge to buy) and classifying it as one of the "impulsive insanities." Only a few case reports and case series have been published in the past two decades. Additional descriptive data are found in the consumer behavior literature, which includes interview and questionnaire studies of self-identified compulsive buyers. The behavior may be considered to fall in the DSM-IV category of Impulse-Control Disorders Not Otherwise Specified (code 312.30) in that it shares the features of impulse-control disorders: preceding tension; repetitive urges that are difficult to resist; and, pleasure or relief following the act.

Diagnosis

In the absence of official diagnostic criteria, McElroy et al. (1994b), suggest diagnostic criteria adapted from the DSM-III-R criteria for obsessive-compulsive, impulse-control and substance use disorders (Table 14.1). The criteria are derived from their series of 20 patients and their review of cases reported in the literature.

The diagnostic criteria suggested by McElroy et al. (1994b) are consistent with the descriptions encountered by Christenson et al. (1994a) in their survey of the psychiatric and consumer behavior literature on compulsive buying. Christenson et al. (1994a) concluded that a consensus exists that compulsive buying is motivated by "irresistible" impulses, characterized by spending that is excessive and inappropriate, has harmful consequences for the individual, and tends to be chronic and stereotyped. Unlike the compulsions of OCD, compulsive buying behavior is pleasurable (until negative consequences develop) and often ego-syntonic.

213

Table 14.1. Diagnostic criteria for compulsive buying

A. Maladaptive preoccupation with buying or shopping, or maladaptive buying or shopping impulses or behavior, as indicated by at least one of the following:
   (1) Frequent preoccupation with buying or impulses to buy that is/are experienced as irresistible, intrusive, and/or senseless.
   (2) Frequent buying of more than can be afforded, frequent buying of items that are not needed, or shopping for longer periods of time than intended.
B. The buying preoccupations, impulses or behaviors cause marked distress, are time-consuming, significantly interfere with social or occupational functioning or result in financial problems (e.g., indebtedness or bankruptcy).
C. The excessive buying or shopping behavior does not occur exclusively during periods of hypomania or mania.

Source: McElroy et al. (1994a). Copyright 1994, Physicians Postgraduate Press. Reprinted by permission.

Prevalence

The prevalence of compulsive buying is unknown, but Faber and O'Guinn (1992) estimated it at 1.8% of the general population in the United States by extrapolating from nearly 300 respondents to a mailed questionnaire sent to a representative sample of 800 residents of Illinois. Studies utilizing structured interviews in larger, more geographically diverse samples are needed to generate more valid prevalence estimates.

Clinical picture

Because the data are limited, only a preliminary sketch of the clinical picture can be drawn. Christenson et al. (1994a) and Schlosser et al. (1994b) studied samples drawn by newspaper advertisements seeking persons with compulsive buying problems. In both series, more than 90% of respondents were women, which is consistent with data in the consumer behavior literature (Faber and O'Guinn, 1992). The age of onset tends to be in the teens or twenties, but a decade may elapse before the adverse consequences force the individual to recognize that a problem exists. The problem is continuous (never absent for a month or more) in most cases, and episodic in about 40%.

The frequency of buying urges and behaviors is quite variable. Urges usually occur every few days to once a week, but may occur from hourly to once a month. Urges may occur in any setting: home; work; stores; or, driving. Most individuals attempt to resist the urges (e.g., by avoiding stores, destroying credit cards), but they often fail (McElroy et al., 1994a). Urges are frequently intensified by negative emotions such as sadness, anger or loneliness, less often by happiness. A feeling of gratification, pleasure or release of tension nearly always follows the compulsive buying, but it is usually short-lived and is followed by feelings of guilt, regret, sadness, anger or indifference to the purchase. The positive attention received from salespeople may also temporarily reward the compulsive buyer.

Several authors have pointed out the similarities between compulsive buying and addictive behaviors, e.g., repetitive urges to engage in immediately pleasurable but ultimately harmful behaviors, preceding buildup of tension, and conditioning of the behavior to internal and external cues (Lejoyeux et al., 1996).

The items purchased most often relate to physical appearance or attractiveness, i.e., clothing, shoes, jewelry and makeup. Less frequently purchased items include collectibles, antiques, records/compact discs, art, cars or auto parts (purchased by males) and household items. Purchased items are not always used – many are returned, stored in their packaging, given away or sold.

Compulsive buying almost always results in guilt, accrual of debt, often beyond the ability to pay, other financial problems, and in marital or familial problems. Occasionally, compulsive buyers resort to passing bad checks or declaring bankruptcy.

Compulsive buyers described in the consumer behavior literature exhibit lower self-esteem and more depression, anxiety and obsessions than comparison groups (Faber and O'Guinn, 1992).

Differential diagnosis

Compulsive buying must be distinguished from excessive spending in *hypomanic* or *manic periods*; *hoarding behaviors* associated with OCD and obsessive-compulsive personality disorder (in which conditions the motive for excessive accumulation is "I might need it sometime," sentimental attachment to items, or the necessity of buying things only when they are on sale); *impulsive buying without adverse consequences*; and, "*revenge spending*" (to deplete another person's funds) (Krueger, 1988).

Assessment instruments

Monahan, Black and Gabel (1996) modified the Yale–Brown Obsessive–Compulsive Scale (Y–BOCS) to measure the severity of compulsive buying obsessions and behaviors and termed the new scale, the YBOCS–Shopping Version (YBOCS–SV). The YBOCS–SV evaluates the five dimensions of the original Y–BOCS – time spent, interference, distress, resistance and control – with regard to shopping thoughts and behaviors. A copy is reprinted in their article. The new instrument demonstrated good interrater reliability and was sensitive to clinical change. For clinical purposes, the clinician can adapt the Y–BOCS form provided in Appendix 2.

Faber and O'Guinn (1992) developed the Compulsive Buying Scale, a reasonably reliable, valid, sensitive and specific screening instrument for compulsive buying. The questionnaire, derived from data collected from individuals writing to a self-help organization and from a systematic sample of the Illinois population, is not designed to measure the severity of compulsive buying behaviors. The questionnaire asks respondents to indicate their degree of agreement/disagreement with seven items that can be paraphrased as:

(1) I must spend money left at the end of a pay period.
(2) I feel my spending habits would horrify others.
(3) I buy things I cannot afford.
(4) I write checks in excess of my bank balance.
(5) I buy things to feel better.
(6) I feel anxious on days I don't shop.
(7) I pay only the minimum on credit card balances.

The weighted scoring algorithm used to classify respondents as compulsive buyers or not has not been validated.

A French language scale for identifying individuals who engage in compulsive buying has been developed by Lejoyeux and Adès (1994).

Comorbidity

The studies of Christenson et al. (1994a), Schlosser et al. (1994b), and Black et al. (1998b) and published case reports suggest that compulsive buyers are likely to suffer from concurrent or past major depression, anxiety disorders, alcohol abuse or bulimia. Impulse control disorders, particularly kleptomania, intermittent explosive disorder and pathological gambling also seem to affect as many as one-third of compulsive buyers. In a study of 20 consecutive psychiatric patients complaining of problematic buying behavior not limited to hypomanic or manic periods, McElroy et al. (1994a) found frequent concurrent disorders: bipolar disorder (35%), bipolar II disorder (35%); OCD (30%); major depression (20%); panic disorder (25%); and, social phobia (25%). Kleptomania (20%), intermittent explosive disorder (10%) and trichotillomania (10%) were less common, as were bulimia (15%) and alcohol abuse (5%). The high comorbidity rate in this group of patients may reflect their having been recruited from psychiatric clinic and hospital settings.

Treatment

No placebo-controlled studies of any treatment have been published. The frequency of comorbid conditions, however, suggests that the clinician must first evaluate the patient carefully for other psychiatric disorders. Treatment of the comorbid condition, especially mood disorders, may ameliorate or cure the compulsive buying. For example, Lejoyeux, Hourtané and Adès (1995) report two depressed patients whose compulsive buying remitted when the depression responded to antidepressant medication (clomipramine, 150 mg/day in case 1; drug unspecified in case 2).

Establishing why the patient engages in compulsive shopping and why he or she has come for treatment will be especially important in treatment planning.

Pharmacotherapy

Of the series of 20 patients reported by McElroy et al. (1994a), nine had partial or full remission of buying behaviors in response to trials of antidepressants, most often selective serotonin reuptake inhibitors, occasionally in combination with a mood stabilizer. In most cases, however, the observation period was limited to a few months. Two of nine patients who had received supportive or insight-oriented psychotherapy before receiving drug treatment found it helpful.

Black (1996) reported positive results in 9 of 10 compulsive shoppers recruited by newspaper advertisements and treated for nine weeks with fluvoxamine, beginning at a dose of 50 mg/day and reaching a mean dose of 205 mg/day. None of the patients had comorbid depression or severe personality disorders. Three patients improved in the first week and the remaining responders by week 5. One patient who discontinued after nine weeks of treatment rapidly relapsed. Two patients followed for six months on fluvoxamine remained well.

Psychotherapy

Krueger (1988) suggests that psychotherapeutic attention to certain psychodynamic issues is important. In his four cases, compulsive shopping was entwined with fragile self-esteem, need for compliments regarding physical appearance, need for reassurance that parent figures would give support (i.e., pay the bills), a need to be rescued, attempts to fill internal emptiness and a sense of power derived from impulsive action.

The place of cognitive and behavioral therapies remains to be established. Lejoyeux et al. (1996) suggest the use of graded exposure to ever more tempting situations with response prevention, and instruction in techniques of impulse and conditioned stimulus control, but these techniques are not described. Bernik et al. (1996) describe two patients with comorbid panic disorder with agoraphobia

Table 14.2. Compulsive buying: treatment planning guidelines

- Assess and treat comorbid mood, anxiety, eating, substance use and other impulse control disorders.
- Assess motivation for treatment.
- Assess motivations for compulsive buying and remove, negate or counteract them.
- Initiate a trial of fluvoxamine or other SSRI or of a tricyclic antidepressant.
- Continue effective medication for at least six months.
- Consider treatment with exposure and response prevention.
- Consider psychodynamic attention to motivations.
- Initiate couple or family therapy for complicity or for resultant strains.
- Utilize bibliotherapy.

Note:
SSRI: selective serotonin reuptake inhibitor.

responsive to clomipramine 150 mg/day, whose compulsive shopping was unaffected. Both patients responded well to three to four weeks of daily exposure to shopping stimuli with response prevention, at first by an accompanying individual, and later by themselves. Long-term outcome data are unavailable.

When compulsive buying affects or has roots in the patient's family situation, family counseling or therapy should be provided to relieve the resultant strains, deal with the financial consequences, or teach the family how to stop facilitating the behavior.

The role of self-help groups has not been studied, but at least two self-help books have been published and can be recommended to patients: *Shopaholics: Serious Help for Addicted Spenders* (Damon 1988) and *Women Who Shop Too Much: Overcoming the Urge to Splurge* (Wesson 1990). In addition, an organization called "Debtors Anonymous" (see Appendix 1) sponsors local chapter meetings and provides printed material modelled on the 12–step program of Alcoholics Anonymous.

Treatment planning guidelines derived from the literature reviewed earlier are shown in Table 14.2.

15

Kleptomania

Yet I lusted to thieve, and did it, compelled by no hunger, nor poverty . . . For I stole that, of which
I had enough, and much better. Nor cared I to enjoy what I stole, but joyed in the theft and sin
itself.

St. Augustine, *Confessions*

Kleptomania was introduced as a diagnostic term in the early nineteenth century
in Esquirol's 1838 textbook, *Des Maladies Mentales* (McElroy et al., 1991a). The
term is derived from the Greek roots for "stealing" and "madness." Since little
research has been published on this condition, only limited data are available.

Diagnosis

DSM-IV diagnostic criteria (312.32)

DSM-IV includes kleptomania with the Impulse-Control Disorders Not Elsewhere
Specified, along with trichotillomania, intermittent explosive disorder, and pyromania (Table 15.1) (American Psychiatric Association, 1994). All of these conditions are characterized by failure to resist an impulse or drive to engage in
pleasurable, but harmful behaviors. Following the behavior, the individual may or
may not experience remorse or guilt.

ICD-10 diagnostic criteria (F63.2)

The ICD-10 diagnostic guidelines for kleptomania (World Health Organization,
1992) differ somewhat from those in DSM-IV. The ICD-10 guidelines include
several aspects that DSM-IV considers Diagnostic Features or Associated Features
rather than Diagnostic Criteria, i.e., attempts at concealment are usually, but not
always, made; no accomplice is involved; and, associated anxiety, despondency or
guilt do not prevent continued stealing. The ICD-10 guidelines include DSM-IV
criterion A (failure to resist the impulse) and criterion B (increasing tension before
the act), mention gratification but not the "relief" in DSM-IV criterion C, and do
not explicitly exclude stealing motivated by anger or psychosis as in DSM-IV criteria D and E. ICD-10 implicitly excludes stealing related to Conduct Disorder or

Table 15.1. DSM-IV diagnostic criteria for kleptomania (312.32)

A. Recurrent failure to resist impulses to steal objects that are not needed for personal use or for their monetary value.
B. Increasing sense of tension immediately before committing the theft.
C. Pleasure, gratification or relief at the time of committing the theft.
D. The stealing is not committed to express anger or vengeance and is not in response to a delusion or a hallucination.
E. The stealing is not better accounted for by Conduct Disorder, a Manic Episode, or Antisocial Personality Disorder.

Source: Reprinted with permission from the *Diagnostic and Statistical Manual of Mental Disorders, Fourth edition.* Copyright 1994, American Psychiatric Association, p. 613.

Antisocial Personality Disorder by distinguishing kleptomania from recurrent shoplifting "when the acts are more carefully planned, and there is an obvious motive of personal gain." ICD-10 also excludes stealing related to an organic mental disorder (F00–F09) or a depressive disorder (F30–F33).

The comparative utility of the DSM-IV and ICD-10 criteria sets for identifying homogeneous groups for research purposes is unknown. The ICD-10 criteria are slightly more restrictive.

Differential diagnosis

Kleptomania is a form of shoplifting. Whether kleptomania is truly a disorder, rather than simply a form of illegal behavior for which the individual should be punished, has been questioned since the concept was introduced into psychiatry. For example, kleptomania was not included in DSM-II. Nonetheless, kleptomania now has a place in both the United States and the international classification systems of diseases and disorders.

Forms of shoplifting from which kleptomania should be distinguished are: *shoplifting by the professional shoplifter,* motivated to steal objects for profit or personal use, and often not bothered by the immorality of the act; *shoplifting by teenagers,* who steal for excitement or to impress peers; *shoplifting by substance abusers or addicts,* who steal in order to support their drug habits; and, *shoplifting by the absent-minded individual,* who inadvertently leaves the store without paying (Murray, 1992). DSM-IV also distinguishes kleptomania from shoplifting associated with *mania, conduct disorder,* and *antisocial personality disorder.* Kleptomania appears to be the proper diagnosis in only a small percentage of arrested shoplifters, but the available data are marred by methodological shortcomings (Goldman, 1991; McElroy et al., 1991a).

A few case reports, reviewed by Goldman (1991), link kleptomania to organic conditions: cortical atrophy (in a 25-year old); a parietal lobe mass associated with blackouts and inability to recall the stealing; narcolepsy; and, severe hypoglycemia caused by an insulinoma.

Three cases of new-onset kleptomania associated with selective serotonin reuptake inhibitor (SSRI) treatment of major depression are reported by Kindler et al. (1997). The kleptomania began 6–12 weeks after starting successful antidepressant treatment with fluoxetine (two cases) or fluvoxamine (one case) and continued while the patients were in a euthymic state. Kleptomania stopped in one case after a month of added lithium; in one case, two months after discontinuing fluoxetine (without recurrence on desipramine); and, in the third case, after six months of lithium and supportive psychotherapy. These isolated cases, though of interest, cannot be taken as having established a causal role for the SSRIs.

Clinical picture

Goldman (1991) and McElroy et al. (1991a) have reviewed the published case reports and case series of individuals with kleptomania. With the caveat that these collections of cases are small and may not reflect accurately those individuals who come to professional attention, a composite clinical picture can be drawn.

In kleptomania, stealing is impulsive and occurs without extensive planning. However, the stealing may resemble compulsive behavior in that it is repetitive, is experienced as irrational and wrong, i.e., ego-dystonic, may be aimed at relieving increasing tension (rather than at obtaining pleasure) and may be resisted, with a resulting increase in anxiety. The stolen items are usually of small value and may not be used. Instead, the individual may return, discard or hoard them.

Stealing begins by age 20 in about half the cases, and is often chronic, although exacerbations and periods of remission may occur. In women, the age at onset ranges from 6 to 44 years; in men, from 25 to 68 years (Goldman, 1991). Most reported cases are of women, but more men are arrested for shoplifting (Murray, 1992). The preponderance of women in reported cases may reflect various selection biases, including the differential treatment by courts of men and women arrested for stealing.

Comorbidity

Affective symptoms were present in more than half of the 56 "possible kleptomania" cases reviewed by McElroy et al. (1991a); about one-third appeared to meet criteria for major depression or bipolar disorder. About one-third had concomitant compulsive behaviors: cleaning, hand-washing, checking and hoarding, among others. Anxiety symptoms were noted in 20% and sexual dysfunction (frigidity, vaginismus, promiscuity and sexual arousal during shoplifting) in 13%. Bulimia nervosa was suspected in 11%. Other antisocial behaviors, e.g., lying, fraud, breaking and entering, embezzlement and torturing animals, were present in 18%. In 20 kleptomania patients recruited from a hospital and its associated clinic, lifetime diagnoses of OCD, panic disorder, social phobia, eating disorder or psychoactive substance use disorder were each present in at least 40% of the subjects (McElroy et al., 1991b). No reliable data on the prevalence of personality disorders are available.

Goldman (1991) points out that the relationship between mood and anxiety symptoms or disorders and kleptomania is poorly described. Which began first is often unclear, and the severity and course of the mood or anxiety symptoms is often unstated.

Eating disorders may be a strong risk factor for kleptomania. A review of data from seven studies encompassing more than 700 patients with anorexia nervosa, bulimia nervosa or both, determined that 21% exhibited stealing or kleptomania (McElroy et al., 1991a). Stealing only food and stealing items other than food were equally prevalent. Bulimia nervosa was more closely associated with stealing than was anorexia nervosa. Major mood disorders, anxiety disorders and alcohol and substance abuse disorders were also common.

Assessing the patient

The patient's motives for seeking treatment will bear heavily on treatment planning. A patient who comes under legal duress may differ considerably from one who seeks care voluntarily.

After clarifying the onset, precipitants and course of the kleptomania, the clinician should explore the patient's motivations for stealing. A host of possibilities have been described and speculated upon. Patients coming voluntarily for treatment may be motivated to shoplift by its transient antidepressant effect, enjoyment of risk, feelings of being neglected, feelings of loss, a need to seek punishment, or other motives (Goldman, 1991). The remote possibility of an organic etiology should be considered.

The presence of comorbid psychiatric disorders, or a past history of mania or panic disorder, will influence the choice of medications, when these are appropriate, and the manner in which they are used (See Chapter 2). SSRIs and other antidepressants, for example, can precipitate mania or panic attacks in patients with a history of these disorders. In patients with a history of mania, a mood stabilizer such as valproate or lithium should be instituted before administering the antidepressant. In patients with a panic attack history, the prophylactic use of a benzodiazepine during the first month of antidepressant treatment is usually indicated (See Chapter 2).

Treatment

In attempting to fashion a treatment plan informed by data, the clinician can draw only on case reports and small, uncontrolled case series. Still, uncontrolled published observations are a reasonable starting point. Antidepressant medications and certain forms of cognitive–behavioral therapy have consistently been reported helpful. Table 15.2 provides treatment planning guidelines derived from the published literature.

Pharmacotherapy

Ten of 20 patients with kleptomania and comorbid disorders as noted above, who were treated with valproate, lithium, fluoxetine, nortriptyline, trazodone or fluoxetine plus imipramine, had a good outcome (McElroy et al., 1991b); seven experienced remissions lasting 3–15 months, and three experienced a partial response. Ten patients were unresponsive to trials of one or more of these medications. Many of the patients who responded positively had comorbid bipolar or unipolar mood disorder, with associated changes in the frequency of stealing, but the relationship between the treatment response of kleptomania and the comorbid conditions is not described. Although 15 patients had been apprehended for stealing, this produced a "permanent" cessation of stealing in only five.

The addition of lithium carbonate (serum level, 0.5 mEq/L) markedly benefitted a woman unresponsive to fluoxetine 40 mg/day (Burstein, 1992). Her stealing urges disappeared within one week. Nonetheless, she stole three times in the next three months (compared to several times a week pre-treatment).

Fluvoxamine, 300 mg/day, brought about remission of stealing in a man with comorbid "compulsive checking and rumination" who had failed to benefit from clomipramine, imipramine, lithium, behavior therapy and psychotherapy (Chong and Low, 1996). Improvement began within two weeks of reaching 200 mg/day; remission occurred and was maintained for nine months at 300 mg/day.

After treatment with valproate 2000 mg/day, a patient's mixed mania, present over 20 years, subsided to mild mood swings while concomitant chronic stealing impulses and kleptomania completely resolved (Kmetz, McElroy and Collins, 1997).

Buspirone 30 mg/day, added after three weeks to fluvoxamine 200 mg/day, reduced the urge to steal to controllable levels in a 29-year-old man with an 18-year history of kleptomania marked by repeated arrests and episodes of major depression with suicidal behaviors (Durst, Katz and Knobler, 1997). The patient had failed to benefit from 15 years of psychodynamic psychotherapy and requested medication trials when he admitted himself to an inpatient unit in a suicidal state. During 10 weeks of treatment with fluvoxamine 250 mg/day and buspirone 30 mg/day, no stealing occurred. Because buspirone was added before a full antidepressant effect of fluvoxamine would be expected, the benefit may have been due to fluvoxamine alone. The brief follow-up period precludes any conclusion about long-term efficacy.

McElroy et al. (1989) report three cases of kleptomania in patients with bulimia nervosa, two of whom also had comorbid depression. The urge to steal and the stealing behavior remitted within two to four weeks of starting treatment with trazodone 300 mg/day, or fluoxetine 60 mg or 80 mg/day, and remained in abeyance during treatment periods of 4–18 months. One patient had a return of urges to steal within two weeks of discontinuing fluoxetine. The treatment response of kleptomania did not always mirror those of the comorbid conditions.

Psychotherapy

Both successful and unsuccessful psychoanalytic cases have been reported (McElroy et al., 1991a,b). One case complicated by both bulimia and borderline personality disorder responded to three years of psychoanalysis combined with fluoxetine 80 mg/day (Schwartz, 1992). In a case unresponsive to psychoanalysis, Fishbain (1988) reported disappearance of kleptomania and comorbid depression in response to amitriptyline (125–150 mg/day) plus perphenazine (10–12 mg/day), with improvement maintained during a two-year treatment period. In this patient, another period of kleptomania associated with depression had responded to electroconvulsive therapy. In a series of 11 patients treated with insight-oriented psychotherapy, none felt that the treatment had helped (McElroy et al., 1991b).

Several behavior therapy approaches are described as beneficial in case reports. Guidry (1969) combined covert sensitization with exposure and response prevention in treating a man in his twenties. In four weekly sessions of covert sensitization followed by three monthly sessions, the patient was instructed to imagine himself stealing and then to imagine in detail the consequences: being observed by the store manager; caught; handcuffed; put in a police car; taken before a judge; embarrassed in front of his family. He was also asked to go to stores and imagine someone watching his behavior surreptitiously. Although the patient continued to have the urge to steal, the frequency of stealing dropped from twice a month to twice during a 10-month follow-up period. The patient reported "a new sense of responsibility" and heightened fear of being caught.

A similar treatment plan was successful with a 30-year-old women, who was motivated to seek treatment by an upcoming trial for shoplifting (Gauthier and Pellerin, 1982). A placebo control week of thought stopping actually worsened the patient's urges. After a 30-minute training session in covert sensitization, the patient was instructed to practice this 10 times per day and whenever the urge to steal occurred. After five weekly sessions, the urge to steal had nearly disappeared.

During 14 months of follow-up, the patient reported an absence of stealing urges and behaviors except for one lapse in month 9.

Covert sensitization was successfully used to treat a woman with a 14-year history of daily kleptomania (Glover, 1985). The patient requested the use of imagery of increasing nausea as she approached tempting objects and of vomiting as she lifted them, with other shoppers then noticing her. Self treatment with images of being caught had been fruitless. The therapist also instructed the patient to adhere to a shopping list when shopping and to leave the bag used for shoplifting at home. After four sessions at two-week intervals, with intervening daily rehearsals of the vomiting scene, the patient had only one lapse in a 19-month follow-up period.

A 25-year-old female patient who had a history of recurrent depression was asked to engage in aversive breath-holding (until mildly painful) whenever she experienced the urge to steal or had an image of herself stealing (Keutzer, 1972). The patient was also instructed to keep a daily log of impulses to steal and of items stolen (including the time, place and value of the item) and bring this to the therapy sessions. The six weekly sessions (including baseline assessment) focussed on review of the log, the patient's thoughts, feelings and behaviors of the past week and problems in implementing the therapeutic instructions. Stealing episodes dropped from daily to one in the fifth week, none in the sixth week, and two confined to the first week of a 10-week follow-up period.

Imaginal desensitization was successful in two patients unresponsive to antidepressants and insight-oriented psychotherapy (McConaghy and Blaszczynski, 1988). During hospitalization (presumably for depression), each was taught progressive muscle relaxation, and in the relaxed state was instructed to imagine each step in a stealing scene while maintaining the relaxed state. The therapist meanwhile gave the suggestions that the patient realized she was engaging in behavior that caused serious troubles, could now control the urge, and should, therefore, end the scene without stealing. After 14, 15–minute sessions administered over five days, no stealing occurred during a two-year follow-up period.

Instead of concentrating on the aversive consequences of stealing, Gudjonsson (1987) focussed on finding alternate sources of satisfaction for a patient whose kleptomania seemed to occur mostly in response to feelings of depression and a need for "excitement" and "purpose." The patient, a married, middle-aged mother, had a 20-year history of shoplifting, and was referred while under a suspended prison sentence for shoplifting. Previous treatment with an aversive conditioning approach had temporarily decreased the frequency of shoplifting, but had not markedly diminished the urge; treatment with antidepressants had brought no benefit. She had comorbid OCD manifest in excessive house cleaning, among other symptoms, and she and her husband communicated poorly. Gudjonsson treated

Table 15.2. Kleptomania: treatment planning guidelines

- Identify the motivation for treatment.
- Identify the motivations for stealing and seek to remove, negate or counteract them.
- Assess and treat comorbid mood, anxiety, eating and substance use disorders.
- Rule out an organic etiology (highly unlikely).
- Try one or more antidepressant trials (tricyclic, SSRI or trazodone).
- Try behavior therapies (covert sensitization, exposure and response prevention, aversive breath holding, log of stealing impulses and items stolen, imaginal desensitization).
- Institute psychotherapy for current life problems.
- Arrange long-term follow-up.

Note:
SSRI: selective serotonin reuptake inhibitor.

her weekly for five months, helping the patient to identify alternative behaviors that could bring self-fulfillment, self-esteem, excitement and pleasure, and instructed her to reduce housework activities gradually and implement relaxation training. The patient's depression markedly improved, her house cleaning markedly decreased, and her urges to shoplift gradually disappeared, remaining in abeyance during two years of follow-up. Gudjonsson believes that "regular but infrequent" sessions during the early part of the follow-up period were important in maintaining the therapeutic gains.

These reported successes with different forms of pharmacotherapy and psychotherapy indicate that kleptomania is treatable. Clinicians wishing to explore in a more controlled fashion the effectiveness of prescribed medications can arrange so-called "*N* of 1" trials in which the patient serves as his own control. Once a stable dose of a seemingly beneficial drug is established, the clinician obtains the patient's consent for one or more double-blind crossover trials. A pharmacy is asked to prepare, and later to dispense, alternate periods of identical-appearing drug and placebo capsules. Double-blind crossover trials of one to two months duration should be instructive.

Whenever possible, psychotherapeutic *N* of 1 trials should use blind raters to assess outcome. Assessing outcome after a year or more is essential when evaluating treatments for this apparently chronic and relapsing disorder. Treatment planning guidelines are shown in Table 15.2.

16

Pathological gambling

The king, sir, hath laid, that in a dozen passes between you and him, he shall not exceed you three hits; he laid on twelve for nine.

Shakespeare, Hamlet

We live in a peculiar age, one in which governments encourage gambling. In the past quarter-century, after decades of suppression, most state governments within the United States and many national governments abroad have legalized gambling in order to generate tax revenues. Lotteries, scratch-off games, riverboat gambling, casinos and video lotteries are but some of the forms progressively legalized (Volberg, 1994). By 1996, six years after the federal Indian Gaming Regulatory Act of 1988 permitted tribes to pursue gambling revenues, 24 states had casinos operating on Native American lands (Westphal and Rush, 1996), bringing both economic benefits and social costs to Native Americans (Zitzow, 1996). Between 1979 and 1995, the amount wagered in legal gambling in the United States increased 28–fold, from US $17 billion to US $482 billion (Westphal and Rush, 1996). Easy availability has entrapped individuals in pathological gambling who would not otherwise have fallen victim (Volberg, 1994; Westphal and Rush, 1996). Rigorous cost-benefit analyses would be valuable guides for future public policy decisions.

Diagnosis

DSM-IV diagnostic criteria (312.31)

Pathological gambling entered the American Psychiatric Association's diagnostic canon in DSM-III, where it was listed as a separate mental disorder. In DSM-III-R, it was grouped with the Disorders of Impulse Control (Not Elsewhere Classified) where it remains in DSM-IV (Table 16.1), along with intermittent explosive disorder, kleptomania, pyromania and trichotillomania (American Psychiatric Association, 1994). The DSM-III-R and DSM-IV diagnostic criteria were intentionally modelled on those for substance dependence. Lesieur and Rosenthal (1991) review the studies of pathological gambling that supported the choice of the DSM-IV diagnostic criteria.

Table 16.1. DSM-IV diagnostic criteria for pathological gambling (312.31)

A. *Persistent and recurrent maladaptive gambling behavior as indicated by five (or more) or the following:*

  (1) is preoccupied with gambling (e.g., preoccupied with reliving past gambling experiences, handicapping or planning the next venture, or thinking of ways to get money with which to gamble);
  (2) needs to gamble with increasing amounts of money in order to achieve the desired excitement;
  (3) has repeated unsuccessful efforts to control, cut back, or stop gambling;
  (4) is restless or irritable when attempting to cut down or stop gambling;
  (5) gambles as a way of escaping from problems or of relieving a dysphoric mood (e.g., feelings of helplessness, guilt, anxiety, depression);
  (6) after losing money gambling, often returns another day to get even ("chasing" one's losses);
  (7) lies to family members, therapist, or others to conceal the extent of involvement with gambling;
  (8) has committed illegal acts such as forgery, fraud, theft, or embezzlement to finance gambling;
  (9) has jeopardized or lost a significant relationship, job, or educational or career opportunity because of gambling;
  (10) relies on others to provide money to relieve a desperate financial situation caused by gambling.

B. *The gambling behavior is not better accounted for by a Manic Episode.*

Source: Reprinted with permission from the *Diagnostic and Statistical Manual of Mental Disorders*, Fourth Edition. Copyright 1994, American Psychiatric Association, p. 618.

The popular term, "compulsive gambling" should be avoided, since gambling behaviors, unlike true compulsions, are associated with pleasure and are not aimed at warding off a negative event.

ICD-10 diagnostic criteria (F63.0)

In ICD-10, the impulse control disorders are termed, "Habit and impulse disorders." Where DSM-IV considers the essential feature of the impulse control disorders to be "the failure to resist" an impulse, urge, or temptation to do something harmful, either to the actor or to others, ICD-10 speaks of impulses "that cannot be controlled." A similar formulation in DSM-III, the term, "irresistible impulse," justified pleas of diminished legal responsibility or not guilty by reason of insanity, and so was abandoned in DSM-IV (Blaszczynski and Silove, 1996).

The ICD-10 diagnostic guidelines are much briefer than the DSM-IV criteria and require only persistently repeated gambling in the face of adverse social consequences. The brief description of pathological gambling of ICD-10 is consistent, however, with the DSM-IV criteria and mentions lying, breaking the law to obtain gambling money, jeopardizing work and family relationships and the exacerbation of gambling by stress.

Differential diagnosis

Both DSM-IV and ICD-10 distinguish pathological gambling from gambling secondary to *mania* as well as from *social gambling*, which does not persist despite adverse effects. DSM-IV suggests that two diagnoses be made when individuals with antisocial personality disorder meet criteria for pathological gambling; ICD-10 excludes gambling by these individuals from the pathological gambling diagnostic category.

Clinical picture

By the time the pathological gambler seeks or is brought to treatment, he or she is likely to be entangled in inter-twined financial, familial, job-related and legal problems. In addition, he or she is highly likely to suffer from a comorbid substance abuse problem or mood disorder (Ciarrocchi and Richardson, 1989; Bland et al., 1993; Murray, 1993). Understanding the three "career phases" of male pathological gamblers can aid the clinician in eliciting the clinical history (Lesieur and Rosenthal, 1991).

In the early, "winning phase," which may persist for years, excitement and financial payoffs reinforce continued gambling. But the pathological gambler becomes "addicted" to the pursuit of "action" (the excitement or euphoria associated with the risk involved in gambling), and continues despite negative consequences. Since male pathological gamblers usually begin gambling in adolescence, the absence of familial or financial obligations permits them to sustain losses relatively easily.

In the "losing phase," the pathological gambler hides his betting and its negative consequences, lies about betting and losses, and engages in "chasing," i.e., continuing to gamble, often with ever larger bets, in vain attempts to win back the money previously lost. As debt increases, the gambler exhausts legal sources of funds such as credit card advances, borrowing from family and friends and asset-backed loans, and his participation in familial, work-related and social roles deteriorates. A Canadian study, for example, found that pathological gamblers were highly likely to have been unemployed for at least six months in the previous five years (Bland et al., 1993). In Spain, however, pathological gamblers are more likely than non-gamblers to be employed (Legarda, Babio and Abreu, 1992). In the Canadian study, nearly one-quarter had hit or thrown things at a spouse or partner more than once, and more than 10% had neglected a child. Throughout the winning and losing phases, family members may enable the pathological gambler to continue gambling by providing loans and paying off debts "one last time."

In the "desperation phase," intense dysphoria, anxiety and social alienation are present, suicidal ideation is common and suicide attempts are not rare (Moran, 1970; McCormick et al., 1984; Schwarz and Lindner, 1992). In this phase, the pathological gambler is highly likely to resort to criminal behavior in order to raise money for gambling (Blaszczynski and Silove, 1996). Rates of criminal acts among gamblers seeking treatment range from 21% to 85% depending on the measure used (self-report, arrest records or conviction records) (Blaszczynski and Silove, 1996). Lesieur (1984) found that pathological gamblers tend to escalate illegal behaviors over time, from lesser crimes, e.g., selling soft drugs or commiting minor forgery, to greater, e.g., embezzlement, tipping burglars for a portion of the take or systematic fraud. Of the 50 gamblers interviewed, none had engaged in crimes of violence against the person, although one had engaged in armed robbery. Brown (1987), studying Scottish and English members of Gamblers Anonymous who volunteered to complete an anonymous questionnaire concerning their criminal records, found that gamblers' crimes were more likely than those of the general population to be income generating (e.g., fraud, forgery, embezzlement and petty theft). Female pathological gamblers may turn to prostitution to raise money (Blaszczynski and Silove, 1996).

Male pathological gamblers engage in many types of gambling in adolescence or very early adulthood and descend into pathological gambling after an eight- to nine-year period of controlled gambling (Ladouceur, 1991). Female pathological gamblers usually begin to gamble later in adult life, but lose control after only three to five years (Rosenthal and Lorenz, 1992). Psychoanalytic views regarding the reasons for this descent are summarized by Bolen and Boyd (1968). Financial motivations for gambling, although prominent initially, often become secondary once pathological gambling sets in. Instead, the pathological gambler gambles to feel excited or euphoric, fight depression or loneliness, escape life problems or combat boredom (Blaszczynski, McConaghy and Frankova, 1990; England and Götestam, 1991). Despite the adverse consequences of pathological gambling, afflicted individuals discovered in community surveys are highly unlikely to have sought treatment (Volberg, 1994).

The pathological gambler holds irrational and often overvalued beliefs about gambling (England and Götestam, 1991). He may believe that he has substantial influence over winning, particularly in situations where estimates of skill can become exaggerated, such as card games or race track betting. He attributes both wins and losses to unrelated factors (e.g., how a slot machine lever was pulled, or the influence of someone standing nearby) rather than to the inexorable laws of chance. He may believe he can predict when a win is imminent or when a string of losses will end, that his (superstitious) behaviors can influence "Lady Luck," that past losses entitle him to win, or that having a chance to win is better than accepting the losses already incurred.

Assessment instruments

The South Oaks Gambling Screen (SOGS), which is based on DSM-III diagnostic criteria, is the most widely used assessment instrument in epidemiological studies (Lesieur and Blume, 1987). The SOGS is a 20-item questionnaire that can be self-administered or administered by a rater. In addition to the DSM-III criteria, the items cover types of gambling, largest amount gambled in a single day, parental history of problematic gambling and the individual's opinion about whether his or her gambling is problematic.

Compared to a clinically established diagnosis of pathological gambling in patients admitted to a drug and alcohol unit of a psychiatric hospital, the SOGS (with score ≥ 5 indicating probable pathological gambling), had a 2% false positive rate and an 8% false negative rate. In a sample of about 200 members of Gamblers Anonymous, the SOGS' sensitivity was 96.7%, false positive rate 1.4%, and false negative rate 0.5% (Lesieur and Blume, 1987). Test–retest reliability for a one-month period was high. Researchers have pointed out that even with a low false positive rate, the SOGS may substantially overestimate the prevalence of pathological gambling, e.g., doubling the estimated rate, if the true prevalence rate is 1% or less (Volberg and Banks, 1990; Westphal and Rush, 1996).

A 20-question screening instrument is available from Gamblers Anonymous chapters, but this generates a high proportion of false negatives (Lesieur and Blume, 1987).

Prevalence

Because most prevalence studies have relied on trained telephone interviewers administering the SOGS, the resulting figures cannot be translated into estimates of cases requiring treatment. Moreover, studies utilizing the SOGS give lifetime rather than point prevalence figures. Still, the available data suggest that more than 10 million people in the United States are affected.

In the United States, a five-state study utilized the SOGS in telephone interviews conducted with 4500 randomly selected individuals aged 18 years and older (Volberg, 1994). The lifetime prevalence of pathological gambling, defined as a SOGS score of at least 5, ranged from 0.1% in Ohio to 2.3% in Massachusetts. The data suggested that the longer a state had legalized gambling, the higher the rate of pathological gambling. The pathological gamblers, whom the authors are careful to identify as "probable pathological gamblers," were statistically significantly more likely than the total study group to be males, non-Caucasian, unmarried and less educated.

Similar figures are reported from a similar telephone interview study of 1818 individuals in Louisiana (Westphal and Rush, 1996). The state had legalized a lottery in 1990 and riverboat casinos and video poker machines in 1991. The investigators found a pathological gambling prevalence rate of 3.1% in adults aged 18 through 21 years, and 1.4% in adults aged 22 years or older. As in Volberg's (1994) study, the pathological gamblers were more likely to be males, non-White, unmarried and less educated. Problem gambling, which is a less severe manifestation of disturbed gambling behavior and has been defined as a SOGS score of 3 or 4, affected 3.0% of adults aged 22 or older and a remarkable 11.2% of those aged 18 through 21.

Studies using translated versions of the SOGS in Quebec (Ladouceur, 1991) and in Seville, Spain (Legarda et al., 1992) produced lifetime prevalence figures similar to those in the United States, 1.2% and 1.7% respectively.

In these epidemiological studies, less than 10% of the pathological gamblers identified by the SOGS had sought help for gambling. Volberg and Steadman (1988) report that only about one-third of individuals identified by the SOGS as pathological gamblers believe they have a gambling problem. The validity of utilizing a SOGS cutoff score of 5 to define individuals needing treatment has not been established.

A Canadian epidemiological study utilized the Diagnostic Interview Schedule to evaluate the prevalence of pathological gambling in more than 7000 randomly selected residents of the city of Edmonton aged 18 years or older (Bland et al., 1993). The investigators found a lifetime prevalence rate of 0.71% among men and 0.23% among women. Six-month prevalence rates were 0.35% for men and 0.11% for women. Only 10% of these individuals had ever told a physician about their gambling behavior.

Comorbidity

Studies of comorbidity in community samples of pathological gamblers are not available. In patients seeking treatment, affective disorders, substance abuse and personality disorders are common (Murray, 1993). For example, McCormick et al. (1984) interviewed 50 men seeking admission to a four-week Veterans Administration inpatient rehabilitation program. Lifetime prevalence rates for comorbid conditions included: major depression 76%; hypomanic episodes 38%; manic episodes 8%; and, alcohol or drug dependence 36%. In addition, 12% had made a potentially lethal suicide attempt in the year before hospitalization and an additional 12% had made preparations for such an attempt. A study of about 150 pathological gamblers seeking inpatient treatment and a similar number drawn from Gamblers Anonymous found that 15% met DSM-III criteria for antisocial personality disorder (Blaszczynski and McConaghy, 1994).

Among 25 men recruited from Gamblers Anonymous, and evaluated with a structured psychiatric interview, 72% had had at least one episode of DSM-III major depression either while gambling or immediately after stopping, and 8% had had manic episodes (Linden, Pope and Jonas, 1986). Lifetime prevalence of alcohol abuse or dependency was 48%, OCD 20% and panic disorder 16%. Major affective disorders and alcohol abuse or dependence were common in first degree relatives. The authors caution that a sample drawn from Gamblers Anonymous is not necessarily representative of all pathological gamblers since few such gamblers are long-term members.

Taken together, these studies suggest that the clinician must be particularly alert for comorbid mood disorders and substance abuse, and that the rate of antisocial personality disorder will exceed that in the general population.

Treatment

Because few controlled clinical trials are available, treatment planning relies primarily on expert opinion and published accounts of clinical experience. As is evident from the clinical picture described earlier, the pathological gambler usually appears for treatment with multiple familial, job-related, financial and legal problems, and often with comorbid mood or substance abuse disorders. A careful and extensive evaluation of these potential problem areas is imperative, taking into account the gambler's likely use of denial and rationalization and possible resort to lying. Compiling a complete problem list is a prerequisite to planning effective interventions. Problems ignored in one biological, psychological or social dimension will compromise treatment efforts in another. Inpatient treatment should be considered when the gambler is suicidal, manic, requires separation from a colluding or provocative support group, persists in gambling or has a severe comorbid mental disorder (including substance abuse) that will interfere with adherence to outpatient treatment (Rosenthal and Lorenz, 1992).

After the problem list is completed and emergent problems have been addressed, one can focus on evaluating the pathological gambling behavior. Why has the patient come for treatment? Is he under familial or legal duress to stop gambling? What is the history of gambling, including age at onset, kinds of gambling, frequencies, motivations, current consequences, financial situation and history of illegal activities in support of gambling? What prior attempts have been made to deal with the problem and with what results?

Psychotherapeutic and multimodal approaches

In our current state of knowledge, one cannot distinguish between the effectiveness of outpatient interventions, brief inpatient stays utilizing behavioral or cognitive techniques and longer inpatient stays deploying multimodal therapies. Until further evidence is available, treatment should combine cognitive therapies with mandatory attendance at Gamblers Anonymous meetings and with family, vocational and social interventions as needed. The choice of an inpatient or an outpatient setting is determined by the factors mentioned earlier.

The literature supports the use of cognitive therapies, derived from theories concerning the role of perceptions, assumptions and cognitions, at least as well as the use of aversive behavioral conditioning therapies, drawn from theories of classical and operant conditioning. Reviewing the literature on cognitive and behavioral therapies applied to pathological gambling, Blaszczynski and Silove (1995) note that small sample sizes and numerous methodological problems prevent one from drawing any firm conclusions about success rates and long-term efficacy.

The most studied cognitive therapy is imaginal desensitization, which was originally implemented in a hospital unit (McConaghy, Blaszczynski and Frankova, 1991). Patients were admitted for five days and after evaluation, received three 20-minute sessions of imaginal desensitization daily, each separated by at least two hours. In each session, the patients spent five minutes achieving a state of relaxation and then visualized themselves sequentially in four situations in which they ordinarily were stimulated to gamble. In the visualized scene, however, they visualized themselves refraining. A state of relaxation was maintained throughout the session, with a break after the first two scenes to re-establish relaxation. In a two- to nine-year follow-up evaluation, limited by including only about half of treated subjects, 79% of 33 patients treated with imaginal desensitization had achieved abstinence or controlled gambling ($\leq$ $10 per week) versus 53% of 30 patients randomly assigned to behavioral interventions (aversive therapy, relaxation or in vivo exposure with response prevention). Since the outcome was determined by means of a structured clinical interview corroborated by an informant designated by the patient, it is reasonably credible. In an earlier one-year follow-up study, 7 of 10 patients treated with imaginal desensitization reported controlled or no gambling compared to only 2 of 10 treated with aversive therapy (McConaghy et al., 1983). Whether the abstinence from gambling enforced by the five-day inpatient stay is a necessary part of the treatment, and whether this required stay selects highly motivated patients, are questions still to be answered. Implementation of this treatment model in an outpatient or partial hospitalization setting should be tried.

Although imaginal desensitization was the focus of treatment in the studies reported, patients also received other forms of cognitive therapy aimed at correcting distorted perceptions, faulty assumptions and maladaptive cognitions (Blaszczynski and Silove, 1995). Educational sessions sought to convey that:

- gambling is an expensive form of entertainment, not a means of earning money;
- gambling serves to raise money for governments and to earn profits for its purveyors;
- the money lost goes to provide cheap food, lodging and entertainment for other patrons, and thus cannot be thought of as an future entitlement;
- gambling creates problems it cannot solve.

In addition, the clinician should attempt to correct the irrational beliefs noted earlier in this chapter.

Behavioral approaches to pathological gambling have shown some success (Blaszczynski and Silove, 1995). In aversive conditioning, the patient, while exposed to gambling stimuli, receives mild electric shocks or brings to mind aversive imagery such as nausea, vomiting or discovery by a spouse. Because aversive conditioning enlists punishment in the service of treatment and because imaginal desensitization appears to be at least, if not more, effective, aversive conditioning has little to recommend it.

Attending Gamblers Anonymous (modeled on the 12–step program of Alcoholics Anonymous) is highly correlated with abstinence from gambling, at least in patients who have completed a multimodal, month-long inpatient treatment program (Russo et al., 1984). One year after discharge, 30 of 31 subjects who had attended at least one meeting were abstinent compared to only 14 of 28 who had not. Of course, willingness to attend may simply indicate strong motivation to abstain, rather than reflecting the effect of attendance. In either case, the patient's reaction to required attendance provides the clinician with valuable information. Unsupervised, patients are not likely to remain in Gamblers Anonymous for long. In a study of 14 Gamblers Anonymous chapters, less than one-third of individuals attending one meeting persisted for 10 or more, and nearly half the drop-outs occurred in the first three weeks (Stewart and Brown, 1988). Spouses or family members can be advised to attend so-called Gam-Anon meetings for information and emotional support.

Experienced clinical investigators recommend other sensible treatment elements aimed at relapse prevention. England and Götestam (1991) and Blaszczynski and Silove (1995) recommend helping the patient to:

- avoid conditioned stimuli for gambling, such as the gambling locale, newspaper sports pages, unstructured leisure time, paychecks and credit cards;
- use budgeting and other techniques to relieve the financial pressures motivating gambling;
- arrange a realistic schedule for repaying debts;
- plan methods other than gambling for dealing with negative mood states, (i.e., stress management techniques);
- develop other methods for achieving excitement and pleasure, particularly at times previously devoted to gambling;

- define lapses as indications for renewed planning, not for condemning oneself as a hopeless failure.

In addition, these authors advise considering:

- marital or family therapy to deal with spousal or familial anger, frustration, despair, mistrust and possible enabling behavior;
- pharmacotherapy for comorbid mood disorders;
- referral to social agencies for help with legal, vocational or other social problems. The clinician should deploy as many of these treatment elements as the needs of the patient indicate.

Whether multimodal month-long inpatient programs that include group psychotherapy methods (Taber and Chaplin, 1988) are more or less effective than the treatment package just described is unknown. These programs were pioneered in Veterans Administration hospitals beginning in 1972 (Russo et al., 1984) and have been established in a few private hospitals (Lesieur and Blume, 1991). Taber et al. (1987) found total abstinence during a six-month follow-up period in 56% of 57 graduates of a multimodal program, along with improvement in psychological and social functioning. The self-reported gambling outcome was corroborated by collateral informants. Lesieur and Blume (1991) report a 64% abstinence rate 6–14 months after multimodal treatment. A German study reports a similar one-year abstinence rate after a four-month multimodal inpatient program (Schwarz and Lindner, 1992).

Pharmacotherapy

No large controlled trials are available. A scant literature is beginning to hint that selective serotonin reuptake inhibitors (SSRIs) may be helpful in treating pathological gambling. For example, a 31-year-old woman with a 12-year history of pathological gambling and comorbid social phobia minimally responsive to double-blind placebo treatment, stopped gambling after three weeks of double-blind treatment with clomipramine, at a sustained dose of 125 mg/day (Hollander et al., 1992a). She remained in remission during seven weeks of continued treatment at this dose and, except for a brief relapse, for seven months of open-label treatment at a dose of 175 mg/day.

In a blind, eight-week-per-treatment, crossover trial of fluvoxamine versus placebo, 7 of 10 fluvoxamine patients were judged much or very much improved after treatment with a mean dose of 210 mg/day (E. Hollander, unpublished data, 1997).

In a 12-week-per-phase, double-blind, placebo-controlled crossover trial, carbamazepine successfully treated a patient with a 16-year history of pathological gambling unresponsive to behavior therapy, psychoanalysis, participation in Gamblers Anonymous or a trial of benzodiazepines (Haller and Hinterhuber,

Table 16.2. Pathological gambling: treatment planning guidelines

- Assess motivation for treatment.
- Assess motivations for pathological gambling and help the patient remove or counteract them.
- Assess financial, familial, occupational and legal problems related to gambling.
- Assess suicide risk and intervene.
- Assess irrational beliefs about gambling.
- Assess gambling activities and venues.
- Identify and treat comorbid mood and substance use disorders.
- Assess for antisocial personality disorder.
- Consider inpatient, multimodal treatment.
- Institute cognitive–behavioral therapy (imaginal desensitization, cognitive restructuring).
- Consider an eight-week trial of fluvoxamine or other SSRI and continue effective drug long-term.
- Consider a four-week trial of carbamazepine or other mood stabilizer and continue effective drug long-term.
- Require attendance at Gamblers Anonymous meetings.
- Institute relapse prevention (budget, schedule debt repayment, use stress management, arrange alternate pleasures, avoid conditioned stimuli).
- Initiate couple or family therapy and recommend Gam-Anon group for spouse or family.
- Refer to social agencies for help with vocational, legal and social problems.

Note:
SSRI: selective serotonin reuptake inhibitor.

1994). Carbamazepine begun at 200 mg/day and increased gradually to 600 mg/day produced a remission by the second week that continued during 2½ years of open-label treatment.

If comorbid major depression or dysthymia is present and requires pharmacotherapy, the clinician should avoid medications easily lethal in overdose. As noted earlier, the pathological gambler is at substantial risk for suicide.

If comorbid generalized anxiety requires pharmacotherapy in a patient with a history of alcohol or substance abuse, buspirone, which is not dependency-producing, is preferred over the benzodiazepines. A tricyclic antidepressant such as nortriptyline represents another effective approach. Comorbid panic disorder, social phobia or OCD can be treated with SSRIs, thereby minimizing the risks associated with intentional overdose.

Controlled trials are needed to define the role of SSRIs, carbamazepine and other modern pharmacotherapeutic agents in the treatment of pathological gambling. Treatment planning guidelines are shown in Table 16.2.

17

Nonparaphilic sexual disorders

A man of pleasure is a man of pain.

Edward Young (1684–1765), *Night*

This chapter explores what is known about "nonparaphilic sexual disorders" (See Table 17.1). Treatment of the paraphilias is discussed elsewhere (Kafka and Coleman, 1991; Gottesman and Schubert, 1993; Zohar, Kaplan and Benjamin, 1994; LoPiccolo and Van Male, 1997). The nonparaphilic sexual disorders included in this chapter, in contrast to paraphilias such as fetishism, exhibitionism and voyeurism, are neither culturally deviant nor illegal. But with genital herpes infection, AIDS and unwanted pregnancy having become prominent public health concerns, these disorders merit more investigation than they have received.

Diagnosis

The nonparaphilic sexual disorders have been variously conceptualized and characterized as "addictions," (Carnes, 1989; Kafka and Prentky, 1992; Goodman, 1993), "compulsions," (Anthony and Hollander, 1992) and disorders of impulse control (Barth and Kinder, 1987). The earlier literature on "hypersexuality," which included some similar cases, is critically reviewed by Orford (1978) and by Levine and Troiden (1988).

DSM-III-R utilized the term, "sexual addiction," and placed nonparaphilic sexual disorders in the subcategory, Sexual Disorders Not Otherwise Specified. DSM-IV (American Psychiatric Association, 1994) abandoned both the addiction terminology and any mention of these behaviors. ICD-10 (World Health Organization, 1992) lists nymphomania and satyriasis, terms abandoned in U.S. nomenclature, within the diagnostic category, Excessive sexual drive (F52.7). Ego-dystonic, compulsive masturbation; chronic, ego-dystonic promiscuity; and, demanding unwanted sexual activity from a partner whose sexual drive is not hypoactive could all fall within this ICD-10 category. These disorders are not limited, however, to the age group to which ICD-10 ascribes most cases of excessive sexual drive – "late teenage or early adulthood."

Table 17.1. Nonparaphilic sexual disorders

• Ego-dystonic, compulsive masturbation.
• Chronic, ego-dystonic promiscuity (compulsive "cruising").
• Dependence for sexual arousal on:
  – pornography;
  – telephone sexual material;
  – sexual accessories (e.g., dildos);
  – drugs (e.g., alcohol, amyl nitrate, cocaine).
• Demanding unwanted sexual activity from a partner whose sexual drive is not hypoactive.
• Fixation on an unobtainable partner.

Sources: Coleman, 1992; Kafka and Prentky, 1997.

A number of organic etiologies can underlie nonparaphilic sexual behaviors. These include diencephalic or frontal lobe lesions or septal injury (Elliot and Biever, 1996; Gorman and Cumming, 1992), temporal lobe epilepsy (postictally or after medical or surgical control of seizures – Savard and Walker, 1965; Blumer and Walker, 1967), dementia, including Alzheimer's disease (Kuhn, Greiner and Arseneau, 1998), stroke involving the temporal lobe (Monga et al., 1986), treatment of Parkinson's disease with dopaminergic agents (Uitti et al., 1989) and the Klüver-Bucy syndrome (caused by bilateral damage to the temporal lobes) (Goscinski et al., 1997).

Nonparaphilic sexual behaviors without an organic cause have been considered addictions, compulsions or impulse control disorders because they partake of many characteristics of these categories. Like addictions (or "substance dependence" in DSM-IV terminology) they cause clinically significant distress or dysfunction in social roles and are characterized by: frequent indulgence more often or longer than intended; unsuccessful efforts to decrease their frequency; preoccupation with the behavior or with preparations for it; continuance of the behavior despite knowledge of its adverse effects; and, the presence of withdrawal symptoms such as restlessness and irritability (Goodman, 1993). Like an addictive chemical, the sexual behavior is often mood-altering and strongly attractive. In ego-dystonic homosexual promiscuity the excitement of the preparatory chase can itself be a powerful reinforcer (Pincu, 1989).

Like compulsions, nonparaphilic sexual behaviors are repetitive, excessive extensions of normal behaviors and may be driven, as true compulsions are, by motives of anxiety reduction rather than by pleasure seeking (Quadland and Shattls, 1987; Coleman, 1992). In contrast to true compulsions, which are never pleasurable in their consummation, compulsive sexual acts are gratifying, however briefly. The conclusion that a sexual behavior is "excessive," cannot depend, however, on frequency alone, since no boundaries of normal (nonpathological) have been established. An idea of the range of the statistically normal frequency of sexual behaviors can be obtained from a modern survey of sexual activity (Seidman and Rieder, 1994), which supplements Kinsey's earlier surveys (Kinsey, Pomeroy and Martin, 1948; Kinsey et al., 1953). Quadland (1985) sensibly suggests that sexual behavior be considered excessive and "compulsive" when the individual complains of a feeling of lack of control. He also notes that the anxiety with which the individual is attempting to cope may stem from a fear of intimacy, low self-esteem or a lack of satisfying relationships. In addition, an individual entangled in homosexual, ego-dystonic promiscuity may fear losing his job, friends or partner if the behavior is discovered (Pincu, 1989).

Like impulse control disorders, nonparaphilic sexual behaviors are often characterized by failure to resist an impulse or temptation that is harmful to the self or others, an increasing sense of tension before initiating the behavior, pleasure or relief in the act, and subsequent remorse or guilt (Barth and Kinder, 1987). This diagnostic category does not, however, capture the preoccupation with sexual behavior or the withdrawal phenomena included within the "addiction" formulation.

Absent any empirically grounded understanding of the etiology of these behaviors, and given their phenomenological resemblance to several current diagnostic categories, the noncommittal terms, nonparaphilic sexual disorders or behaviors seem appropriate. The label used by the clinician will have important effects on the patient's self-image and his or her expectations regarding the treatment (Coleman, 1992). Because an addiction label is the most stigmatizing and the most likely to engender hopelessness, clinicians may wish to avoid it.

Prevalence

Nothing useful is known of the prevalence or familial patterns of these disorders. Men come more often for treatment, but the gender distribution of these unwanted sexual behaviors in the community is unknown.

Comorbidity

Comorbidity is reported in two case series. Since the included cases were obtained by advertisement or from clinic attenders, the findings cannot be generalized to all individuals with nonparaphilic sexual disorders. Moreover, the numbers are so small within a given category that they cannot be regarded as accurate estimates of population figures. Still, these case series suggest that certain disorders will be found frequently in individuals who present for treatment.

In the first series, 26 men, primarily self-referred to a specialized treatment program, were examined by means of a sexual inventory and a psychiatric interview (Kafka and Prentky, 1994). The most common nonparaphilic sexual disorders were compulsive masturbation (85%), dependence on pornography (73%), heterosexual (50%) or homosexual (35%) ego-dystonic promiscuity, and less commonly, dependence on telephone sex (31%), dependence on accessories (12%) or incompatible levels of desire (4%). The same nonparaphilic sexual disorders were common in a simultaneously examined group of 34 men with paraphilias. Lifetime histories of major depression and early-onset dysthymia were found in three-fifths of the men with nonparaphilic sexual disorders, social phobia in nearly half, alcohol abuse in about two-fifths, marijuana abuse in one-sixth, and OCD in 12%. Only 2 of the 26 men had histories of an impulse control disorder.

The second series describes 36 subjects who answered an advertisement for persons troubled by "compulsive sexual behavior" (Black et al., 1997). The subjects were assessed by means of a semi-structured psychiatric interview, a computerized version of the NIMH Diagnostic Interview Schedule, the Structured Interview for DSM-III-R Personality Disorders, Revised, and several self-report questionnaires. The subjects' mean age was 27 years, 26 (72%) were single and 8 (22%) were women. The most common nonparaphilic sexual behaviors were compulsive "cruising" (22%), compulsive seeking of multiple lovers (22%), compulsive masturbation (17%) and compulsive sex within a relationship (14%). Because the university's committee for the protection of human subjects asked the investigators to instruct subjects not to report illegal sexual behaviors, no estimate of the frequency of comorbid paraphilias was possible. The computerized diagnostic assessment suggested that the most common current (six-month) comorbid conditions were major depression or dysthymia (31%), phobic disorder (25%), alcohol abuse or dependence (19%), and mania, OCD and generalized anxiety disorder (each 14%). Panic disorder (11%) and bulimia (8%) were less common. The pattern of lifetime prevalence of comorbid conditions was similar except that alcohol abuse or dependence was the most common disorder (58%). A semi-structured interview revealed a significant prevalence of impulse control disorders: compulsive buying (14%); kleptomania (14%); pathological gambling (11%); compulsive exercise (8%); and, pyromania (8%). DSM-IV Cluster B personality disorders were present in 44%, Cluster C in 39% and Cluster A in 28%, with the single most common disorders being Histrionic and Passive–Aggressive (both 28%).

The case literature cited by the authors of these two studies also suggests that the comorbid conditions most common in individuals with nonparaphilic sexual disorders are mood disorders, anxiety disorders and substance abuse disorders.

Assessment and assessment instruments

Critical to good treatment planning is obtaining a careful description of the behaviors to be treated. What are they? When and how did they begin? What is the patient's understanding of their original and current motivation? How often do they occur? Under what circumstances? With what positive and negative consequences? Unfortunately, embarrassment, mistrust and ambivalence about giving up the behaviors will all interfere with obtaining this information quickly. Since sexuality is a prominent strand in the fabric of an individual's life, the clinician will want to explore the patient's sexual experiences in early life before narrowing the therapeutic focus to the here-and-now. These experiences include not only early sexual encounters, but also the attitudes of the patient's family toward sex.

In many cases, the patient will be troubled by more than one nonparaphilic sexual behavior (Kafka and Prentky, 1994), which may be episodic rather than constant (Black et al., 1997). Repetitive, intrusive fantasies may be just as disturbing to the patient as repetitive behaviors and should be inquired about. Mood states before, during and immediately after the sexual behavior should be carefully ascertained, both for their motivational relevance and because they may require separate treatment. Depression, anxiety, loneliness, frustration, anger and happiness are often present before the act and remorse and guilt afterwards (Black et al., 1997). Negative consequences can also include criticism by others, marital discord, financial drain, inordinate expenditure of time, work impairment and sexually transmitted diseases (Black et al., 1997). Past histories of sexual or physical abuse and of suicide attempts should be actively sought – they may be more common than in the general population (Black et al., 1997).

When the patient complains of an unresponsive partner, the clinician must determine whether the partner exhibits hypoactive desire and whether the patient's demands fall within the range of "normal," tasks made difficult by the wide range this concept embraces (Kinsey et al., 1948; Kinsey et al., 1953; Seidman and Rieder, 1994). When the behavior involves any harm to the partner, one has moved into the realms of paraphilias or of illegal behaviors.

Assessment instruments

No validated assessment instrument has been published. Kafka, however, has developed and utilized a Sexual Outlet Inventory that documents the frequency of well-defined "conventional" and "unconventional" sexual fantasies, urges and activities during a given week (Kafka and Prentky, 1992).

Treatment

No well-controlled trials of pharmacotherapies or psychotherapeutic methods are available. Nonetheless, a number of case reports and case series support pharmacological interventions, and expert opinion is available regarding approaches to psychotherapy.

If a comorbid condition is present, especially alcohol or substance abuse, a depressive disorder, hypomania or mania, social phobia or a severe personality disorder, treating the comorbid condition is prerequisite to helping the patient with the presenting sexual problem (Goodman, 1993). Since selective serotinin reuptake inhibitors (SSRIs) seem effective or helpful for some nonparaphilic sexual disorders and are effective for many of the potential comorbid conditions, initiating a trial will be a reasonable course of action in many circumstances.

When physical or sexual abuse in childhood is uncovered, its effects on the patient's sexual life must be mitigated. This may require techniques of supportive psychotherapy such as ventilation, sympathy, education, relief of guilt and expression of caring, as well as the specific techniques recommended by various psychotherapeutic schools (Klerman and Weissman, 1993; Linehan, 1993; Gabbard, 1994; Beck, 1995).

Psychotherapeutic considerations

The psychotherapeutic plan should take into account not only the sexual complaint and possible comorbid conditions, but equally importantly, the cultural background and the past and present life experience of the complaining individual. Feelings, attitudes, beliefs and experiences will shape the patient's abilities and willingness to cooperate in any attempt to change behavior. While the goal of therapy is changed behavior, the therapist must first help the patient change the intervening feelings, attitudes and beliefs. The patient must also be taught to recognize risky situations, engage in alternative behaviors in response to pathological urges and prevent isolated behavioral lapses from becoming prolonged relapses (Goodman, 1993).

Experienced therapists such as Carnes (1989), who follows an addiction model, and Schwartz (1992), who utilizes a post-traumatic stress paradigm, offer detailed descriptions of psychotherapeutic approaches to unwanted sexual behaviors. Like drug treatments, however, psychotherapeutic approaches to these disorders await large, carefully controlled trials to separate opinion from fact. In the absence of well-controlled clinical trials, psychodynamic psychotherapies, cognitive–behavioral techniques, interpersonal therapy and couple and family therapies all remain reasonable approaches for clinicians to tailor to the circumstances.

If a psychodynamic approach is elected, the therapist will focus on helping the patient learn to manage feelings, change maladaptive beliefs, resolve inner and interpersonal conflicts, and get needs met adaptively (Goodman, 1993). Therapists of all schools, however, will often witness behaviors consistent with the psycho-dynamically defined defense mechanisms of denial (minimizing the magnitude of the problem and its harmful consequences) and rationalization (providing excuses for the behavior) (Pincu, 1989).

Recommended cognitive-behavioral techniques include:

- analyzing during treatment sessions the patient's daily diary of the circumstances surrounding urges for the symptomatic sexual behavior;
- developing contingency plans to prevent lapses from progressing to full relapse;
- cognitive reframing of a lapse as an indication for adding to the management strategy rather than an occasion for self-castigation (Goodman, 1993).

A randomized trial found that imaginal desensitization (ID) was more effective than covert sensitization (CS) in patients with either a paraphilia ($n = 15$) or compulsive homosexuality ($n = 5$) (McConaghy, Armstrong and Blaszczynski, 1985). In ID, the patient imagines, while relaxed, situations leading to unwanted sexual behavior, but ends the scenes with successful avoidance of the behavior because he does not feel "impelled to complete the activity." In CS, the patient imagines a self-designed aversive situation, e.g., vomiting or being surprised in the act by relatives, that prevents the scenes from ending in the unwanted behavior; the therapist describes the aversive situation when the patient signals the appropriate moment in the visualized scene. Patients were randomly assigned to 14 ID or CS treatment sessions administered during a one-week inpatient stay. During the one-year follow-up period, each patient was interviewed four to six times by the therapist to assess need for further treatment, and three CS patients received aversive therapy. At one-year follow-up, a blind rater rated the anomalous sexual behaviors of seven ID and four CS subjects as improved; the ID patients reported a significantly greater mean reduction in anomalous sexual urges (89%) than the CS patients (55%).

Expert opinion suggests that certain feelings and core conflicts often underlie nonparaphilic sexual behaviors, including low self-esteem, social inadequacy or generalized anxiety (Coleman, 1992). Core life issues underlying dysfunctional sexual behaviors may involve conflicts between the fear of being controlled and the wish for intimacy, or the fear of being abandoned and the wish to be independent (Goodman, 1993). As the patient gives up sexual means of coping with life problems, depression or anxiety may emerge or worsen. In either case, the clinician should consider pharmacological treatment (Goodman, 1993).

Couple therapy

When a spouse or partner is present, his or her participation in therapy is indicated (Coleman, 1992). This individual may be suffering along with the patient or contributing to the continuance of the sexual disorder. Facilitating mutual conventional sexual fulfillment and understanding why the sexual relationship is not satisfying one or both partners can be critical treatment elements.

Group psychotherapy

Models of group psychotherapy are offered by Carnes (1989), who adapted the 12-step methods of Alcoholics Anonymous (substituting healthful sex for the AA goal of abstinence), and by Schwartz and Brasted (1985), who describe a six-stage model encompassing behavior modification techniques, overcoming denial, anxiety reduction techniques, modifying irrational beliefs and social skills training. These models await empirical evaluation. Goodman (1993) believes that groups can help patients deal with fears of closeness, difficulties with intimate relationships, low self-esteem and shame. He notes that the philosophy and structure of 12-step groups prevent the emergence of abusive leaders. Groups organized under the aegis of Sex Addicts Anonymous, Sexual Compulsives Anonymous and Sex and Love Addicts Anonymous were reportedly helpful to his patients, but their availability varies from locale to locale and no quality control exists. (See Appendix 1 for self-help groups and Internet educational sites.) Because societal checks on the quality of local groups are absent, the clinician should either be quite familiar with a group in his or her locale before recommending it or ask the patient for detailed reports of group meetings.

Quadland (1985) reports changed sexual behavior in 30 "compulsive" homosexual and bisexual males who attended an average of 20 group psychotherapy sessions focussed on understanding and changing the motives for unwanted sexual behaviors. The therapy methods are not described. Six months after completing the group, the men had significantly reduced their number of partners, the proportion of partners seen only once, the use of drugs or alcohol in conjunction with sex, and the proportion of encounters in public settings.

Pharmacotherapy

The small open-label trials and case reports that are available consistently suggest the utility of SSRIs.

A 12-week, open trial investigated the effectiveness of fluoxetine, begun at 20 mg/day and titrated every four weeks to 60 mg/day (mean dose about 40 mg/day) (Kafka and Prentky, 1992). An indeterminate number of the 10 subjects received concomitant psychotherapy. At baseline, all subjects apparently were dysthymic and five had major depression. The seven patients who completed the trial exhibited, on average, significant decreases in unconventional sexual urges and behaviors and in depression scores, but the relationship between these symptomatic improvements is not described. The treatment effect, present by week 4, did not

Table 17.2. Nonparaphilic sexual disorders: treatment planning guidelines

---

- Assess the patient's motivations for treatment.
- Assess and treat comorbid disorders (especially, mood disorders, anxiety disorders and substance abuse).
- Obtain a full description of the troubling behaviors and their contexts.
- Inquire about a past history of physical or sexual abuse and implement appropriate psychotherapy.
- If harm to a partner is involved, legal responsibilities supervene.
- Institute psychotherapy (psychodynamic, cognitive–behavioral, interpersonal or eclectic).
- Consider four- to six-week trials of several SSRIs.
- Consider couple therapy.
- Consider referral to a 12-step group therapy program.
- Utilize Internet sites for patient education.

Note:
SSRIs: selective serotonin reuptake inhibitors.

diminish conventional sexual behaviors. Four of these patients may have been described in Kafka's earlier (1991) series of fluoxetine-treated patients.

In a case series, five patients, four with comorbid OCD (and comorbid major depression, substance abuse or social phobia) and one with comorbid major depression and polysubstance abuse, were treated with fluoxetine 20–80 mg/day for at least four weeks (Stein et al., 1992). One patient with OCD experienced an improvement in compulsive masturbation and OCD; the patient with major depression and polysubstance abuse experienced an improvement in compulsive masturbation and depression. Two patients had an improvement in OCD without change in their sexual symptoms. The unwanted sexual promiscuity of one patient with OCD worsened when fluoxetine caused anorgasmia.

A 25-year-old man who complained of compulsive masturbation, frequent visits to prostitutes and preoccupation with pornography markedly improved within one week of starting treatment with clomipramine 125 mg/day (Rubey, Brady and Norris, 1993). When he stopped treatment after two months because of anorgasmia, his symptoms returned. When clomipramine was restarted, he improved again, rapidly and markedly. His comorbid dysthymia did not respond to clomipramine.

An open-label trial of sertraline was conducted in 12 men with nonparaphilic sexual disorders (and 14 with paraphilias) (Kafka, 1994). Sertraline was begun at 25 mg/day and increased every two weeks (minimum) as necessary and as tolerated. The mean duration of treatment was about 18 weeks and the mean final dose 99 ± 62 mg/day. One patient dropped out. Four were very much improved, two much improved; one patient became worse as measured by the Clinical Global Impressions scale. On average, total unconventional sexual outlet (orgasms per day) dropped by nearly half, and conventional sexual outlet was not adversely affected. Response was independent of a baseline measure of depression. Of five patients unresponsive to sertraline and crossed over to fluoxetine 20–80 mg/day for 3–15 months, one was much and one very much improved.

Randomized, double-blind, placebo-controlled trials of SSRIs in nonparaphilic sexual disorders are sorely needed. Observations must extend for six months or more to assure the stability of any response. Treatment planning guidelines are shown in Table 17.2.

18

Obsessive–compulsive personality disorder

The perfect is the enemy of the good.

Anonymous

Much less is known about personality disorders than about the disorders placed on Axis I of DSM-IV. Great uncertainty exists, moreover, about whether the current grouping of maladaptive traits into "disorders" is a valid map of this domain of psychopathology. Stone (1990), for example, lists more than 500 maladaptive traits reducible to 66 "dimensions," and wonders whether the categories comprising our current personality disorders are valid (Stone, 1993). He also notes that culture plays a large role in defining desirable and maladaptive behavioral traits.

Even if our current personality disorder categories are valid, our methods of determining their presence or absence are severely wanting. Reviewing eight studies that compared different methods of diagnosing the same personality disorders, Perry (1992) concluded that no two methods agreed sufficiently about the presence of individual personality disorders to consider any method "scientifically acceptable." His conclusion was the same when he compared structured interview methods with one another, and similarly, self-report questionnaires.

The level of uncertainty regarding how to conceptualize personality disorders is well illustrated by the disagreements between DSM-IV and ICD-10 in their diagnostic criteria for obsessive–compulsive personality disorder (OCPD).

Diagnosis

DSM-IV diagnostic criteria (301.4)

Because the DSM-IV criteria (Table 18.1) represent a substantial change from those in DSM-III, comparing studies that utilized these differing versions is problematic. DSM-IV added four diagnostic criteria to those of DSM-III and discarded one – emotional constriction. The new criteria are: miserliness; excessive conscientiousness; inability to discard worn-out or worthless objects; and, the need to have things done exactly one's way.

Table 18.1. DSM-IV diagnostic criteria for obsessive compulsive personality disorder (301.4)

A pervasive pattern of preoccupation with orderliness, perfectionism, and mental and interpersonal control, at the expense of flexibility, openness and efficiency, beginning by early adulthood and present in a variety of contexts, as indicated by four (or more) of the following:

(1) is preoccupied with details, rules, lists, order, organization, or schedules to the extent that the major point of the activity is lost;

(2) shows perfectionism that interferes with task completion (e.g., is unable to complete a project because his or her own overly strict standards are not met);

(3) is excessively devoted to work and productivity to the exclusion of leisure activities and friendships (not accounted for by obvious economic necessity);

(4) is overconscientious, scrupulous, and inflexible about matters of morality, ethics, or values (not accounted for by cultural or religious identification);

(5) is unable to discard worn-out or worthless objects even when they have no sentimental value;

(6) is reluctant to delegate tasks or to work with others unless they submit to exactly his or her way of doing things;

(7) adopts a miserly spending style toward both self and others; money is viewed as something to be hoarded for future catastrophes;

(8) shows rigidity and stubbornness.

Source: Reprinted with permission from the *Diagnostic and Statistical Manual of Mental Disorders,* Fourth Edition. Copyright 1994, American Psychiatric Association, pp. 672–3.

ICD-10 diagnostic criteria (F60.5)

The overlap between the diagnostic criteria for OCPD in DSM-IV and ICD-10 is modest, suggesting that the essence of this maladaptive personality style is a matter of debate. DSM-IV, but not ICD-10, includes miserliness and difficulty discarding worn-out or worthless objects. ICD-10, but not DSM-IV, includes excessive doubting, excessive pedantry and insistent, unwelcome thoughts or impulses. DSM-IV requires that four of its eight trait criteria be present; ICD-10 requires only three. Finally, ICD-10 prefers the diagnostic label, "Anankastic personality disorder" (from the Greek, *anankastos,* compelled).

Prevalence

Given the uncertainty regarding how to define this disorder and the limited validity of the available assessment instruments (Perry, 1992), little can be said definitively about its prevalence. Only one community survey is available. Nestadt et al. (1991) surveyed a representative sample of the population of Eastern Baltimore, USA.

Subjects were examined by psychiatrists, who utilized a semi-structured interview protocol. The estimated prevalence of DSM-III OCPD for this population was 1.7%. OCPD was five times as prevalent in men as in women, more common in Caucasians than in African Americans, and in the highly educated than in the uneducated.

Comorbidity

A number of studies have examined the co-occurrence of OCPD and OCD. OCPD prevalence estimates reported from structured interview studies of patients with OCD range, for DSM-III criteria, from 16% (Baer, et al., 1992) and 19% (Cassano, Del Buono and Catapano, 1993a) to 28% (Black, et al., 1993a). For DSM-III-R criteria, which closely resemble those of DSM-IV, the estimates range from 8% (Crino and Andrews, 1996) and 17% (Torres and Del Porto, 1995) to 28% (Stanley, Turner and Borden, 1990) and 31% (Diaferia et al., 1997). In three of the four DSM-III-R studies (Stanley et al., 1990; Crino and Andrews, 1996; Diaferia et al., 1997), OCPD was the most common personality disorder in the OCD patients, but avoidant and dependent personality disorders were also common. The occurrence of OCD in childhood, however, does not predispose to developing OCPD. Children with OCD are not more likely than controls to develop OCPD (Thomsen and Mikkelsen, 1993).

These studies suffer from the possible confusion of state variables with trait variables. That is, behavioral expressions of OCD may be confused with traits linked to an OCPD diagnosis. For example, several OCPD diagnostic criteria may be confused with symptoms of OCD – hoarding, scrupulosity and preoccupation with rules, order and lists. Consistent with this possibility, Ricciardi et al. (1992) noted that OCPD, established by a structured clinical interview, disappeared in five of six OCD patients whose OCD was successfully treated.

Treatment

The genesis and psychological function of the traits comprising OCPD have been the subject of much speculation over the past century. Fears concerning the negative consequences of losing control – emotional, intellectual and interpersonal – have repeatedly been identified as the source of OCPD traits (Pollak, 1987; Simon and Myer, 1990). Perfectionism, preoccupation with rules, being overly conscientious, the need to control others, inability to discard worthless objects, rigidity and stubbornness, procrastination and indecisiveness, all can be conceptualized as anxiety-induced defensive strategies designed to avoid making mistakes. When these strategies cause excessive conflict at home or at work, the patient with OCPD reluctantly comes for help. No controlled studies of psychotherapeutic approaches are available to guide the clinician, and only one controlled drug trial has been reported.

Psychotherapy

In the absence of empirical studies to guide the choice of a psychotherapeutic method, I prefer the cognitive–behavioral approach outlined by Simon and Myer (1990), which is based on methods developed by Aaron Beck (1976). Readers who prefer a psychodynamic approach will find a detailed guide in the work of Salzman (1980, 1983) and a useful summary in Gabbard's (1994) text.

At the patient's initial visit, the questions noted in Chapter 2, "Approach to the Patient," are particularly germane. Why has the patient come to you, and why now? How do his beliefs about his condition affect what he wants or expects? Who else is affected by the patient's disorder? How will you measure the outcome of your treatment?

After taking the history, the clinician should focus on the presenting problem. Simon and Myer (1990) believe that rapport is best established by adopting a rather formal, businesslike approach, not by offering emotional support. The patient is educated to understand that the assumptions, perceptions and meanings that he assigns to events bring about his feelings and behaviors. These underlying assumptions, perceptions and meanings have to be examined, and where appropriate changed, so that feelings and behavior can change. The clinician and the patient together select circumscribed behavioral goals to work on, taking into account their difficulty and how directly they will relieve the presenting problem.

Simon and Myer (1990) suggest the use of a number of cognitive–behavioral techniques. First, the therapist should negotiate an agenda for the session to prevent rumination, indecision and procrastination from sabotaging productive work. The initial agenda includes setting priorities for which problems are to be worked on and in what order. Next, the patient should be asked to collect examples of the chosen problematic behavior outside the session and to keep a record (termed a "Dysfunctional Thought Record") that notes:

- the situation;
- how the patient felt in the situation;
- the assumptions, perceptions and meanings that gave rise to the problematic behavior;
- the behavior's negative consequences.

The record is reviewed at each session and the therapist helps the patient to think of alternative assumptions and behaviors. The potential benefits of these alternative assumptions and behaviors are explored. In addition, exploring how the patient came to hold his problematic views, and how family and other experiences may have shaped them, can help the patient realize that alternative views and different behavioral styles are available.

The clinician should expect to encounter certain presenting problems, derived from the patient's automatic thoughts (Simon and Myer, 1990). Common automatic thoughts include:

Feelings, decisions and behaviors are either morally right or wrong. The naturalness of feelings such as anger, jealousy and dislike is denied. Stringent morality condemns their presence. The rich mixture of an act's positive and negative consequences is distilled and only the positive or negative portion passes into awareness.

Making mistakes means that I am bad, worthless or a failure. Alexander Pope's observation that "To err is human," (*An Essay on Criticism*) escapes the patient with OCPD. Mistakes and imperfect decisions bring feelings of guilt and depression. Seeking perfect outcomes, the patient dismisses as worthless those that are merely good. Anxiety about making mistakes may provoke any of the behavioral traits noted earlier.

Certainty and predictability are necessary to avoid mistakes; therefore, I must always be in control. The patient's hypertrophied need to control the environment and others creates conflict. Yet the patient is likely to perceive the conflict as due to others' failure to adhere to his high standards, rather than to his unreasonable demands for control. Psychoanalytical writers believe that the need to control masks yearnings for dependence and nurturance, and that anxiety over being in control prevents the OCPD patient from achieving mutual nurturance in a satisfying intimate relationship (Gabbard, 1994, pp. 592–3). If others' reactions to the patient's controlling behaviors are a presenting problem, the clinician should explore why the patient finds it difficult to depend on others and to allow others to care for him.

Worrying about things helps to prevent bad events from occurring. While planning, attention to detail and rehearsal in imagination are adaptive, the patient with OCPD transmutes these into excessive rumination, magical thinking and superstitious rituals. Worrying occupies the psychological space and sidereal time that should be devoted to iterative steps in problem solving.

Doing nothing, hesitating, is better than making a mistake or producing something imperfect. Herein lies the rationale for procrastination. The patient fails to grasp that employers, clients and associates will appreciate a good product delivered on time and will punish delivery of a "perfect" product presented late or not at all.

Without the rules and rituals I live by, I won't know how to function. Since flexibility, choice and openness to novelty carry the risk of making mistakes, they terrify the patient. Small behavioral experiments with new assumptions and behaviors can gradually increase the patient's tolerance of spontaneity.

The Dysfunctional Thought Record provides the material for identifying these unfortunate assumptions. Reviewing this material, the clinician should challenge the patient's operative assumptions and gently confront the patient with their failure to bring about desired outcomes. In helping the patient develop alternatives, one can use techniques such as asking, "What are the advantages and disadvantages of the approach you are taking?" "What is the evidence for your view (assumption, interpretation)?" The clinician should invite the patient to imagine the likely outcome of alternate approaches to the problematic situation or of approaches that respected colleagues or friends might take. Then, the clinician can suggest an experiment with an actual change in behavior and instruct the patient to record the outcome in terms of his feelings and the degree of correspondence between desired and actual results. Behavioral change is divided into small steps to keep anxiety manageable, allow progressive approach to a goal and illustrate to the patient that all-or-none thinking is not necessary for success.

When worrying is a major problem, the clinician can suggest that it be assigned to a particular time of day or specific part of each hour rather than being allowed to pervade the day. Only a minority of patients, however, are able to achieve this segregation. In these circumstances, anxiolytic medications may be beneficial.

Psychotherapy for procrastination

Burns (1990) has written a self-instructional manual that applies these cognitive–behavioral techniques to procrastination, among other problems. Burka and Yuen (1983) have written a more detailed self-help book for procrastinators. I find it helpful to assign one or the other of these books to my procrastinating patients. I advise them to read only a section or chapter (in order to prevent the assignment from seeming overwhelming) and then return to discuss their reactions.

In the course of these discussions, I encourage the patient to implement a step-by-step approach to overcoming procrastination. The steps (as laid out in Burns, 1990) are:

- Identify a task affected by procrastination.
- List and apply weights to the advantages and disadvantages of procrastinating on this task. I use a scale of 1 to 3, which translates into "small," "medium" and "large."
- Compare the weighted sum of advantages against that of the disadvantages. Reserve judgment until after taking the next step.
- Prepare an analogous list of weighted advantages and disadvantages for starting work today, or if necessary, tomorrow (not of completing the work). The emphasis on starting precludes feeling overwhelmed, which frequently accompanies thoughts about completing a task. If the advantages of starting outweigh the disadvantages, proceed with the remaining steps. If not, the patient can conclude with relief that the task can be abandoned.
- Pick a time to start the task and write it down. Then, make a written list of all the

hindrances to starting at that time and work out a solution for each. Hindrances include other tasks, aversive feelings and negative thoughts. Cognitive distortions, such as all or none thinking, emotional reasoning (e.g., "I have to feel like doing something in order to start doing it."), and dwelling on negative, untested expectations, should be neutralized by means of rational analyses.

- Divide the task into small parts and commit only to completing one part or to spending a limited time on the task, say 15 to 30 minutes. Eschew "perfection" and commit to accepting "good."
- Give oneself credit for each portion of the task completed rather than criticizing oneself for not having completed the entire task.

Teaching OCPD patients these techniques requires patience and time. Three or four sessions at weekly intervals are often needed to establish their regular use.

Techniques for dealing with hoarding and the inability to discard objects, both of which can be symptomatic of OCPD, are described in Chapter 3.

Although the cognitive–behavioral approach to problematic behaviors of OCPD patients seems reasonable and has met with moderate success in my hands, the effectiveness of individual techniques and of this approach in general remain to be demonstrated in controlled trials.

Pharmacotherapy

Two reports begin to suggest that medications may alleviate symptoms of this personality disorder. Ansseau and Tilman (unpublished data, 149th Annual Meeting of the American Psychiatric Association, New York, 1996) conducted a 12-week double-blind trial of fluvoxamine 100 mg/day versus placebo in 24 patients with DSM-IV OCPD. The fluvoxamine group showed a 26% drop in mean score (from 18.6 to 13.7) on a 0–4 scale applied to each of the eight DSM-IV criteria for OCPD, compared to a 4% drop in the placebo group. The report does not state why the patients came for treatment or whether any no longer met OCPD diagnostic criteria.

Ricciardi et al. (1992) report that OCPD disappeared in five of six OCD patients following four months of behavioral and/or pharmacological treatment (not further described). Although the authors asked patients to distinguish between symptoms of OCD and unrelated behavioral traits in responding to a structured interview instrument, they caution that symptoms and traits may have been conflated.

For patients who are willing to take medication, the clinician should institute a 12-week trial of fluvoxamine or another selective serotonin reuptake inhibitor (SSRI) at the highest dose tolerated comfortably. The trial can begin after symptoms have been carefully explored or when several months of cognitive–behavioral or other therapy have produced little benefit. Since control is a particular issue with

Table 18.2. Obsessive compulsive personality disorder: treatment planning guidelines

- Assess the patient's motivation for seeking treatment.
- Identify problematic behaviors.
- Apply techniques of cognitive-behavioral therapy:
  - select circumscribed behavioral goals;
  - negotiate an agenda at each session;
  - prioritize problems to work on;
  - show the patient how his assumptions, perceptions and meanings bring about his feelings and behaviors;
  - ask the patient to keep a Dysfunctional Thought Record;
  - examine "automatic thoughts" and resulting problems;
  - challenge the patient's assumptions;
  - ask the patient to imagine alternative approaches to problematic situations;
  - have the patient experiment with changes in behavior;
- If worrying is a major problem, consider a trial of an anxiolytic medication.
- Consider a 12-week trial of an SSRI.

Note:
SSRI: selective serotonin reuptake inhibitor.

OCPD patients, the medication should be offered with the suggestion that it represents a way for patients to have more control over choosing responses to situations than their driven behavioral style has heretofore allowed.

Studies of the effectiveness of the SSRIs alone and combined with psychotherapies are needed. The possibility that time-limited use of an anti-anxiety medication, such as a benzodiazepine or buspirone, may be beneficial in certain circumstances also deserves exploration. Meanwhile, the limited state of our knowledge favors maintaining the flexibility and openness to new ideas that we seek to impart to patients with OCPD. Treatment planning guidelines are shown in Table 18.2.

Accessing patient education materials

Educated patients are more effective allies in the battle with their ailments. Moreover, educated patients join advocacy groups, whose work is so important to us all: lessening stigma through public education; lobbying government for research funds, work place protections and equitable insurance coverage; and, providing social support for mentally ill individuals and their families.

This Appendix is a guide to educational resources, grouped into four sections: US advocacy and informational organizations, international advocacy and information organizations, self-help and patient education materials, and Internet (world wide web) resources. In the 'international' list, the countries shown are those for which we could discover relevant organizations; the list should not therefore be taken as exhaustive.

US advocacy and informational organizations

Alcoholics Anonymous
P.O. Box 459 Grand Central Station
New York, NY 10163
Telephone: 212/870–3400
Provides educational materials, information on starting local support groups, and contact information for local support groups.

ANAD-National Association of Anorexia Nervosa and Associated Disorders
Box 7
Highland Park, IL 60035
Telephone: 708/831–3438;
Fax: 708/433–4632
National and international chapters. Provides information and advocates for services and research.

Anorexia Nervosa and Related Eating Disorders
P.O. Box 5102
Eugene, OR 97405
Telephone: 503/344–1144
Collects and disseminates information, maintains local chapters, provides medical referrals, conducts educational and training sessions for educators, civic organizations and professionals.

Anxiety Disorders Association of America
6000 Executive Blvd., Suite 513
Rockville, MD 20852
Telephone: 301/231–9350;
Fax: 301/231–7392
Provides a directory of self-help groups and a newsletter summarizing recent developments in the treatment of anxiety disorders.

Association for the Advancement of Behavior Therapy
305 7th Avenue, Suite 1601
New York, NY 10001–6008
Telephone: 212/647–1890
Provides a membership list of mental health professionals who focus on behavior therapy.

Children and Adults with Attention Deficit Disorders (CHADD)
8181 Professional Place, Suite 201
Landover, MD 20785

Telephone: 800/233–4050; 301/306–7070;
Fax: 301/306/–7090

Provides educational materials, sponsors local chapters and lobbies government for education policies that appropriately accommodate individuals with attention deficit disorder.

Council on Compulsive Gambling of New Jersey

1315 W. State Street
Trenton, NJ 08618
Telephone: 609/599–3299;
Fax: 609/599–5383

Provides education and training, and referrals nationwide for the treatment of compulsive gambling. Referral service at: 1–800/GAM-BLER (1–800/426–2537).

Debtors Anonymous

P.O. Box 400
Grand Central Station
New York, NY 10163–0400
Telephone: 212/642–8220

Provides printed material modelled on the 12-step program of Alcoholics Anonymous. Sponsors local chapter meetings.

Gam-Anon

P.O. Box 157
Whitestone, NY 11357
Telephone: 718/352–1671;
Fax: 718/352–1671

Acts as an educational and referral resource for relatives and close friends of compulsive gamblers.

Gamblers Anonymous

P.O. Box 17173
Los Angeles, CA 90017
Telephone: 213/386–8789;
Fax: 213/386–0030

Organizes local support groups for compulsive gamblers and publishes educational material. Modelled on the Alcoholics Anonymous 12-step model.

National Alliance for the Mentally Ill

200 North Globe Road, Suite 1015
Arlington, VA 22203–3754

Telephone: 800/950–6264, or 703/524–7600;
Fax: 703/524–9094

Advocates for increased funding of mental health services and research, offers educational materials including books, pamphlets and videotapes, and has local support groups.

National Depressive and Manic-Depressive Association

730 N. Franklin, Suite 501
Chicago, IL 60610
Telephone: 800/826–3632
(or, 800/82–NDMDA)

Sells an extensive list of scientific article reprints and self-help books; lobbies on behalf of patients with mood disorders.

National Mental Health Association

1021 Prince St.
Alexandria, VA 22314–2971
Telephone: 703/684–7722, or 800/969–6642;
Fax: 703/684–5968

Lobbies the federal and state governments for adequate provision of mental health care and for research funding; publishes educational pamphlets and has local chapters.

OC Foundation, Inc.

P.O. Box 70
Milford, CT 06460–0070
Telephone: 203/878–5669;
Fax: 203/874–2826

Provides an educational newsletter, publications, videotapes, list of obsessive–compulsive disorder (OCD) support groups across the United States and referral to mental health professionals with a special interest in OCD.

Obsessive Compulsive Information Center

c/o Madison Institute of Medicine
7617 Mineral Point Road, Suite 300
Madison, WI 53717
Telephone: 608/827–2470;
Fax: 608/827–2479

Provides educational publications regarding OCD, trichotillomania, body dysmorphic disorder and other mental disorders; conducts searches of the scientific literature.

Sexaholics Anonymous
P.O. Box 111910
Nashville, TN 37222
Telephone: 615/331–6230;
Fax: 615/331–6901
A recovery program modelled on the principles of Alcoholics Anonymous. Provides a kit for starting a local group, educational materials and listing of local meeting sites.

Tourette Syndrome Association, Inc.
42–40 Bell Boulevard
New York, NY 11361–2874
Telephone: 718/224–2999
Provides reprints of scientific articles, a quarterly newsletter, offers local support groups and lobbies for research funds and health benefits.

Trichotillomania Learning Center
1215 Mission St., Suite 2
Santa Cruz, CA 95060
Telephone: 831/457–1004;
e-mail: trichster@aol.com
Provides members with an information packet and a bimonthly newsletter. Sponsors educational conferences.

International advocacy and informational organizations

Mutual help groups and educational organizations for obsessive–compulsive and selected disorders, by country

We have not investigated the individuals or organizations listed here and do not endorse their competence or expertise. Unless otherwise indicated (e.g., by the organization's title), the organizations shown include a focus on obsessive–compulsive disorder.

Argentina
Asociacion Argentina de Grupos de Autoayuda
Gonzalo Laje-Rivademar, M.D.
Paraguay, 1307 4 "38"
1057 Buenos Aires
Telephone: 1/ 813 4698

Australia
New South Wales:
Mental Health Information for Rural and Remote Australia
60–62 Victoria Road
Gladsville, New South Wales 2111
Telephone: 1300/ 785 005 or 02/ 9879 5341;
Fax: 02/ 9816 4056

NSW Mental Health Information Service (INC)
60–62 Victoria Road
Gladsville, New South Wales 2111
Telephone: 1800/ 674 200 or 02/ 9816 5688;
Fax: 02/ 9816 4056

Anxiety Disorders Foundation of Australia
P.O. Box 6198 Shopping World,
New South Wales 2060
Telephone: 016/ 282 897; Fax: 02/ 9716 0416

Northern Territory:
Northern Territory Association for Mental Health
Suite 2, Mallan Chambers
26 Mitchell Street
Darwin, NT 0800
Telephone 08/ 8981 4128; Fax: 08/ 8981 4933

Queensland:
Queensland Association for Mental Health
20 Balfour Street
New Farm, Queensland 4005
Telephone: 07/ 3358 4988; Fax: 07/ 3254 1027

South Australia:
Obsessive–Compulsive Disorders Support
Service
Room 318, Epworth Building
33 Pirie Street
Adelaide, South Australia 5000
Telephone: 08/ 8231 1588

Tasmania:
The Mental Health Community Resource
Centre
97 Campbell Street
Hobart, TAS 7000
Telephone: 03/ 6233 4041

Victoria:
Obsessive Compulsive & Anxiety Disorders
Foundation of Victoria (Inc)
600 Orrong Road
Armadale, VIC 3143
Telephone: 03/ 9576 2477;
Fax: 03/ 9576 2499

Mental Health Centre
1 Cookson Street
Camberwell, VIC 3124
Telephone: 03/ 813 3736

Mental Health Foundation Victoria
270 Church Street
Richmond, VIC 3121
Telephone: 03/ 9427 0407;
Fax: 03/ 9427 1294

Western Australia:
Co-ordinator
Western Australia OCD Group
Telephone: 09/ 385 7081

Western Australian Association for Mental
Health
305/79 Stirling Street
Perth, WA 6000
Telephone: 08/ 9228 2250;
Fax: 08/ 9228 2253

Austria
Club D & A [for depression and manic
depression]
Ms. Carla Stanck
Schwindgasse 5
Vienna
Telephone: 1/ 5044 4680

Belgium
Mr. Stefaan Theeuus
Vlaanse Vereniging Manisch Depressieven
Maria Theristrasstrasse 53
B 3000 Leuven
Telephone: 16/ 205 749

Brazil
ASTOC
Associado de Portadores de Sindrome de
Tourette, Tiques E
Trastornos Obsessivo Compulsivo
c/o: Maria C. De Luca Pereira, Presidente
Rua Dr. Ovidio Pires de Campos S/NE
30 A Sala 4025
Sao Paolo
Telephone: 11/ 280 9198; Fax: 11/ 280 0842

Canada
Manitoba:
OC Information and Support Center
c/o Manitoba Clearinghouse
Telephone: 204/ 772–6979;
Fax: 204/ 786–0860

Ontario:
Obsessive–Compulsive Disorders Network
P.O. Box 151
Markham, Ontario L3P 3J7
Telephone: 905/ 472–0494

Free from Fear or The Anxiety Disorders
Network
1848 Liverpool Road, Suite 199
Pickering, Ontario L1V 6M3
Telephone: 905/ 831–3877

Czech Republic

No patient organization exists. Treatment centers:

Medical Faculty of Charles University
Department of Psychiatry
500 05 Hradec Králové
Telephone: 49/ 583 2228; Fax: 49/ 551 1677

Prague Psychiatric Center
Ùstavhí 91
181 03 Prague 8
Telephone: 2/ 6600 3361; Fax: 2/ 6600 3366

1st Medical Faculty of Charles University
Department of Psychiatry
Ke Karlovu 11
128 21 Prague 2
Telephone: 2/ 2491 4120; Fax: 2/ 2491 0577

Egypt

No patient organization exists. Contact:
A. Okasha, M.D.
3, Shawarby Stret
Kasr El Nil
Cairo
Telephone: 2/ 710 233 or 710 605;
Fax: 2/ 348 1786

France

Association Française des Troubles
Obsessionnels Compulsifs
24, rue Léon Gambetta
59790 Ronchin
France
Telephone: 03/ 20 85 96 42;
Fax: 03/ 20 85 96 42

Ms. Agnès Lecarpentier, Présidence
Association Française de personnes atteintes
de Troubles Obsessionnels et Compulsifs
Cidex 15
14610 Villons les Buissons
Telephone: 02/ 31 44 03 81;
e-mail: aftoc@mail.cpod.fr

Germany

OCA Group
c/o Ms. Cordula Muller
Bornheimer Strasse 130
Bonn, Germany
Telephone: 02241/336 424

Deutsche Gesellschaft Zwangserkrankungen
E.V.
Post Fach 1545
49005 Osnabruck
Telephone: 0541/409 66 33

Hungary

No patient organization exists. Contact:
Atila Németh, M.D.
Haynal Imre University of Health
Nyéki út 10–12
1021 Budapest
Telephone: 1/ 176 3406; Fax: 1/ 393 0281

A Kényszerbeteg Ambulancia és Információs
Központ
1525 Budapest 114, Pf.: 864
Telephone: 115–8606 or 115–8466

Israel

No patient organization exists. Contact:
Professor Joseph Zohar, M.D.
Departmnet of Psychiatry
Chaim Sheba Medical Center
Tel-Hashomer 56261
Telephone: 3/ 530 3300; Fax: 3/ 535 2788

Italy

No patient organization exists. Contact:
Stefano Pallanti, M.D.
Istituto di Neuroscienze
Viale Ugo Bassi 1
50137 Firenze
Telephone: 055/ 587 889; Fax: 055/ 581 051;
e-mail: s.pallanti@agora.stm.it

Paolo L. Morselli, M.D.
IDEA
via Statuto 8
20121 Milano
Telephone: 02/ 65 3994; Fax: 02/ 65 4716

Donatella Marazziti, M.D.
Instituto di Clinica Psichiatrica
Universitá degli Studi di Pisa
Via Roma, 67
56100 Pisa
Telephone: 050/ 553 388; Fax: 050/ 21581

L. Ravizza, M.D.
Isituto di Clinica Psichiatrica
Universitá degli Studi di Torino
Via Cherasco 11
Torino 10126
Telephone: 011/ 634 848; Fax: 011/ 673 473

Netherlands
Mr. Fred Bos
NSMD (depression and manic depression)
P.O. Box 380
NL 1115 ZH Duivendrecht
Telephone: 20/ 69 00 710; Fax: 20/ 69 57 496

New Zealand
O.C.D.S.G.
P.O. Box 4195
Christchurch
Telephone: 366 0560

Norway
Ananke Norway (in Norwegian)
e-mail: ananke@geocities.org
website: *http://www.bounce.to/ananke*

Puerto Rico
NAMI III of Puerto Rico
P.O. Box 902
2569 Viejo San Juan
Puerto Rico 00902
Telephone: 787/ 745 1760;
Fax: 787/ 743 8475;
e-mail: prami5185@aol.com

Singapore
Singapore Association for Mental Health
Block 69, Lorong 4, Toa Payoh #01–365
Singapore 1231
Telephone: 255 3222

South Africa
Ms. Janet Serebro, Chairperson
OCD Association of South Africa
P.O. Box 87127 Houghton,
2041, Johannesburg
Telephone: 11/ 786 6617; Fax: 11/ 887 3678

Sweden
Föreningen ANANKE
Box 7070
S-720 25 Västeras
Telephone: 08/ 628 30 30; e-mail:
eriksson@ananke.org
website: *http://www.ananke.org/information.*
   html

Ms. Barbro Gill-Larsson, Chairman
Rikstoreningen Ananke
Box 7003
S-172 07 Sundbyberg
Telephone: 08/ 628 3030; Fax: 08/ 628 3030

Switzerland
Mr. John Kummer
SHG Depression/Zug
Zimmelstrasse 48
CH-6314, Unteraegeri
Telephone: 41/ 750 0004; Fax: 41/ 750 0245

United Kingdom
England:
Ms. Celia Bonham Christie
Telephone: 0225/ 314 129
Meets at: Royal National Hospital for
Rheumatic Diseases,
(Main Upper Boro Walls), Bath

Ms. Kathleen Savory
Telephone: 091/ 389 1765
Meets at: Durham Health Center, Chester

Phobic Action
Hornbeam House, Claybury Grounds
Manor Road
Woodford Green
Essex IG8 8PR
Provides a national telephone helpline
service

Ms. Michelle Rowett
Manic Depressive Fellowship
8–10 High Street
Kingston upon Thames
Surrey, KT1 1EY
Telephone: 81/ 974–6550; Fax: 81/ 974–6600

Support People
Ms. Laura Olivieri, Administrator/Editor
P.O.Box 6097
London W2 1WZ

Mr. Rodney Elgie
Depression Alliance
309 The Chandlery
50 Westminster Bridge Road
London SE1 7QY
Telephone: 0171/ 721 7411;
Fax: 0171/ 721 7629

No Panic
92 Brands Farm Way
Randlay, Telford
Shropshire TF3 2JQ
Telephone: 01952/ 590 005;
Fax: 01952/ 270 962

Ms. Terri Conley
Wallsend Self-Help Group
P.O.Box 5
Wallsend
Tyne and Wear NE28 6DZ

First Steps to Freedom
22 Randall Road
Kenilworth
Warwickshire CV8 1JY
Telephone: 01926/ 851 608

Ms. Sue Scerri
Worcester Park,
Surrey
Telephone: 081/ 337 2362

Scotland:
Mr. Rob Hughes
Carer's Centre, Belmont Street
Aberdeen
Telephone: 404/ 057 01224

Ms. Jamie Booth
1277 Dumbarton Road
Glasgow G1R 9VY

Mr. James McGinley
Time Out Scotland (depression and manic
depression)
c/o GCVS,
11 Queens Crescent
Glasgow G4 9AS
Telephone: 0141/ 337 2521;
Fax: 0141/ 958 0379

Wales:
Manic Depression Fellowship Wales
St. Cadoc's Hospital
Caerleon, Newport
Gwent NP6 1XQ
Telephone: 01633/ 430 430;
Fax: 01633/ 430 353

D.M. Bonney
Meets at: The Elms Centre, Four Elms Street
Cardiff, S. Glamorgan
Telephone: 01446/ 722 941

Zimbabwe

Department of Psychiatry
University of Zimbabwe
P.O. Box A 178
Avondale
Harare
Telephone: 4/ 791 631; Fax: 4/ 724 912

Tourette Syndrome Association: international contacts

Argentina

Oscar Gershanik, M.D.
Fundacion Thomson
La Rioja 951
Capital Federal
Buenos Aires

Lic. Luisa Osdoba
Donato Alvarez 205
Cap. Fed (1406) 2°C
Buenos Aires

Guillermo Tyberg
Fax: +54 1/773 3147

Australia
Tourette Syndrome Association of Victoria Inc.
34 Jackson Street
Toorak 3142, Victoria
Tel. +03/9828 7218;
Fax: +03/9826 9054

Tourette Syndrome Association of Australia
PO Box 1173
Maroubra, NSW 2035
Tel/Fax: +02 9311 2745

Western Australian Tourette Syndrome Organisation, Inc.
Paul M. Smith, President
Neurological Lotteries House
320 Rokeby Road
Subiaco, W.A. 6008
Tel: +61 8/9388 3486; Fax: +61 8/9382 1149;
e-mail: ncwa@cygnus.uwa.edu.au

Dr. Michael Beech
Raymond Terrace, South Brisbane,
Queensland 4101
Tel: 07/3840 8188; Fax: 07/3840 8333

Austria
Mara Stamenkovic, M.D.; Schindler Shird, M.D.
Department of General Psychiatry
Vienna University Hospital of Psychiatry
Wahringergurtel 18–20
A-1090 Vienna
Tel: +43 140/400 3526;
Fax: +43 140/400 3560

Belgium
Gilles de la TOURETTE
Vera Casier Cassimon, Pres. (Flemish)
Vlaamse Vereniging Gilles de la Tourette
v.z.w. – J. Nauwelaertstraat, 7
2210 Wijnegen
Tel: +32 3/354 3669; Fax: +32 3/353 6791

Patricia Seminerio (French)
17 Avenue Bel Horizon
1301 Bierges/Wavre
Tel/Fax: +32 10/41 7052

Bermuda
Carmen Phillips
27 Clarendon Road
Smiths FL04

Brazil
Euripedes C. Miguel, MD, Ph.D.
PROTOC do IPQ-HCFMUSP
Rua Ovidio Pires de Campos, s/n° -sala 4025
05403-010 Sao Paulo, SP
Tel/Fax: +55 11/853 3531

Christina de Luca/Maura de Carvallo
Rua Bras Cardoso 201
Sao Paulo
Cep. 04510-030
Fax: 5511/822 0023

Bulgaria
Dr. Dimiter Terziev
Child Psychiatric Clinic
33, Prohlada Street
16169 – Sofia

Canada
TS Foundation of Canada
Rosie Wartecker, Executive Director
194 Jarvis Street, Suite 206
Toronto, Ontario M5B 2B7
Tel: 416/861 8398; Fax: 416/861 2472;
e-mail: tsfc.org@sympatico.ca

Chile
Carla Hendee
Casilla 342
Maipu

China
Dr. Liu Zhisheng
Department of Neurology
Wuhan Children's Hospital
No. 213 Qiu Chang Road
Hubei 430016

Zhang Shi Ji, M.D.
Beijing Child and Adolescent Mental Health
Center
5, Ankang Avenue, De Sheng Men Wai
Beijing 100088
Tel: +86 10 6425 5034

Shu-Yin Chen
No. 7-1, Lane 49, Ming Chung Street
Hsin Chung City, Taipei Hsien
Taiwan, R.O.C.
Fax: +886 2/993 4984

Colombia
Maria Alicia Irequi
Apartado Ae'reo 250914
Bogota
Tel: +57 1/310 6616

Croatia
Dubravka Kocijan
Clinic Hospital Dubrava
Aleja Izvidsca 6
10000 Zagreb

Cyprus
Angela Charalambous
Adrocleous 15
Flat 102
Nicosia
Tel: +003/572 466750; Fax: +003/572 362488

Denmark
Kjeld Christensen, President
Dansk Tourette Forening
Prestehusene 31
DK 2820
Tel: +45 43/96 57 09

Kirsten Kristensen
Sollerodvej 7B
DK 2840 Holte
Tel: +45 45/80 07 53

Ecuador
Vicente Maldonado
Lizardo Garcia
328 y 6 de Diciembre
Quito

Finland
Eila Niemi
Project Secretary
The Finnish MS-Society
Seppalantie 90, Masku
PO Box 15, SF-21251 Masku
Tel: +358 21/439 2111;
Fax: +358 21/439 2112

Kenneth Carlberg
Manager, Kurscentret Hogsand
FS 10 820 Hogsand
Tel: +358 19/244 3800;
Fax: +358 19/244 3740

France
Bridget Haardt
Aftoc-Tourette
17, rue Paule Borghese
F 92200 Neuilly Sur Seine
Tel: +33-1-47-38-29-08;
Fax: +33-1-47-38-18-10

Germany
Prof. Dr. A. Rothenberger, Vice President
Tourette Gesellschaft Deutschland
Universitat Gottingen
Abteilung fur Kinder und
Jugendpsychiatrie
von-Siebold-Str. 5
D 37075 Gottingen

Karl Joseph
Stolting Hof 1
D 30 455 Hannover
Tel: +49-511-486-262

Johannes Hebebrand, M.D.
Dept. of Child & Adolescent Psychiatry
Philipps University of Marburg
Mans-Sachs-Str. 6
D-35033, Marburg
Tel: +49-6421-286-466;
Fax: +49-6421-283-056;
e-mail: jonas@mvkjp2.kjp.uni.marburg.de

Christian Hempel
Am Sande 40/41
Lueneburg, D
e-mail: chempel@uni-lueneburg.de

Iceland

Elisabeth K. Magnusdottir, President
Tourette Samtokin a Islandi
Postholf 3128
IS 123 Reykjavik
Tel: +354/588-8581; Fax: 354/551-4580

India

Mrs. Jaishri Iyer
No. 154, S.F.S. (208), G.K.V.K. Post
Yelahanka, Bangalore-560065
Tel: +91-80-846-2392

Iraq

Ali Maziad Abd. Al. Azeez
P.O. Box 46114
Postal code 12506
Al-Mustansiriya University
Baghdad
Tel: +964-1-541-5591 (work),
+964-1-425-7119 (home)

Ireland

John Owens
Chief Psychiatrist, St. Darnetts Hospital
Monaghan
Tel: +353-47-81-822; Fax: +353-47-81-527

Tourette Syndrome Association of Ireland
39, Elderwood Road
Palmerstown, Dublin 20
Tel: +01-626-4564

Mrs. Una Finucane
29 Granville Road
Dun Laoghaire
Co Dublin
Tel: +353-1-285-2193;
Fax: 353-1-808-2578 (c/o Brendan)

Israel

TSA of Israel
P.O. Box 7018
Ramat Gan 52170
Tel: +740-8478

Nahum Muskat
Fax: +00972-6-341466

Italy

Prof. Michele Zappella
Department of Child Neuropsychiatry
Via Mattioli 10
53100 Siena

Japan

Masako Kaji
Dystonia Support Group of Japan
2-1917 Sencho
Ohtsu-City Shiga 520
Tel: +81-775-33-0297; Fax: +81-775-33-0297

Dr. Masaya Segawa/Dr. Yoshiko Nomura
Segawa Neurological Clinic for Children
2-8 Surugadai, Kanda
Chiyoda-Ku, Tokyo 101
Tel: +81-3-294-0317; Fax: +81-3-294-0290

Mr. and Mrs. J. Dando
Yagoto Shataku East A401
4-17 Yamate Dori, Showa Ku
Nagoya Shi, Aichi 466
Tel: +052-834-4670

Korea (South)

Professor Michael Hong
Seoul National Univ/ Children's Hospital
Div. of Child & Adolescent Psychiatry
28 Yongon-Dong, Chongno-gu
Seoul 110-744
Tel: +82-2-760-3647; Fax: +82-2-747-5774

Soo Churl Cho, M.D.
Dept. of Neuropsychiatry
College of Medicine
Seoul National University
#28 Yeongun-Dong, Chongro
Seoul 110-744

Young-Suk Paik, M.D.
Wonkwang Univ. Neuropsychiatric Hospital
144-23 Dongsan-dong, Iksan
Chonpuk 570-060
Tel: +(653) 840-6005; Fax: +(653) 840-6069

Libya

Dr. A. Alsanossi
P.O. Box 20240, Sebha

Lithuania

Valmantes Budrys, MD, Ph.D.
Vilnius University Hospital
Santariskiu Klinikos
Santariskiu gatve 2
LT 2600 Vilnius

Mexico

Dr. Jesus Gomez-Plascencia
Eclipse 2745 J. Del Bosque
Guadalajara, Jal 44520
Tel: +3-684-3337; e-mail:
jgomezp@udgserv.cencar.udg.mx

Mozambique

Galen Carey and Delia Realmo
Caixa Postal 680
Maputo, Mozambique
Tel: +258-1-49-29-67 or +258-1-49-27-25;
Fax: +258-1-49-29-74;
e-mail: carey@zebra.uem.mz

Netherlands

Hans Eijsacher, President
Stichting Gilles de la Tourette
de Schans 20
3144 ET Maassleus
Tel: +31-10-591-5278

Ben B.J.M. van de Wetering, MD, Ph.D.
Dept. of Psychiatry - Outpatient Service
Univ. Hospital Rotterdan-Dijkzigt
Dr. Molewaterplein 40
3015 GD Rotterdam
Tel: +31-10-463-5871; Fax: +31-10-463-5867

New Zealand

David and Caroline Ashby
258 Kennedy Road
Napier

Norway

H.C.A. Melbye, International Contact
Munkerudasen 33
N 1165 Oslo
Tel/Fax: +47-22-285-043

Tom A. Wulff, President
Norsk Tourette Forening
Brolandsveien 19 B
N-0980 Oslo
Tel: +47-22-216-506; Fax: +47-22-109-921;
e-mail: tomwulff@online.no

Paraguay

Jose Raul Torres Kirmser
Avenida General Santos u-330
Ansuncion

Peru

Norka Lopez
La Chalanaa 225
La Molina
Lima 12
Fax: +51-1-479-0430

Luisa Fernanda L. de Romana, Gen. Sec.
Associacion Sindrome de Tourette del Peru
Las Golondrinas #390
Lima 27
Fax: +51-1-224-7567

Poland

Kalina Michalkiewicz
ul. Plocka 12 m 51
01-231 Warszawa

Ewa Boguszewska
ul. Kostrzewskiego 1 m. 58
00-768 Warszawa
Tel: +48-22-651-4154

Puerto Rico

Flora Santiago
Esmerelda #52, Villa Blanca
Caguas 00725

Russia

Janna Baranovskaja
Tel: +7-095-267-7083 (work),
+7-095-218-6566 (home);
Fax: +7-501-940-2310

South Africa

Johan van der Westhuizen, President
South Africa Tourette Syndrome Institute
(SATSI)
228 Oak Avenue
Ferndale, 2194
Tel: +27-11-886-6353

Izelda Pelser
Neurogenetic Clinic
Institute for Pathology Building
P.O. Box 2034
Pretoria 0001
Tel: +27-12-324-5060; Fax: +27-12-323-2788

George S. Gericke, MBChB. MMed.
Prof. and Head, Dept. of Human Genetics
and Developmental Biology
Univeristy of Pretoria
P.O. Box 2034, Pretoria 0001
Tel: +012-329-1111; Fax: +012-329-1343

Ellen Nortje
P.O. Box 26529, Hout Bay 7872
Cape Province
Tel: +27-21-790-2502

Spain

Eduardo Tolosa, M.D.
Neurology Service, Hospital Clinico
1 Provincial de Barcelona
Villaroel, 170-08036 Barcelona
Tel: +34-3-227-5400; Fax: +34-3-227-5454

Jaime Diaz Guzman, M.D.
Servicio de Neurologia
Hospital Universitario Doce de Octubre
Carretera de Andalucia Km 5,400
28041 Madrid

Sweden

Ulf Christiansson
The Swedish Tourette Association
Soerkroken 2,
S-440 74 Hjaelteby
Tel: +46-304-678-130; Fax: +46-304-678-130; e-mail: ulf.c@kpab.se

Svensk Tourette Forening
Kungsgardets sjukhus
St. Johannesgatan 28
S-752 33 Uppsala
e-mail: info@tourette.se

Marie Ashker, President
Svenskk Tourette Forening
Stora Askeron 8271
S-471 75 Hjalteby
Tel: +46-303-77-20-96;
e-mail: asker@ebox.tninet.se

Switzerland

Guido Hilfiker, President
Tourette Gesellschaft Schweiz
Dorfstrasse 64
CH 8912 Obfelden
Tel: +41-1-760-0265

Jurg Timm
Tel: +41-71-722-2506

Gigi Kundert
Tel: +41-52-376-1077

Turkey

M. Yanki Yazgan, M.D.
Marmara University
Faculty of Psychiatry
Altunizade, Istanbul 81190
Tel: +90-216-332-2553

United Kingdom

Paul Smith, National Coordinator
Iain Steedman, General Secretary
Tourette Syndrome (UK) Association
1st Floor Offices, Old Bank Chambers
London Road, Crowborough
East Sussex
TN6 2TT
Tel: +44/1892 669 151; Fax: +44/1892 663
649; e-mail: 101667.3131@compuserve.com

Chris Mansley
Watling Street, Fulwood
Preston, Lancs

Zimbabwe

Peter Perry
P.O. Box M187
Mabelreign, Harare
Tel/Fax: +263-4-741-884

Self-help and patient education materials

Information published by the federal government's National Institute of Mental Health (NIMH) is available at no cost by writing:

Information Resources and Inquiries Branch
National Institute of Mental Health
5600 Fishers Lane, Room 7C-02
Rockville, MD 20857
Telephone: 888/826–9438 (or, 88–88–ANXIETY)

See also the NIMH World Wide Web address: *www.nimh.nih.gov/publicat/*

Books for patients with specific disorders

Body dysmorphic disorder

Phillips, K.A. (1996). *The Broken Mirror: Understanding and Treating Body Dysmorphic Disorder.* New York: Oxford University Press.

Compulsive buying

Damon, J.E. (1988). *Shopaholics: Serious Help for Addicted Spenders.* Los Angeles: Price Stein Sloan.
Wesson, C. (1990). *Women Who Shop too Much: Overcoming the Urge to Splurge.* New York: St. Martin's Press.

Compulsive gambling

Berman, L. and Siegel, M. (1992). *Behind the 8-ball: A guide for Families of Gamblers.* New York: Fireside/Parkside.

Hypochondriasis

Cantor, C. and Fallon, B.A. (1996). *Phantom Illness: Shattering the Myth of Hypochondria.* Boston: Houghton Mifflin Company.

Mood disorders

Burns, D.D. (1989). *The Feeling Good Handbook.* New York: Plume (Penguin).
Greist, H.H. and Jefferson, J.W. (1992). *Depression and Its Treatment.* Washington DC: American Psychiatric Press, Inc.
Papolos, D. (1996). *Overcoming Depression.* 3rd. edn. New York: Harper Collins.

Obsessive–compulsive disorder

Baer, L. (1991). *Getting Control: Overcoming Your Obsessions and Compulsions.* New York: Plume (Penguin).
Ciarrocchi, J.W. (1995). *The Doubting Disease: Help for Scrupulosity and Religious Compulsions.* Mahwah, NJ: Paulist Press.
Foa, E.B. and Wilson R. (1991). *Stop Obsessing! How to Overcome Your Obsessions and Compulsions.* New York: Bantam Books.
Schwartz, J.M. (1996). *Brain Lock: Free Yourself from Obsessive–Compulsive Behavior.* New York: Harper Collins.
Stekatee, G. and White, K. (1990). *When Once Is Not Enough: Help for Obsessive Compulsives.* Oakland, CA: New Harbinger Publications, Inc.

Panic disorder

Sheehan, D.V. (1986). *The Anxiety Disease.* New York: Bantam Books.

Procrastination

Burka, J. and Yuen, L. (1983). *Procrastination: Why You Do It, What To Do About It.* Reading, MA: Addison-Wesley.

Social phobia

Schneier, F. and Welkowitz, L. (1996). *The Hidden Face of Shyness: Understanding and Overcoming*

Social Anxiety. New York: Avon Books (Hearst Corporation Press).

Zimbardo, P.G. (1987). *Shyness, What It Is, What To Do About It*. Reading, MA: Addison-Wesley.

Trichotillomania

Salazar, C. (1996). *You Are Not Alone: Compulsive Hair Pulling, The Enemy Within*. Carmichael, CA: Rophe Press.

A review of selected books for patients and families can be found in:

Reavis, P.A., Epstein, B.A. and Piotrowicz, L.M. (1995). Selected books on mental illness and treatment for patients and their families. *Psychiatr. Serv.*, **46**:1292–302.

Internet (world wide web) resources

Patients with access to the Internet can tap into a nearly limitless sea of information. Since anyone with a modicum of technological expertise can post on the Web whatever information, assertion or opinion he or she wishes, the Web reader must be prepared to be cautious and skeptical. While truth overwhelms falsehood and error in the long-run, in the short-run the Internet browser must beware. We cannot vouch for the accuracy of all of the information on any site listed, either at the time of this writing or when this Appendix is read. Still, we believe that the following sites will be found to be useful and, in the main, trustworthy. The sites for patients are organized by mental disorder categories. The clinician is urged to visit a site before recommending it to a patient.

Sites providing broad access or information more suited to clinicians than patients

http://www.mentalhealth.com
An online encyclopedia concerning the most common mental disorders and the most commonly prescribed psychotropic drugs. The information about treatments reflects the biases of the psychiatric author. The site's Mental Health Magazine contains news from other Internet newspapers and magazines and online booklets from professional organizations and support groups. The site has good links to other mental health sites.

Mental Health Net
http://www.cmhc.com
http://www.mhnet.org (same organization as above.)
One of the largest and most comprehensive guides to mental health information and resources online, featuring about 6000 resources on the Internet. Also includes self-help resources, a reading room, discussion groups and a searchable calendar of events related to specific mental disorders.

Mental Health Information Center
http://www.mhsource.com/
Published by CME Inc., the site contains an ask-the-expert forum, a chat room for discussing psychiatric topics, educational material and an alphabetical directory of World Wide Web links organized by topic. The site's OCD page,
http://www.mhsource.com/disorders/ocd.html,
features answers by experts to questions about OCD-related problems.

Mental Health Resources at Western Psychiatric Institute, Pittsburgh
http://www.wpic.pitt.edu/psychiat.htm
The site lists Internet directories, access to U.S. government research sites, online text of the *British Medical Journal*, slides prepared by members of the Department of Psychiatry for lectures on selected mental disorders, and information about ongoing research at Western Psychiatric Institute and Clinic.

National Library of Medicine Hyperdoc
http://www.nlm.nih.gov
The federal government's National Library of Medicine site provides access to the Library's book catalogue and to Medline and other online databases, allowing bibliographic searches of the world's published medical journal articles.

Pharminfonet,
http://www.pharminfo.com/
The site contains information about drug uses and side effects, with a focus on news releases regarding new drug therapies. The site has links to various information centers regarding classes of medications and specific drugs.

Psychopharmacology
http://uhs.bsd.uchicago.edu/dr-bob/tips/tips.html
From the University of Chicago, Department of Psychiatry. The site contains psychopharmacology tips posted by the Interpsych psychopharmacology discussion groups run by Ivan Goldberg, M.D., and access to detailed drug monographs. The site's search engine can search for a specific category of drugs or a side effect posted on its bulletin board.

Psychopharmacology
http://www.psycom.net/depression.central.html
This site, which is devoted to mood disorders, is managed by Ivan Goldberg, M.D., and is an excellent source of online psychopharmacology articles, psychopharmacology tips e-mailed in by clinicians, and links to other psychopharmacology sites.

Sites that can be recommended to patients

National Alliance for the Mentally Ill
http://www.nami.org
NAMI's site contains information about mental illnesses in general, an online helpline, summaries of recent news stories and news releases, an online bookstore and a list of local affiliates and family support groups.

National Mental Health Association
http://www.nmha.org
The site provides a list of local affiliates, titles of free educational pamphlets and of pamphlets and books for sale, and a current list of issues before the federal and state governments, with the names and addresses of public officials to write.

Alcohol and substance abuse

Alcoholics Anonymous
http://www.alcoholics-anonymous.org
This site provides a description of Alcoholics Anonymous, a list of available literature, and descriptions of AA philosophy, the 12-step method, and AA meetings.

Online AA Resources
http://www.recovery.org/aa/homepage.html
This site is not endorsed by Alcoholics Anonymous World Services, Inc., but provides information on AA, online AA literature, regional AA resources, event information, AA Intergroup telephone numbers for locating local groups, and links to AA sites.

Anxiety disorders

Mental Health Net
http://www.cmhc.com
http://www.mhnet.org (the same organization)
One of the largest and most comprehensive guides to mental health information and resources online, featuring about 6000 resources on the Internet. Also includes self-help resources, a reading room, discussion groups, a searchable calendar of events related to specific mental disorders.

National Anxiety Foundation
http://www.lexington-on-line.cme/naf.html
This site provides limited but accurate information on panic disorder and obsessive–compulsive disorder screened by a professional board of advisors.
NPAD, Inc.
http://www.npadnews.com

This site offers a subscription to *NPAD News*, a periodical offering lay audiences current summaries of research; book reviews; articles about medications and behavioral therapies; and, self-help resources, all reviewed by a professional advisory board. The site contains an index to articles published in *NPAD News*.

Royal College of Psychiatrists
http://www.ex.ac.uk/CIMH/help/help.htm
The British Royal College of Psychiatrists offers online educational pamphlets on a variety of mental disorders, termed the "Help is at Hand," leaflet series.

Attention deficit disorder

Children and Adults with Attention Deficit Disorders (CH.A.D.D.)
http://www.chadd.org/
Children and Adults with Attention Deficit Disorders (CH.A.D.D.) is a nonprofit, parent-based organization formed to better the lives of individuals with attention deficit disorders and those who care for them. The site offers online information, access to chapters, a bookstore, full text of U.S. government publications on attention deficit disorder and links to other sources of information.

National Attention-Deficit Disorder Association
http://www.add.org
The site offers information, a bookstore, a calendar of events and access to support groups.

Depressive disorders

Mental Health Net
http://www.cmhc.com
http://www.mhnet.org (same organization)
See description under 'Anxiety disorders'.

National Depressive and Manic Depressive Association
http://www.ndmda.org
The site offers an overview of depressive and bipolar disorders, online educational booklets, an online bookstore and access to local chapters.

Royal College of Psychiatrists
http://www.ex.ac.uk/CIMH/help/help.htm
The British Royal College of Psychiatrists offers online educational pamphlets on a variety of mental disorders, termed the "Help is at Hand," leaflet series.

Eating disorders

Mental Health Net
http://www.cmhc.com/guide/eating.htm
See description under 'Anxiety disorders'.

Nonparaphilic sexual disorders

Sexaholics Anonymous
http://www.sa.org
The site provides access to meetings across the United States which are modelled on the 12-step groups of Alcoholics Anonymous. The site also offers publications in English and Spanish.

Sexual Addicts Anonymous
http://www.sexaa.org
The site provides access to local chapter meetings and literature.

Sexual Compulsives Anonymous (SCA)
http://www.sca-recovery.org/
The site provides a calendar, a list of meetings of the society, information about how to organize local meetings and a pen pal program controlled by SCA.

The National Council on Sexual Addiction and Compulsivity,
http://www.ncsac.org/
The site provides information about sexual compulsions, their symptoms, diagnosis and treatment; addresses of 12-step programs for support and treatment; and, recommendations for reading.

Obsessive compulsive disorder

Obsessive–Compulsive Foundation
http://www.ocfoundation.org
The site provides comprehensive information about OCD, access to informational booklets, a list of OCD support groups across the United States, an online calendar of OCD-related events, the *OCF Newsletter* online and a list of OCF publications, which can be

ordered by mail. The site also provides information on trichotillomania.

OCD
http://www.fairlite.com/ocd/
The Fairlite OCD site includes an OCD and a tri-chotillomania page, quotes on OCD and links to other Internet resources on OCD. The site discusses anti-OCD medications, contains abstracts from medical journals (not necessarily current), articles on OCD written by people with the disorder, and a useful bulletin board on which patients can chat online with others interested in OCD. The site includes information about organizations that help people who cannot afford medications.

Obsessive Compulsive Anonymous (OCA)
http://members.aol.com/west24th/index.html
The homepage of OCA, a support organization, pro-vides access to local chapter meetings and links to other OCD-related sites.

National Institute of Mental Health (NIMH), OCD page,
http://www.nimh.nih.gov/publicat/ocd.htm
The NIMH is part of the National Institutes of Health (NIH), the federal Government's primary agency for biomedical and behavioral research. The Web site contains information on OCD and other common psychiatric disorders. The OCD page describes the definition, biology, presentation and treatment of OCD as well as case examples. The site also contains addresses for support groups and government offices dealing with job accommoda-tion for OCD patients.

Pathological gambling
Gamblers Anonymous
http://www.gamblersanonymous.org
The Web site of Gamblers Anonymous provides access to local meetings, which are modelled on the 12-step methods of Alcoholics Anonymous. The site provides limited information about pathological gambling, describes the 12-step program and has a self-test.

http://www.mentalhealth.com/mag1/p5h-gam1.html
A 1996 article from the Harvard Mental Health Letter describing pathological gambling and its treatment. Somewhat formal, but useful.
http://www.800gambler.org/
This site, sponsored by the Council On Compulsive Gambling Of New Jersey, provides related articles for the lay public, a directory of other state Councils on Compulsive Gambling and links to related sites.

Social phobia
Mental Health Net
http://www.cmhc.com
http://www.mhnet.org (same organization)
See description under 'Anxiety disorders'.

Trichotillomania
The Trichotillomania Learning Center
http://www.trich.org
The site provides basic information about tri-chotillomania, a calendar of events related to the dis-order, access to a videotape made by sufferers to explain their experiences, information about Learning Center membership, and links to other sites.

Trichotillomania
http://www.fairlite.com/trich/
This site within the fairlite site contain information on trichotillomania and a bulletin board, where people who wish to can share their experiences and ideas.

Autosubscription to a trichotillomania mailing list.
http://www.cmhcsys.com/guide/trich.htm
If a patient wishes to become a member of a mailing list that specifically focuses on trichotillomania and to participate in the online exchange, this site pro-vides the means to subscribe.

Tourette's syndrome
National Tourette Syndrome Association, Inc.
http://tsa.mgh.harvard.edu
This site, maintained at the Harvard-affiliated Massachusetts General Hospital, contains a brief

description of the syndrome, a glossary, frequently asked questions in English, Spanish and French, descriptions of famous individuals who have had Tourette's syndrome, a calendar of events and access to chapters around the United States.

> *Tourette in Mentalhealth*
> *http://www.mentalhealth.com/book/p40–gtor. html*

The site offers information on diagnosis and treatment, videotapes and books about Tourette's syndrome (TS), an annual review of published scientific articles and journal abstracts grouped by subject (e.g. TS and stimulants). The site also contains the National TSA's quarterly *Newsletter*, which features references to scientific articles related to TS, OCD and attention deficit disorder. There is also page about insurance benefits and TS organizations working on this issue.

Usenet groups

Usenet is an international and extremely large, decentralized information utility. It hosts well over 1200 newsgroups, and several thousand pages of new technical articles, news and discussion are added daily. Because of this daily volume, the messages cannot be kept indefinitely for online access and expire after a time. The information in Usenet groups has not been filtered or verified for accuracy by experts or professionals. It simply represents the opinions of the individuals who post the information and should not be relied upon as if it were professional medical advice.

Usenet groups can be 'unmoderated' (anyone can post a message) or 'moderated' (submissions are automatically directed to a moderator, who edits and then posts the results). Some newsgroups have parallel mailing lists for Internet users with no netnews access; the postings to the group are automatically propagated to the e-mail list and vice versa. More than anything else, Usenet is an electronic community. A patient can browse through a news group or search it using one of the search engines.

One must have an Internet access and a news group server (provided by a local Internet service provider) to be able to read or post messages on most newsgroups. Look for the keyword "usenet" on the server. Unlike mailing lists, one does not have to subscribe to a Usenet newsgroup to read it or post messages to it. To read and search the Usenet News groups, one can use any of the popular search engines:

> *http://www.altavista.com*
> *http://www.hotbot.com*
> *http://www.excite.com*
> *http://www.lycos.com*
> *http://www.dejanews.com*

(Using dejanews, an individual can post messages to a newsgroup.)

To access Usenet, select the term Usenet in the search engine's selection box and enter the search keyword. When one enters the title of the news group, the search engine displays the latest messages posted for that specific newsgroup.

The following newsgroups may be of interest to patients with particular conditions or to their significant others.

Attention deficit disorder:
alt.support.attn-deficit

Body dysmorphic disorder:
alt.support.ocd
alt.support.anxiety-panic
alt.support.depression

Clutterers anonymous:
alt.recovery.clutter
alt.recovery.procrastinatn

Compulsive personality disorder:
alt.support.ocd
alt.support.depression
sci.psychology.personality

Hypochondriasis:
alt.med.fibromyalgia
alt.med.cfs
alt.support.anxiety-panic
sci.med.diseases.lyme
alt.support.ibs
sci.psychology.psychotherapy

alt.support.crohns-colitis
alt.support.ocd

Kleptomania:
alt.support.depression
soc.support.depression.manic

Nonparaphilic sexual disorders:
alt.recovery.addiction.sexual
alt.recovery.sexual-addiction
sci.psychology.psychotherapy

Obsessive–compulsive disorder:
alt.support.ocd
alt.support.anxiety-panic
sci.med.psychobiology

Pathological gambling:
soc.support.depression.manic
alt.suicide
alt.abuse.recovery
alt.gambling
alt.recovery
alt.recovery.codependency
alt.support.abuse-partners

Tourette's syndrome:
alt.support.tourette

Trichotillomania:
alt.baldspot
alt.support.ocd

Rating scales for clinical use

Montgomery–Åsberg Depression Rating Scale	276
Yale–Brown Obsessive–Compulsive Scale (Y–BOCS) – brief instructions	280
Yale–Brown Obsessive–Compulsive Checklist	281
Yale–Brown Obsessive–Compulsive Scale (Y-BOCS) interview questions	286
Yale–Brown Obsessive–Compulsive Scale (Y–BOCS)	288
Yale Global Tic Severity Scale	290
Whiteley Index (hypochondriasis)	293
Liebowitz Social Anxiety Scale	295
Sheehan Disability Scales	296
Clinical Global Impressions Scales	297
MOS 36-item Short-Form Health Survey (SF-36) (quality of life)	298

Montgomery–Åsberg Depression Rating Scale

| (1) | Apparent sadness | Score |

Representing despondency, gloom and despair (more than just ordinary transient low spirits) reflected in speech, facial expression, and posture. Rate by depth and inability to brighten up.

0. No sadness
1.
2. Looks dispirited but does brighten up without difficulty
3.
4. Appears sad and unhappy most of the time
5.
6. Looks miserable all the time. Extremely despondent

| (2) | Reported sadness | Score |

Representing reports of depressed mood, regardless of whether it is reflected in appearance or not. Includes low spirits, despondency, or the feeling of being beyond help and without hope. Rate according to the intensity, duration, and the extent to which the mood is reported to be influenced by events.

0. Occasional sadness in keeping with the circumstances
1.
2. Sad or low but brightens up without difficulty
3.
4. Pervasive feelings of sadness or gloominess. The mood is still influenced by external circumstances
5.
6. Continuous or unvarying sadness, misery, or despondency

| (3) | Inner tension | Score |

Representing feelings of ill-defined discomfort, edginess, inner turmoil, mental tension mounting to either panic, dread, or anguish. Rate according to intensity, frequency, duration, and the extent of reassurance called for.

0. Placid. Only feeling inner tension
1.
2. Occasional feelings of edginess and ill-defined discomfort
3.
4. Continuous feelings of inner tension or intermittent panic which the patient can only master with some difficulty
5.
6. Unrelenting dread or anguish. Overwhelming panic

(4)   Reduced sleep   Score _____

Representing the experience of reduced duration or depth of sleep compared to the subject's own normal pattern when well.

0.   Sleeps as usual
1.
2.   Slight difficulty dropping off to sleep or slightly reduced, light or fitful sleep
3.
4.   Sleep reduced or broken by at least two hours
5.
6.   Less than two or three hours sleep

(5)   Reduced appetite   Score _____

Representing the feeling of a loss of appetite compared with when well. Rate by loss of desire for food or the need to force oneself to eat.

0.   Normal or increased appetite
1.
2.   Slightly reduced appetite
3.
4.   No appetite. Food is tasteless
5.
6.   Needs persuasion to eat at all

(6)   Concentration difficulties   Score _____

Representing difficulties in collecting one's thoughts mounting to incapacitating lack of concentration. Rate according to intensity, frequency, and degree of incapacity produced.

0.   No difficulties in concentrating
1.
2.   Occasional difficulties in collecting one's thoughts
3.
4.   Difficulties in concentrating and sustaining thought which reduces ability to read or hold a conversation
5.
6.   Unable to read or converse without great difficulty

(7)   Lassitude   Score _____

Representing a difficulty getting started or slowness initiating and performing everyday activities.

0.   Hardly any difficulty in getting started. No sluggishness
1.
2.   Difficulties in starting activities
3.
4.   Difficulties in starting simple routine activities which are carried out with effort
5.
6.   Complete lassitude. Unable to do anything without help

(8)   Inability to feel   Score _____

Representing the subjective experience of reduced interest in the surroundings, or activities that normally give pleasure. The ability to reach with adequate emotion to circumstances or people is reduced.

0.   Normal interest in the surroundings and in other people
1.
2.   Reduced ability to enjoy usual interests
3.
4.   Loss of interest in the surroundings. Loss of feelings for friends and acquaintances
5.
6.   The experience of being emotionally paralyzed. Inability to feel anger, grief, or pleasure and a complete or even painful failure to feel for close relatives and friends

(9)   Pessimistic thoughts   Score _____

Representing thoughts of guilt, inferiority, self-reproach, sinfulness, remorse, and ruin.

0.   No pessimistic thoughts
1.
2.   Fluctuating ideas of failure, self-reproach or self-deprecation
3.
4.   Persistent self-accusations, or definite but still rational ideas of guilt or sin. Increasingly pessimistic about the future
5.
6.   Delusions of ruin, remorse, or unredeemable sin. Self-accusations which are absurd and unshakable

(10) Suicidal thoughts   Score _____

Representing the feeling that life is not worth living, that a natural death would be welcome, suicidal thoughts and preparations for suicide. Suicidal attempts should not in themselves influence the rating.

0. Enjoys life or takes it as it comes
1.
2. Weary of life. Only fleeting suicidal thoughts
3.
4. Probably better off dead. Suicidal thoughts are common, and suicide is considered as a possible solution, but without specific plans or intention
5.
6. Explicit plans for suicide when there is an opportunity. Active preparations for suicide

TOTAL

_____

                                                             Rater's Signature

Yale–Brown Obsessive Compulsive Scale (Y–BOCS) – brief instructions

Before doing a Y–BOCS rating with a new patient, the clinician should explain to the patient the meaning of the terms "obsession" and "compulsion." For example, "Obsessions are recurrent, intrusive, unwelcome, persistent thoughts, impulses or images. Compulsions are repetitive behaviors that you feel compelled to perform, often according to certain rules, in order to reduce anxiety or prevent something bad from happening. Compulsions include mental rituals like counting, reviewing lists and praying." Once the patient has become familiar with the ratings, the definitions need not be repeated.

The *Y–BOCS Symptom Checklist* identifies current and past symptoms. The clinician should be aware of past symptoms because they may re-occur. Before starting a Y–BOCS rating, the clinician and the patient should select several symptoms as the major targets of treatment. The score for each scale item, however, should take into account all of the patient's obsessions or compulsions.

Y–BOCS Symptom Checklist

Check all that apply, but clearly mark the principle symptoms with a "P".

Current	Past	AGGRESSIVE OBSESSIONS
_____	_____	Fear might harm self
_____	_____	Fear might harm others
_____	_____	Violent of horrific images
_____	_____	Fear of blurting out obscenities or insults
_____	_____	Fear of doing something else embarrassing*
_____	_____	Fear will act on unwanted impulses (e.g., to stab a friend)
_____	_____	Fear will steal things
_____	_____	Fear will harm others because not careful enough (e.g., hit/run motor vehicle accident)
_____	_____	Fear will be responsible for something else terrible happening (e.g., fire, burglary)
_____	_____	Other

		CONTAMINATION OBSESSIONS
_____	_____	Concerns or disgust with bodily waste or secretions (e.g., urine, feces, saliva)
_____	_____	Concern with dirt or germs
_____	_____	Excessive concern with environmental contaminants (e.g., asbestos, radiation, toxic waste)
_____	_____	Excessive concern with household items (e.g., cleaners, solvents)
_____	_____	Excessive concern with animals (e.g., insects)
_____	_____	Bothered by sticky substances or residues

Current	Past	
		CONTAMINATION OBSESSIONS (*cont.*)
_____	_____	Concerned will get ill because of contaminant
_____	_____	Concerned will get others ill by spreading contaminant
_____	_____	No concern with consequences of contamination other than how it might feel
		SEXUAL OBSESSIONS
_____	_____	Forbidden or perverse sexual thoughts, images, or impulses
_____	_____	Content involves children or incest
_____	_____	Content involves homosexuality
_____	_____	Sexual behavior towards others
_____	_____	Other
		HOARDING/SAVING OBSESSIONS
_____	_____	Distinguish from hobbies and concern with objects of monetary or sentimental value
		RELIGIOUS OBSESSIONS (Scrupulosity)
_____	_____	Concerned with sacrilege and blasphemy
_____	_____	Excess concern with right/wrong morality
_____	_____	Other
		OBSESSION WITH NEED FOR SYMMETRY OR EXACTNESS
_____	_____	Accompanied by magical thinking (e.g., concerned that mother will have an accident unless things are in the right place)
_____	_____	Not accompanied by magical thinking

Current	Past	MISCELLANEOUS OBSESSIONS
_____	_____	Need to know or remember
_____	_____	Fear of saying certain things
_____	_____	Fear of not saying just the right thing
_____	_____	Fear of losing things
_____	_____	Intrusive (non-violent) images
_____	_____	Intrusive nonsense sounds, words, or music
_____	_____	Bothered by certain sounds/noises*
_____	_____	Lucky/unlucky numbers
_____	_____	Colors with special significance
_____	_____	Superstitious fears
_____	_____	Other
		SOMATIC OBSESSIONS
_____	_____	Concern with illness or disease*
_____	_____	Excessive concern with body parts or aspect of appearance (e.g., dysmorphophobia)*
_____	_____	Other

Current	Past	CLEANING/WASHING COMPULSIONS
_____	_____	Excessive or ritualized handwashing
_____	_____	Excessive or ritualized showering, bathing, tooth brushing, grooming or toilet routine
_____	_____	Involves cleaning of household items or other inanimate objects
_____	_____	Other measures to prevent or remove contact with contaminants
_____	_____	Other

		CHECKING COMPULSIONS
_____	_____	Checking locks, stoves, appliances, etc.
_____	_____	Checking that did not/will not harm others
_____	_____	Checking that did not/will not harm self
_____	_____	Checking that nothing terrible did/will happen
_____	_____	Checking that did not make mistake
_____	_____	Checking tied to somatic obsessions
_____	_____	Other

		REPEATING RITUALS
_____	_____	Re-reading or re-writing
_____	_____	Need to repeat routine activities (e.g., in/out door, up/down from chair)
_____	_____	Other

		COUNTING COMPULSIONS
_____	_____	Specify

Current	Past	
		ORDERING/ARRANGING COMPULSIONS
_____	_____	Specify
		HOARDING/COLLECTING COMPULSIONS
_____	_____	Distinguish from hobbies and concerns with objects of monetary or sentimental value, (e.g., carefully reads junkmail, piles up old newspapers, sorts through garbage, collects useless objects)
_____	_____	Specify
		MISCELLANEOUS COMPULSIONS
_____	_____	Mental rituals (other than checking/counting)
_____	_____	Excessive listmaking
_____	_____	Need to tell, ask, or confess
_____	_____	Need to touch, tap, or rub*
_____	_____	Rituals involving blinking or staring*
		Measures (not checking) to prevent:
_____	_____	harm to self
_____	_____	harm to others
_____	_____	terrible consequences
_____	_____	Ritualized eating behaviors*
_____	_____	Superstitious behaviors
_____	_____	Trichotillomania*
_____	_____	Other self-damaging or self-mutilating behaviors*
_____	_____	Other

* May or may not be obsessive–compulsive phenomena.

Y–BOCS interview questions

The following questions may be helpful in eliciting the information needed to make Y–BOCS ratings. These wordings tend to prevent patients from being paralyzed by the need to give exact answers. These probes are intended for clinical use and are not identical to those used in research studies.

Rating time occupied

How much time, in an average day in the last week, roughly, did you have obsessions in your mind?

[Additional probe: Can you guesstimate?]

[Additional probe: Count the time that obsessions were either the focus of your attention or noticeably present in the background while you were thinking of something else].

If the patient has a problem making an estimate, ask:

'How many hours do you sleep each night?' 'Of the ## hours you're awake, during how many are obsessions present?' 'In those hours, roughly how much time do you generally lose to obsessing?'

With these data, the interviewer then calculates the approximate amount of time spent obsessing.

Rating interference

In the past week, how did the obsessions interfere with your functioning? How did they interfere with work, taking care of your home, your relationships, having fun with hobbies or leisure activities? Did the obsessions prevent you from doing certain things?

Rating distress

When the obsessions were there, how distressing or disturbing were they? How much discomfort or anxiety did they cause you?

Rating resistance

Of all the times that obsessions were present, in what proportion, roughly, did you try to push them out of your mind or suppress or ignore them? Whether or not you succeeded, how often did you try?

We use the following numerical conventions to get a reliable Resistance score:

4 = ≤ 10% of the time
3 = 11–25% of the time
2 = 26–74% of the time
1 = 75–89% of the time
0 = 90–100% of the time

Rating success

Of all the times that you tried to get rid of the obsessions, in what proportion, roughly, did you succeed? That is, how often could you get rid of the obsessions within about 30 seconds of trying and keep them away for 15 minutes or more?

We use the following numerical convention to get a reliable Success score:

$4 = \leq 10\%$ of the time, or has a Resistance score of 4. That is, a patient who is resisting $\leq 10\%$ of the time cannot be considered to have control.

$3 = 11–25\%$ of the time tried, but the patient must be trying at least 11% of the time (Resistance ≤ 3)

$2 = 26–74\%$ of the time tried, but the patient must be trying at least 26% of the time (Resistance ≤ 2)

$1 = 75–89\%$ of the time tried, but the patient must be trying at least 50% of the time

$0 = 90–100\%$ of the time tried, but the patient must be trying at least 75% of the time

Similar questions are asked in the process of rating compulsions. However, in rating distress, one would ask: "How distressed would you be if you couldn't perform your compulsions? How anxious or uncomfortable would you be?" If the patient would be less distressed if his or her compulsions were prevented, one can ask, "How anxious do you generally get while you are doing your compulsions?"

Yale–Brown Obsessive Compulsive Scale (Y–BOCS)

Note: Scores should reflect the composite effect of all the patient's obsessive and compulsive symptoms. Rate the average occurrence of each item during the prior week up to and including the time of interview.

Obsession rating scale (circle appropriate score)

Item	Range of severity				
1. Time spent on obsessions	0 h/day	>0–1 h/day	>1–3 h/day	>3–8 h/day	>8 h/day
Score	0	1	2	3	4
2. Interference	None	Mild	Definite	Substantial	Incapacitating
Score	0	1	2	3	4
3. Distress from obsessions	None	Little	Moderate but manageable	Severe	Near constant, disabling
Score	0	1	2	3	4
4. Resistance to obsessions	Always resists	Much resistance	Some resistance	Often yields	Completely yields
Score	0	1	2	3	4
5. Control over obsessions	Complete control	Much control	Some control	Little control	No control
Score	0	1	2	3	4

Obsession subtotal (add items 1–5) _____

Compulsion rating scale (circle appropriate score)

Item	Range of severity				
6. Time spent on compulsions	0 h/day	>0–1 h/day	>1–3 h/day	>3–8 h/day	>8 h/day
Score	0	1	2	3	4
7. Interference from compulsions	None	Mild	Definite but manageable	Substantial impairment	Incapacitating
Score	0	1	2	3	4
8. Distress from compulsions	None	Mild	Moderate but manageable	Severe	Near constant, disabling
Score	0	1	2	3	4
9. Resistance to compulsions	Always resists	Much resistance	Some resistance	Often yields	Completely yields
Score	0	1	2	3	4
10. Control over compulsions	Complete control	Much control	Some control	Little	No control
Score	0	1	2	3	4

Compulsion subtotal (add items 6–10) _____

Y–BOCS total (add items 1–10) _____

Total Y–BOCS score: range of severity for patients who have both obsessions and compulsions – 0–7 subclinical; 8–15 mild; 16–23 moderate; 24–31 severe; 32–40 extreme.

Yale Global Tic Severity Scale

Instructions: This clinical rating scale is designed to rate the overall severity of tic symptoms across a range of dimensions (number, frequency, intensity, complexity and interference). The final rating is based on all available information and reflects the clinician's overall impression for each of the items rated.

The clinician should first compile a list of motor and phonic tics present during the past week as reported by the patient and observed during the evaluation. Then, the clinician proceeds with the questions concerning each rating dimension, using the content of the anchor points as a guide.

As reproduced here, the scale is intended for clinical rather than research use.

NUMBER OF TICS   Motor score_____   Phonic score_____

0   = None.
1   = Single tic.
2   = Multiple discrete tics (2–5).
3   = Multiple discrete tics (>5).
4   = Multiple discrete tics plus at least one orchestrated pattern of multiple simultaneous or sequential tics where it is difficult to distinguish discrete tics.
5   = Multiple discrete tics plus several (>2) orchestrated paroxysms of multiple simultaneous or sequential tics where it is difficult to distinguish discrete tics.

FREQUENCY   Motor score_____   Phonic score_____

0   = None, no evidence of specific behaviors.
1   = Rarely, specific tic behaviors have been present during previous week. These behaviors occur infrequently, often not on a daily basis. If bouts of tics occur, they are brief and uncommon.
2   = Occasionally, specific tic behaviors are usually present on a daily basis, but there are long tic-free intervals during the day. Bouts of tics may occur on occasion and are not sustained for more than a few minutes at a time.
3   = Frequently, specific tic behaviors are present on a daily basis. Tic-free intervals as long as 3 hours are not uncommon. Bouts of tics occur regularly, but may be limited to a single setting.
4   = Almost Always, specific tic behaviors are present virtually every waking hour of every day, and periods of sustained tic behaviors occur regularly. Bouts of tics are common and are not limited to a single setting.
5   = Always, specific tic behaviors are present virtually all the time. Tic-free intervals are difficult to identify and do not last more than 5 to 10 minutes, at most.

INTENSITY   Motor score_____   Phonic score_____

0   = Absent.
1   = Minimal intensity, tics not visible or audible (based solely on patient's private experience) or tics are less forceful than comparable voluntary actions and are typically not noticed because of their intensity.
2   = Mild intensity, tics are not more forceful than comparable voluntary actions or utterances and are typically not noticed because of their intensity.
3   = Moderate intensity, tics are more forceful than comparable voluntary actions, but are not

outside the range of normal expression for comparable voluntary actions or utterances. They may call attention to the individual because of their forceful character.

4   = Marked intensity, tics are more forceful than comparable voluntary actions or utterances and typically have an "exaggerated" character. Such tics frequently call attention to the individual because of their forceful and exaggerated character.

5   = Severe intensity, tics are extremely forceful and exaggerated in expression. These tics call attention to the individual and may result in risk of physical injury (accidental, provoked or self-inflicted) because of their forceful expression.

COMPLEXITY   Motor score_____   Phonic score_____

0   = None, if present, all tics are clearly "simple" (sudden, brief, purposeless) in character.

1   = Borderline, some tics are not clearly "simple" in character.

2   = Mild, some tics are clearly "complex" (purposive in appearance) and mimic brief "automatic" behaviors, such as grooming, syllables or brief meaningful utterances such as "ah huh," "hi," that could be readily camouflaged.

3   = Moderate, some tics are more "complex" (more purposive and sustained in appearance) and may occur in orchestrated bouts that would be difficult to camouflage, but could be rationalized or "explained" as normal behavior or speech (picking, tapping, saying "you bet" or "honey," brief echolalia).

4   = Marked, some tics are very "complex" in character and tend to occur in sustained orchestrated bouts that would be difficult to camouflage and could not be easily rationalized as normal behavior or speech because of their duration and/or their unusual, inappropriate, bizarre, or obscene character (a lengthy facial contortion, touching genitals, echolalia, speech atypicalities, longer bouts of saying "what do you mean" repeatedly, or saying "fu" or "sh").

5   = Severe, some tics involve lengthy bouts of orchestrated behavior or speech that would be impossible to camouflage or successfully rationalize as normal because of their duration and/or extremely unusual, inappropriate, bizarre or obscene character (lengthy displays or utterances often involving copropraxia, self-abuse behavior or coprolalia).

INTERFERENCE   Motor score_____   Phonic score_____

0   = None

1   = Minimal, when tics are present, they do not interrupt the flow of behavior or speech.

2   = Mild, when tics are present, they occasionally interrupt the flow of behavior or speech.

3   = Moderate, when tics are present, they frequently interrupt the flow of behavior or speech.

4   = Marked, when tics are present, they frequently interrupt the flow of behavior or speech, and they occasionally disrupt intended action or communication.

5   = Severe, when tics are present, they frequently disrupt intended action or communication.

IMPAIRMENT (Rate overall impairment for motor and phonic tics)

0   = None

10   = Minimal, tics associated with subtle difficulties in self-esteem, family life, social acceptance, or school or job functioning (infrequent upset or concern about tics vis-a-vis the future, periodic, slight increase in family tensions because of tics, friends or acquaintances may occasionally notice or comment about tics in an upsetting way).

20   = Mild, tics associated with minor difficulties in self-esteem, family life, social acceptance, or school or job functioning.

30   = Moderate, tics associated with some clear problems in self-esteem, family life, social acceptance, or school or job functioning (episodes of dysphoria, periodic distress and upheaval in the family, frequent teasing by peers or episodic social avoidance, periodic interference in school or job performance because of tics).

40   = Marked, tics associated with major difficulties in self-esteem, family life, social acceptance, or school or job functioning.

50   = Severe, tics associated with extreme difficulties in self-esteem, family life, social acceptance, or school or job functioning (severe depression with suicidal ideation, disruption of the family, separation, divorce, residential placement), disruption of social ties—severely restricted life because of social stigma and social avoidance, removal from school or loss of job).

Reprinted with permission from Leckman et al. (1989). Copyright 1989, *Journal of the American Academy of Child and Adolescent Psychiatry.*

The Whiteley Index (hypochondriasis)

Below is a list of questions about your health. For each one, please circle the number indicating how much this is true for you.

	Not at all	A little bit	Moderately	Quite a bit	A great deal
(1) Do you worry a lot about your health	1	2	3	4	5
(2) Do you think there is something seriously wrong with your body?	1	2	3	4	5
(3) Is it hard for you to forget about yourself and think about all sorts of other things?	1	2	3	4	5
(4) If you feel ill and someone tells you that you are looking better, do you become annoyed?	1	2	3	4	5
(5) Do you find that you are often aware of various things happening in your body?	1	2	3	4	5
(6) Are you bothered by many aches and pains?	1	2	3	4	5
(7) Are you afraid of illness?	1	2	3	4	5
(8) Do you worry about your health more than most people?	1	2	3	4	5
(9) Do you get the feeling that people are not taking your illnesses seriously enough?	1	2	3	4	5
(10) Is it hard for you to believe the doctor when he/she tells you there is nothing for you to worry about?	1	2	3	4	5
(11) Do you often worry about the possibility that you have a serious illness?	1	2	3	4	5
(12) If a disease is brought to your attention (through the radio, TV, newspapers, or someone you know), do you worry about getting it yourself?	1	2	3	4	5
(13) Do you find that you are bothered by many different symptoms?	1	2	3	4	5
(14) Do you often have the symptoms of a very serious disease?	1	2	3	4	5

Key to the Whitely Index.

Disease conviction is reflected in questions (2), (4) and (9).

Disease fear is reflected in questions (3), (7), (8), (10) and (12).

Bodily preoccupation is reflected in questions (1), (5), (6), (11), (13) and (14).

Source: Reprinted with permission from Barsky, Wyshak and Klerman (1986). Copyright 1986, American Medical Association.

Liebowitz Social Anxiety Scale

Please rate your fear or anxiety and your avoidance of situations using the numbers shown below.

Fear or anxiety:
0 = none, 1 = mild, 2 = moderate, 3 = severe

Avoidance:
0 = never (0%), 1 = occasionally (1–33%), 2 = often, (34–66%), 3 = usually (67–100%)

		Fear or anxiety	Avoidance
1.	Telephone in public (P)		
2.	Participating in small groups (P)		
3.	Eating in public places (P)		
4.	Drinking with others in public places (P)		
5.	Talking to people in authority (S)		
6.	Acting, performing, or giving a talk in front of an audience (P)		
7.	Going to a party (S)		
8.	Working while being observed (P)		
9.	Writing while being observed (P)		
10.	Calling someone you do not know very well (S)		
11.	Talking with people you do not know very well (S)		
12.	Meeting strangers (S)		
13.	Urinating in a public bathroom (P)		
14.	Entering a room when others are already seated (P)		
15.	Being the center of attention (S)		
16.	Speaking up in a meeting (P)		
17.	Taking a test (P)		
18.	Expressing a disagreement to people you do not know well (S)		
19.	Looking at people you do not know very well in the eyes (S)		
20.	Giving a report to a group (P)		
21.	Trying to pick up someone (P)		
22.	Returning goods to a store (S)		
23.	Giving a party (S)		
24.	Resisting a high-pressure salesperson (S)		
	Total score		
	Performance (P) subscores		
	Social (S) subscores		

Sheehan Disability Scales

Please mark ONE box for each scale.

DISABILITY SCALES

Work
The symptoms have disrupted your work

Not at all		Mildly			Moderately			Markedly			Extremely
0	1	2	3	4	5	6	7	8	9	10	

Social Life
The symptoms have disrupted your social life

Not at all		Mildly			Moderately			Markedly			Extremely
0	1	2	3	4	5	6	7	8	9	10	

Family Life/Home Responsibilities
The symptoms have disrupted your family life/home responsibilities

Not at all		Mildly			Moderately			Markedly			Extremely
0	1	2	3	4	5	6	7	8	9	10	

Source: Adapted with permission from Sheehan (1983). Copyright 1983, Charles Scribner and Sons.

Clinical Global Impressions Scales

Severity of illness

Considering your total clinical experience with this particular population, how mentally ill is the patient at this time?

0 = Not assessed

1 = Normal, not at all ill

2 = Borderline mentally ill

3 = Mildly ill

4 = Moderately ill

5 = Markedly ill

6 = Severely ill

7 = Among the most extremely ill patients

Global improvement

Rate total improvement whether or not, in your judgment, it is due entirely to drug treatment.

Compared to his condition at admission to the project, how much has he changed?

0 = Not assessed

1 = Very much improved

2 = Much improved

3 = Minimally improved

4 = No change

5 = Minimally worse

6 = Much worse

7 = Very much worse

Source: Guy (1976).

The MOS 36–item Short-Form Health Survey (SF-36)

Instructions: This survey asks for your views about your health. This information will help keep track of how you feel about, and how well you are able to do, your usual activities.

Answer every question by marking the answer as indicated. If you are unsure about how to answer a question, please give the best answer you can.

1. In general, would you say your health is: (circle one)

    Excellent. 1

    Very Good 2

    Good 3

    Fair 4

    Poor 5

2. Compared to one year ago, how would you rate your health in general now?   (circle one)

    Much better now than one year ago 1

    Somewhat better now than one year ago 2

    About the same as one year ago. 3

    Somewhat worse now than one year ago 4

    Much worse now than one year ago 5

3. The following items are about activities you might do during a typical day. Does your health now limit you in these activities? If so, how much?   (circle one number on each line)

	Activities	Yes, limited a lot	Yes, limited a little	No, not limited at all
(a)	Vigorous activities, such as running, lifting heavy objects, partici pating in strenuous sports	1	2	3
(b)	Moderate activities, such as moving a table, pushing a vacuum cleaner, bowling or playing golf	1	2	3
(c)	Lifting or carrying groceries	1	2	3
(d)	Climbing several flights of stairs	1	2	3

	Activities	Yes, limited a lot	Yes, limited a little	No, not limited at all
(e)	Climbing one flight of stairs	1	2	3
(f)	Bending, kneeling, or stooping	1	2	3
(g)	Walking more than a mile	1	2	3
(h)	Walking several blocks	1	2	3
(i)	Walking one block	1	2	3
(j)	Bathing or dressing yourself	1	2	3

4. During the past 4 weeks, have you had any of the following problems with your work or other regular daily activities as a result of your physical health?   (circle one number on each line)

		YES	NO
(a)	Cut down on the amount of time you spent on work or other activities	1	2
(b)	Accomplished less than you would like	1	2
(c)	Were limited in the kind of work or other activities	1	2
(d)	Had difficulty performing the work or other activities (for example, it took extra effort)	1	2

5. During the past 4 weeks, have you had any of the following problems with your work or other regular daily activities as a result of any emotional problems (such as feeling depressed or anxious?)

(circle one number on each line)

		YES	NO
(a)	Cut down the amount of time you spent on work or other activities	1	2
(b)	Accomplished less than you would like	1	2
(c)	Didn't do work or other activities as carefully as usual	1	2

6. During the past 4 weeks, to what extent has your physical health or emotional problems interfered with your normal social activities with family, friends, neighbors or groups?   (circle one)

Not at all 1

Slightly. 2

Moderately 3

Quite a bit 4

Extremely 5

7. How much bodily pain have you had during the past 4 weeks? (circle one)

None 1

Very mild. 2

Mild 3

Moderate 4

Severe. 5

Very severe. 6

8. During the past 4 weeks, how much did pain interfere with your normal work (including both work outside the home and housework?) (circle one)

Not at all 1

A little bit. 2

Moderately 3

Quite a bit 4

Extremely 5

9. These questions are about how you feel and how things have been with you during the past 4 weeks. For each question, please give the one answer that comes closest to the way you have been feeling. How much of the time during the past 4 weeks: (circle one number on each line)

		All of the time	Most of the time	A good bit of the time	Some of the time	A little of the time	None of the time
(a)	Did you feel full of pep?	1	2	3	4	5	6
(b)	Have you been a very nervous person?	1	2	3	4	5	6
(c)	Have you felt so down in the dumps that nothing could cheer you up?	1	2	3	4	5	6
(d)	Have you felt calm and peaceful?	1	2	3	4	5	6
(e)	Did you have a lot of energy?	1	2	3	4	5	6
(f)	Have you felt down-hearted and blue?	1	2	3	4	5	6
(g)	Did you feel worn out?	1	2	3	4	5	6

		All of the time	Most of the time	A good bit of the time	Some of the time	A little of the time	None of the time
(h)	Have you been a happy person?	1	2	3	4	5	6
(i)	Did you feel tired?	1	2	3	4	5	6

10. During the past 4 weeks, how much of the time has your physical health or emotional problems interfered with your social activities (like visiting with friends, relatives, etc.?)   (circle one)

   All of the time. 1

   Most of the time. 2

   Some of the time 3

   A little of the time 4

   None of the time. 5

11. How TRUE or FALSE is each of the following statements for you?   (circle one number on each line)

		Definitely true	Mostly true	Don't know	Mostly false	Definitely false
(a)	I seem to get sick a little easier than other people	1	2	3	4	5
(b)	I am as healthy as anybody I know	1	2	3	4	5
(c)	I expect my health to get worse	1	2	3	4	5
(d)	My health is excellent	1	2	3	4	5

Source: Reprinted with permission from Ware, Snow, Kosinski and Gandek (1993).

SF-36 scoring

Scoring the SF-36 for research purposes requires recoding the precoded numerical response items according to "Final Item Values" provided in the *SF-36 Manual and Interpretation Guide*. For clinical purposes, reasonable indicators of the quality of life in the eight dimensions measured by the SF-36 can be obtained by simply reversing the numerical values for items 1, 6, 7, 8, 9(a) and 9(e), 9(d) and 9(h), 11(b) and 11(d) and then summing the scores as indicated. Taking item 1 as an example, a circled $1=5$, $2=4$, $3=3$, $4=2$, and $5=1$. Once the item scores have been calculated, the Scale scores are made up of the following item values:

Scale	Sum of items	Lowest and highest possible raw score	Raw score range
Physical functioning	3a through 3j	10–30	20
Role impairment due to physical factors	4a through 4d	4–8	4
Bodily pain	7+8	2–12	10
General health	1+11a through 11d	5–25	20
Vitality	9a+9e+9g+9i	4–24	20
Social functioning	6+10	2–10	8
Role impairment due to emotional factors	5a through 5c	3–6	3
Mental health	9b + 9c + 9d + 9f + 9h	5–30	25

Except for Bodily Pain and General Health, scores obtained in this way can be compared, after transformation, to norms for the U.S. population, which are provided in the *SF-36 Manual and Interpretation Guide*. To transform a raw scale score, one uses the following formula:

$$\text{Transformed score} = \left[\frac{(\text{Actual raw score} - \text{lowest possible score})}{\text{Raw Score Range}} \right] \times 100$$

For example, a mental health raw score of 20 becomes a transformed score of 60: $\{[20-5]/[25]\} \times 100 = 60$.

Trademark drug names — an international list

Abbreviations

A	Austria	ICL	Iceland
B	Belgium	ISR	Israel
CH	Switzerland	ITA	Italy
DK	Denmark	JPN	Japan
EG	Egypt	NL	Netherlands
ESP	Spain	NOR	Norway
F	France	PORT	Portugal
FIN	Finland	SAR	South African Republic
G	Germany	SG	Singapore
GR	Greece	SWE	Sweden
HK	Hong Kong	TH	Thailand
HUNG	Hungary	UK	United Kingdom
		USA	United States of America

Alphabetized list of trademark drug names by class

Anti-anxiety drugs

alprazolam

Alprox	DK, FIN
Mialin	ITA
Pazolam	PORT
Tafil	DK, G, ICL
Trakimazin	ESP
Unilan	PORT
Valeans	ITA
Xanax	B, CH, F, ITA, NL, PORT, UK, USA
Xanor	A, FIN, SAR, SWE

clonazepam

Iktoviril	SWE
Klonopin	USA
Rivotril	A, B, CH, CK, ESP, F, G, GR, ITA, NL, SAR, UK
Rivatril	FIN, NOR, PORT

diazepam

Aliserum	ITA
Alupram	UK
Aneurol	ESP
Ansiolin	A
Ansium	ESP
Apollonset	GR
Apozepam	DK, FIN, SWE
Atarvitron	GR
Atensine	UK
Audium	GR
Bentapam	SAR
Benzopin	SAR
Bialzepam	PORT
Valiquid	G
Valium	A, B, CH, DK, ESP, F, FIN, G, GR, ICL, ITA, NL, NOR, PORT, SAR, SWE, UK, USA

lorazepam

Albium	GR
Almazine	UK
Ansilor	PORT
Aripax	GR

Ativan	SAR, UK, USA
Control	ITA
Dorm	GR
Durazolam	G
Indalpram	ESP
Lauracalm	B
Laubeel	G
Lorabenz	DK
Lorans	PORT
Loriden	B
Lorsedal	PORT
Merlit	A
Modium	GR
Nifalin	GR
Noan-Gap	GR
Novhepar	GR
Orfidal	ESP
Placinoral	ESP
Por Dorm	G
Punktyl	A, G
Sebor	GR
Sedapon	A
Sedozin	CH
Serenase	B
Somagerol	G
Somnium	CH
Tavor	G, GR, ITA
Temesta	B, CH, DK, F, FIN, NL, SWE
Temesta Expidet	B, SWE
Thymal	GR
Titus	GR
Tolid	G
Trankilium	GR
Tranquipam	SAR
Tran-Quil	SAR

buspirone

Ansial	ESP
Ansised	ESP
Axoren	ITA
Bespar	G
Buscalm	PORT
Buspar	B, CH, CK, ESP, FIN, ITA, NL, NOR, PORT, SAR, SWE, UK, USA
Buspimen	ITA
Buspisal	ESP
Narol	ESP

Anticonvulsants

carbamazepine

Carbapin	FIN
Carbymal	NL
Carpaz	SAR
Degranol	SAR
Hermolepsin	SWE
Nordotol	DK
Neurotol	FIN, ICL
Neurotrop	A
Sirtal	G
Tardotal	DK, ICL
Tardotol	DK
Tegretal	ICL, ITA, PORT, SAR
Tégrétol	A, B, CH, DK, ESP, F, FIN, GR, NL, NOR, SWE, UK
Tégrétol LP	F
Timonol	G

valproic acid

Convulex	A, B, CH, G, NL, SAR
Depakin	ITA
Depakine	B, CH, ESP, F, GR, ICL, NL
Depakine Chrono	PORT
Depakine Zuur	NL
Depakote	USA
Deprakin	DK, FIN, NOR
Epilim	UK
Ergenyl	A, G, SWE
Leptilan	A, DK, FIN, G
Leptilen	A, SWE
Orfilept	SWE
Orfiril	CH, DK, FIN, G, ICL, NOR
Orfiril Retard	ICL
Propynal	NL
Valcote 250	G

Antidepressant drugs

citalopram

Celexa	USA
Cipram	EG, HK, SG, TH
Cipramil	DK, EST, FIN, ICL, SAR, SWE
Elopram	ITA
Prisdal	ESP

Seralgan	A
Seropram	A, CA, CH, F, GR, HUNG, ITA

desipramine

Norpramin	USA
Nortimil	ITA
Pertofran	A, B, CH, CK, F, G, NL, SAR, UK
Pertofrin	SWE
Sertofren	NOR

fluoxetine

Adofen	ESP
Fontex	DK, FIN, ICL, SWE
Fluctin	G
Fluctine	CH
Fluoxeren	ITA
Fluoxin	ICL
Flutin	DK
Fonzac	DK
Lorien	SAR
Mutan	A
Orthon	GR
Prozac	B, ESP, F, ITA, NL, PORT, SAR, UK, USA
Prozyn	SAR
Reneuron	ESP
Seronil	FIN

fluvoxamine

Dumirox	ESP, PORT
Faverin	UK
Fevarin	G, DK, FIN, ITA, NL, NOR, SWE, SAR, UK
Floxyfral	A, B, CH, F
Luvox	SAR, USA
Maveral	ITA

imipramine

Deprinol	DK, ICL
Depramine	GR
Ethipramine	SAR
Imavate	USA
Imipramin	DK, NOR
Sedacoroxen	GR
SK-Pramine	USA
Tofranil	A, B, CH, DK, ESP, F, FIN, G, GR, ICL, ITA, NL, NOR, PORT, SWE, SAR, UK, USA
Tofranil pamoata	ESP

Tofranil-PM	USA
Venefon	GR

mirtazapine

Remeran	A, FIN, NL, SWE, USA
Zisprin	UK

nefazodone

Dutonin	G, UK
Nefadar	ITA, SWE
Reseril	ITA
Serzone	USA

nortriptyline

Allegron	B, UK
Aventyl	SAR, UK, USA
Benpon	A, G
Dominans	ITA
Martinil	ESP
Motipress	UK
Motival	F, GR, SAR, UK
Norfenazine	ESP
Noritren	DK, FIN, ITA, NOR, SWE
Nortrilen	A, B, CH, G, GR, ICL, NL
Nortrix	PORT
Pamelor	USA
Paxtibi	ESP
Sensaval	SWE
Sensival	DK
Tropargal	ESP

paroxetine

Aropax	B, NL, SAR, UK
Deroxat	CH, F, SAR
Frosinor	ESP
Paxil	USA
Sereupin	ITA
Seroxat	CK, ESP, FIN, G, GR, ICL, ITA, NOR, NL, SWE
Tagonis	G

phenelzine

Nardelzine	B, ESP
Nardil	UK, USA

selegiline/L-deprenyl

Déprenyl	F
Eldepryl	B, DK, FIN, ICL, NL, NOR, SAR, SWE, UK, USA

Jumex	A, ITA, PORT
Jumexal	CH
Movergan	G
Plurimen	ESP

sertraline

Aremis	ESP
Besitran	ESP
Gladem	CH
Lustral	UK
Serad	ITA
Serlain	B, SWE
Tatig	ITA
Zoloft	DK, CH, FIN, ITA, NL, SAR, SWE, USA

trazodone

Azona	FIN
Deprax	ESP
Desyrel	USA
Molipaxin	SAR, UK
Pragmarel	F
Tramensan	FIN
Trazodone	PORT
Trazolan	B, NL
Thombran	G
Trittico	A, CH, GR, ITA

Neuroleptics

clozapine

Alemoxan	G
Clozaril	USA
Leponex	A, CH, DK, ESP, F, FIN, G, ICL, NL, NOR, PORT, SWE

fluphenazine

Anatensol	NL
Cardilac	GR
Cenilene	PORT
Dapotum	A, CH, G
Dapotum Acutum	A, CH, G, SAR
Flufenazin	CK, FIN, ICL, NOR, SWE
Lyogen	A, CH, G
Moditen	B, F, ICL, NL, UK
Omca	G
Pacinol	DK
Permitil	B

Prolixin	USA
Sevinol	B, GR
Siqualone	FIN, NOR, SWE

haloperidol

Alased	GR
Aloperidin	GR
Buteridol	G
Cereen	SAR
Dozic	UK
Duraperidol	G
Fortunan	UK
Haldol	A, B, CH, F, G, ICL, ITA, NL, NOR, PORT, SWE, UK, USA
Halperin	FIN
Safrionol	GR
Serenace	CK, FIN, ITA, SAR, UK
Serenelfi	PORT
Sevium	GR
Sigaperidol	CH, G
Sylador	CK

pimozide

Orap	A, CH, DK, ESP, FIN, G, ICL, ITA, NL, PORT, NOR, SAR, UK, USA
Opiran	F
Pirium	GR

risperidone

R 64.766	B
Risperdal	A, CK, G, NL, SWE, SAR, UK, USA
Rispolin	A, CK

sulpiride

Aiglonyl	F
Alimoral	GR
Ansium	ESP
Arminol	G
Belivon	SWE
Calmoflorine	GR
Championyl	ITA
Darleton	GR
Dixibon	ESP
Dobren	ITA
Dogmatil	A, B, CH, DK, F, G, GR, NL
Dolmatil	UK
Dresent	GR
Eclorion	GR

Eglonyl	SAR
Enimon	GR
Equilid	ITA
Eusulpid	ITA
Fardalan	GR
Fidelan	GR
Guastil	ESP
Libopride	ESP
Mariastel	GR
Meresa	A, G
Mirbanil	ESP
Neogama	G
Neoride	ESP
Noneston	GR
Norestran	GR
Normum	ITA
Nufarol	GR
Omaha	GR
Omiryl	GR
Ozoderpin	GR
Paratil	FIN
Restful	GR
Sulpril	CK
Sulpitil	UK
Suprium	FIN
Synédil	F
Synédil Fort	F
Tepavil	ESP
Tepazepam	ESP
Valirem	GR
Zemorcon	GR
Zymocomb	GR

Stimulant drugs

methylphenidate

Ritalin	DK, G, GR, ICL, ITA, NL, NOR, UK, USA
Ritaline	B, CH
Rubifen	ESP

pemoline

Anform	B
Cylert	USA
Dynalert	SAR
Hyton Asa	CK, ICL

Ronyl	UK
Stimul	B, CH
Tradon	G
Volital	UK

Miscellaneous drugs

amantadine

Amantadine	ESP
Amantan	B
Antadine	SAR
Aturin	FIN
Glucuronide	RUS
Hofcommant	A
Mantadix	B, F
Mantadan	ITA
PK-Merz	A, CH, G
Symmetrel	A, CH, ICL, NL, NOR, SAR, UK, USA
Virofral	ICL, SWE

cetirizine

Virlix	F
Zyrtec	B, DK, G, NL, USA
Zyrlec	SWE

clonidine

Barclid	F
Catapres	UK, USA
Catapressan	B, F
Caprysin	FIN
Clonisin	FIN
Dixarit	B, G, NL, UK
F\Paracefan	B, NL
Tenso-Timelets	G

cyproheptadine

Adekin	GR
Betoliman	GR
Istam Far	GR
Kulinet	GR
Nuran	G
Periactin	B, CH, DK, GR, NL, NOR, SWE, UK, USA
Périactine	F
Periactinol	G
Sialotin	GR
Vinorex	GR

naltrexone

Antaxone	ESP, ITA
Celupan	ESP
Nalorex	F, ITA, NL, UK
Nemexin	CH
Revia	USA

propranolol

Alfaxical	GR
Avlocardyl	F
Bedranol	UK
Berkolol	UK
Betadrenol	GR
Beta-Tablinen	G
Beta-Timelets	G
Dociton	G
Dorizan	GR
Efektolol	G
Elbrol	G
Frekven	DK
Inderal	B, DK, FIN, GR, NL, NOR, SWE, UK, USA
Indobloc	G
Kiteran	GR
Kostalerg	G
Prandol Retard	NL
Prano-Puren	G
Pronovan	NOR
Propabloc	G
Reducor	FIN
Sagittal	G
Tenomal	GR

tryptophan

Ardeytropin	G
Atrimon	G
Bikalm	G
Biotin	G
Kalma	G
Neurocalm	G
Optimax	UK
Optimax Powder	UK
Optimax WV	UK
Pacitron	UK
Sedanoct	G
Tryptocompren	G

Source: DePrins, L. (1995).

Bibliography

Abbey, S.E. and Garfinkel, P.E. (1991). Neurasthenia and chronic fatigue syndrome: The role of culture in the making of a diagnosis. *Am J Psychiatry*, **148**: 1638–46.

Achamallah, N.S. and Decker, D.H. (1991). Mania induced by fluoxetine in an adolescent patient. (Letter.) *Am J Psychiatry*, **148**: 1404.

Ackerman, D.L., Greenland, S. and Bystritsky, A. (1998). Clinical characteristics of response to fluoxetine treatment of obsessive–compulsive disorder. *J Clin Psychopharmacol*, **18**: 185–92.

Ackerman, D.L., Greenland, S., Bystritsky, A., Morgenstern, H. and Katz, R.J. (1994). Predictors of treatment response in obsessive compulsive disorder: Multivariate analyses from a multi-center trial of clomipramine. *J Clin Psychopharmacol*, **14**: 247–54.

Adam, B.S. and Kashani, J.H. (1990). Trichotillomania in children and adolescents: Review of the literature and case report. *Child Psychiatry Hum Dev*, **20**: 159–67.

Ahles, T.A., Khan, S.A., Yunus, M.B., Spiegel, D.A. and Masi, A.T. (1991). Psychiatric status of patients with primary fibromyalgia, patients with rheumatoid arthritis, and subjects without pain: A blind comparison of DSM-III diagnoses. *Am J Psychiatry*, **148**: 1721–6.

Aizenberg, D., Zemishlany, Z. and Weizman, A. (1995). Cyproheptadine treatment of sexual dysfunction induced by serotonin reuptake inhibitors. *Clin Neuropharmacol*, **18**: 320–4.

Akhtar, S., Wig, N., Varma, V., Dwarka, P. and Verma, K. (1975). A phenomenological analysis of symptoms in obsessive–compulsive neurosis. *Br J Psychiatry*, **127**: 342–8.

Alden, L. (1989). Short-term structured treatment for avoidant personality disorder. *J Consult Clin Psychology*, **57**: 756–64.

Alexander, R.C. (1991). Fluoxetine treatment of trichotillomania. (letter.) *J Clin Psychiatry*, **52**: 88

Allen, L. and Tejera, C. (1994). Treatment of clozapine-induced obsessive–compulsive symptoms with sertraline. (Letter.) *Am J Psychiatry*, **151**: 1096–7.

Altemus, M., Swedo S.E., Leonard, H.L., Richter, D., Rubinow, D.R., Potter, W.Z. and Rapoport, J.L. (1994). Changes in cerbrospinal fluid neurochemistry during treatment of obsessive–compulsive disorder with clomipramine. *Arch Gen Psychiatry*, **51**: 794–803.

Altshuler, L.L., Cohen, L, Szuba, M.P., Burt, V.K., Gitlin, M and Mintz, J. (1996). Pharmacologic management of psychiatric illness during pregnancy: Dilemmas and guidelines. *Am J Psychiatry*, **153**: 592–605.

Altshuler, L.L., Pierre, J.M., Wirshing, W.C. and Ames, D. (1994). Sertraline and akathisia. (Letter.) *J Clin Psychopharmacol*, **14**: 278–9.

Alzaid, K. and Jones, B. (1997). A case report of risperidone-induced obsessive–compulsive symptoms. (Letter.) *J Clin Psychopharmacol*, **17**: 58–9.

American Academy of Pediatrics, Committee on Drugs. (1994). Transfer of drugs and other chemicals into human milk. *Pediatrics*, **93**: 137–50.

American Psychiatric Association. (1993). Practice guideline for major depressive disorder in adults. *Am J Psychiatry*, **150**(4)(suppl): 1–26.

American Psychiatric Association. (1994). *Diagnostic and Statistical Manual of Mental Disorders*, 4th edn. Washington DC: American Psychiatric Association.

Ames, D., Cummings, J.L., Wirshing, W.C., Quinn, B. and Mahler, M. (1994). Repetitive and compulsive behavior in frontal lobe degenerations. *J Neuropsychiatry Clin Neurosci*, **6**: 100–13.

Amsterdam, J.D., Hornig-Rohan, M. and Maislin, G. (1994). Efficacy of alprazolam in reducing fluoxetine-induced jitteriness in patients with major depression. *J Clin Psychiatry*, **55**: 394–400.

Ananth, J., Burgoyne, K., Smith, M. and Swartz, R. (1995). Venlafaxine for treatment of obsessive–compulsive disorder. (letter.) *Am J Psychiatry*, **152**: 1832.

Ananth, J. and Elmishaugh, A. (1991). Hair loss associated with fluoxetine treatment. (Letter.) *Can J Psychiatry*, **36**: 621.

Andreasen, N.C. and Bardach, J. (1977). Dysmorphophobia: Symptom or disease? *Am J Psychiatry*, **134**: 673–6.

Andrews, G., Stewart, G., Allen, R. and Henderson, A.S. (1990). The genetics of six neurotic disorders: A twin study. *J Affective Disord*, **19**: 23–9.

Ansseau, M., Legros, J.J., Mormont, C., Cerfontaine, J.L., Geenen, V., Adam., F. and Franck, G. (1987). Intranasal oxytocin in obsessive–compulsive disorder. *Psychoneuroendocrinology*, **12**: 231–6.

Anthony, D.T. and Hollander, E. (1992). Sexual compulsions. In *Obsessive–Compulsive-Related Disorders*, ed. E. Hollander, pp. 139–50. Washington, DC: American Psychiatric Press.

Anthony, J.C., Folstein, M., Romanoski, A.J., Von Korff, M.R., Nestadt, G.R., Chahal, R., Merchant, A., Brown, C.H., Shapiro, S., Kramer, M. and Gruenberg, E.M. (1985). Comparison of the lay Diagnostic Interview Schedule and a standardized psychiatric diagnosis: Experience in Eastern Baltimore. *Arch Gen Psychiatry*, **42**: 667–75.

Apter, A., Pauls, D.L., Bleich, A., Zohar, A.H., Kron, S., Ratzoni, G., Dycian, A., Kotler, M., Weizman, A., Gadot, N. and Cohen, D.J. (1993). An epidemiological study of Gilles de la Tourette's syndrome in Israel. *Arch Gen Psychiatry*, **50**: 734–8.

Arnott, S. and Nutt, D. (1994). Successful treatment of fluvoxamine-induced anorgasmia by cyproheptadine. *Br J Psychiatry*, **164**: 838–9.

Artigas, F., Perez, V. and Alavarez, E. (1994). Pindolol induces a rapid improvement of depressed patients treated with serotonin reuptake inhibitors. (letter.) *Arch Gen Psychiatry*, **51**: 248–51.

Arya, D.K. (1994). Extrapyramidal symptoms with selective serotonin reuptake inhibitors. *Br J Psychiatry*, **165**: 728–33.

Arya, D.K. and Szabadi, E. (1993). Dyskinesia associated with fluvoxamine. (Letter.) *J Clin Psychopharmacol*, **13**: 365–6.

AuBuchon, P.G. and Malatesta, V.J. (1994). Obsessive compulsive patients with comorbid personality disorder: Associated problems and response to comprehensive behavior therapy. *J Clin Psychiatry*, **55**: 448–53.

Ault, A. (1998). US FDA warns doctors to use cisapride as last resort only. (Letter.) *Lancet* **352**: 120.

Azrin, N.H., Nunn, R.G. and Frantz, S.E. (1980). Treatment of hairpulling (trichotillomania): A comparative study of habit reversal and negative practice training. *J Behav Ther Exp Psychiatry*, **11**: 13–20.

Bach, M. and Bach, D. (1993). Psychiatric and psychometric issues in acné excoriée. *Psychother Psychosom*, **60**: 207–10.

Bacher, N.M. (1990). Clonazepam treatment of obsessive compulsive disorder. (Letter.) *J Clin Psychiatry*, **51**: 168–9.

Baer, L. (1994). Factor analysis of symptom subtypes of obsessive compulsive disorder and their relation to personality and tic disorders. *J Clin Psychiatry*, **55**(suppl 3): 18–23.

Baer, L., Jenike, M.A., Black, D.W., Treece, C., Rosenfeld, R. and Greist, J. (1992). Effect of Axis II diagnoses on treatment outcome with clomipramine in 55 patients with obsessive–compulsive disorder. *Arch Gen Psychiatry*, **49**: 862–6.

Baer, L. and Minichiello, W.E. (1990). Behavior therapy for obsessive–compulsive disorder. In *Obsessive–Compulsive Disorder: Theory and Management*, ed. M.A. Jenike, L. Baer and W.E. Minichielo, pp. 203–32. Chicago: Yearbook Medical Publishers.

Baer, L., Rauch, S.L., Ballantine, H.T., Martuza, R., Cosgrove, R., Cassem E., Giriumas, I., Manzo, P.A., Dimino, C. and Jenike, M.A. (1995). Cingulotomy for intractable obsessive–compulsive disorder: Prospective long-term follow-up of 18 patients. *Arch Gen Psychiatry*, **52**: 384–92.

Baker, R.W. (1992). Fluoxetine and schizophrenia in a patient with obsessional thinking. (Letter.) *J Neuropsychiatry Clin Neurosci*, **4**: 232–3.

Baker, R.W., Ames, D., Umbricht, D.S.G., Chengappa, K.N.R. and Schooler, N.R. (1996). Obsessive–compulsive symptoms in schizophrenia: A comparison of olanzapine and placebo. *Psychopharmacol Bull*, **32**: 89–93.

Baker, R.W., Bermanzohn, P.C., Wirshing, D.A. and Chengappa, K.N.R. (1997). Obsessions, compulsions, clozapine, and risperidone. *CNS Spectrums*, **2**: 26–31, 34–6.

Baker, R.W., Chengappa, R., Baird, J.W., Steingard, S., Christ M.A.G. and Schooler, N.R. (1992). Emergence of obsessive–compulsive symptoms during treatment with clozapine. *J Clin Psychiatry*, **53**: 439–42.

Baliga, R.R. and McHardy, K.C. (1993). Syndrome of inappropriate antidiuretic hormone secretion due to fluvoxamine therapy. *Br J Clin Practice*, **47**: 62–3.

Ball, S.G., Baer, L. and Otto, M.W. (1996). Symptom subtypes of obsessive–compulsive disorder in behavioral treatment sutdies: a quantitative review. *Behav Res Ther*, **34**: 47–51.

Ballenger, J.C. (1997). Panic disorder in the medical setting. *J Clin Psychiatry*, **58**(suppl 2): 13–17.

Balogh, S., Hendricks, S.E. and Kang, J. 1992. Treatment of fluoxetine-induced anorgasmia with amantadine. (Letter.) *J Clin Psychiatry*, **53**: 212–13.

Balon, R. (1994). Sexual obsessions associated with fluoxetine. (Letter.) *J Clin Psychiatry*, **55**: 496.

Balon, R., Yeragani, V.K., Pohl, R. and Ramesh, C. (1993). Sexual dysfunction during antidepressant treatment. *J Clin Psychiatry*, **54**: 209–12.

Barabasz, M. (1987). Trichotillomania: A new treatment, *Int J Clin Exper Hyp*, **3**: 146–54.

Bark, N. and Lindenmayer, J.P. (1992). Ineffectiveness of clomipramine for obsessive–compulsive symptoms in a patient with schizophrenia. (Letter.) *Am J Psychiatry*, **149**: 136–7.

Barkley, R. A. (1990). *Attention Deficit Hyperactivity Disorder: A Handbook for Diagnosis and Treatment*. New York: Guilford Press.

Barlow, D.H. (1997). Cognitive-behavioral therapy for panic disorder: Current status. *J Clin Psychiatry*, **58**(suppl 2): 32–6.

Barr, L.C., Goodman, W.K., Anand, A., McDougle, C.J. and Price. L.H. (1997). Addition of desipramine to serotonin reuptake inhibitors in treatment-resistant obsessive–compulsive disorder. *Am J Psychiatry*, **154**: 1293–5.

Barr, L.C., Goodman, W.K. and Price, L.H. (1992). Acute exacerbation of body dysmorphic disorder during tryptophan depletion. (Letter.) *Am J Psychiatry*, **149**: 1406–7.

Barr, L.C., Goodman. W.K. and Price, L.H. (1994). Physical symptoms associated with paroxetine discontinuation. (Letter.) *Am J Psychiatry*, **151**: 289.

Barsky, A.J. (1992). Hypochondriasis and obsessive–compulsive disorder. *Psychiatr Clin North Am*, **15**: 791–801.

Barsky, A.J., Barnett, M.C. and Cleary, P.D. (1994). Hypochondriasis and panic disorder: Boundary and overlap. *Arch Gen Psychiatry*, **51**: 918–25.

Barsky, A.J., Cleary, P.D., Wyshak, G., Spitzer, R.L., Williams, J.B.W. and Klerman, G.L. (1992a). A structured diagnostic interview for hypochondriasis: A proposed criterion standard. *J Nerv Ment Dis*, **180**: 20–7

Barsky, A.J. and Klerman, G.L. (1983). Overview: Hypochondriasis, bodily complaints, and somatic styles. *Am J Psychiatry*, **140**: 273–83.

Barsky, A.J., Wyshak, G. and Klerman, G.L. (1986). An evaluation of the DSM-III criteria in medical outpatients. *Arch Gen Psychiatry*, **43**: 493–500.

Barsky, A.J., Wyshak, G. and Klerman, G.L. (1990). Transient hypochondriasis. *Arch Gen Psychiatry*, **47**: 746–52.

Barsky, A.J., Wyshak, G. and Klerman, G.L. (1992b). Psychiatric comorbidity in DSM-III-R hypochondriasis. *Arch Gen Psychiatry*, **49**: 101–8.

Barth, R.J. and Kinder, B.N. (1987). The mislabeling of sexual impulsivity. *J Sex Marital Ther*, **13**: 15–23.

Bartlik, B.D., Kaplan, P. and Kaplan, H.S. (1995). Psychostimulants apparently reverse sexual dysfunction secondary to selective serotonin re-uptake inhibitors. *J Sex Marital Ther*, **21**: 262–8.

Barton, R. (1965). Diabetes insipidis and obsessional neurosis: A syndrome. *Lancet*, **1**: 133–5.

Bauer, M., Hellweg, R. and Baumgartner, A. (1996a). Fluoxetine-induced akathisia does not reappear after switch to paroxetine. (Letter.) *J Clin Psychiatry*, **57**: 593–4.

Bauer, M., Linden, M., Schaaf, B. and Weber, H.J. (1996b). Adverse events and tolerability of the combination of fluoxetine/lithium compared with fluoxetine. *J Clin Psychopharmacol*, **16**: 130–4.

Baxter, L.R. (1994). Positron emission tomography studies of cerebral glucose metabolism in obsessive compulsive disorder. *J Clin Psychiatry*, **55**(suppl 10): 54–9.

Baxter, L.R., Schwartz, J.M., Bergan, K.S., Szuba, M.P., Guze, B.H., Mazziotta, J.C., Alazraki, A., Selin, C.E., Ferng, H.K. and Phelps, M.E. (1992). Caudate glucose metabolic rate changes with both drug and behavior therapy for obsessive–compulsive disorder. *Arch Gen Psychiatry*, **49**: 681–9.

Bear, D.M. and Fedio, P. (1977). Quantitative analysis of interictal behavior in temporal lobe epilepsy. *Arch Neurol*, **34**: 454–67.

Beck, A.T. (1976). *Cognitive Therapy of the Emotional Disorders.* New York: International Universities Press.

Beck, J. and Padefsky, C. (1990). Avoidant personality disorder. In *Cognitive Therapy of Personality Disorders*, ed. A.T. Beck, A. Freeman and Associates, pp. 257–82. New York: Guilford Press.

Beck, J.S. (1995). *Cognitive Therapy: Basics and Beyond.* New York: Guilford Press.

Bergeron, R. and Blier, P. (1994). Cisapride for the treatment of nausea produced by selective serotonin reuptake inhibitors. *Am J Psychiatry*, **151**: 1084–6.

Bergman, U., Rosa, F.W., Baum, C., Wiholm, B.E. and Faich, G.A. (1992). Effects of exposure to benzodiazepine during fetal life. *Lancet*, **340**: 694–6.

Berman, I., Kalinowski, A., Berman S.M., Lengua, J. and Green, A.I. (1995a). Obsessive and compulsive symptoms in chronic schizophrenia. *Compr Psychiatry*, **36**: 6–10.

Berman, I., Sapero, B.H., Chang, H.H.G., Losonczy, M.F., Schmildler, J. and Green, A.I. (1995b).

Treatment of obsessive compulsive symptoms in schizophrenic patients with clomipramine. *J Clin Psychopharmacol*, **15**: 206–10.

Berman, R.M., Darnell, A.M., Miller, H.L., Anand, A. and Charney, D.S. (1997). Effect of pindolol in hastening response to fluoxetine in the treatment of major depression: A double-blind, placebo-controlled trial. *Am J Psychiatry*, **154**: 37–43.

Bernik, M.A., Akerman, D., Amaral, J.A.M.S. and Braun, R.C.D.N. (1996). Cue exposure in compulsive buying (Letter.) *J Clin Psychiatry*, **57**: 90.

Berrios, G.E. (1996). *The History of Mental Symptoms: Descriptive psychopathology since the nineteenth century*. Cambridge, England: Cambridge University Press.

Bethier, M.L., Kulisevsky, J., Gironell, A. and Heras, J.A. (1996). Obsessive compulsive disorder associated with brain lesions: Clinical phenomenology, cognitive function, and anatomic correlates. *Neurology*, **47**: 353–61.

Bhandary, A.N., Fernandez, F., Gregory, R.J., Tucker, P. and Masand, P. (1997). Pharmacotherapy in adults with ADHD. *Psychiatr Ann*, **27**: 545–55.

Bhatara, V.S., Gupta, S. and Freeman, J.W. (1996). Fluoxetine-associated paresthesias and alopecia in a woman who tolerated sertraline. (Letter.) *J Clin Psychiatry*, **57**: 227.

Bhatia, M.S., Singhal, P.K., Rastogi, V., Dhar, N.K., Nigam, V.R. and Taneja, S.B. (1991). Clinical profile of trichotillomania. *J Indian Med Assoc*, **89**: 137–9.

Biederman, J., Farone, S.V., Spencer, T., Wilens, T., Norman, D., Lapey, K.A., Mick, E., Lehman, B.K. and Doyle, A. (1993). Patterns of psychiatric comorbidity, cognition, and psychosocial functioning in adults with attention deficit hyperactivity disorder. *Am J Psychiatry*, **150**: 1792–8.

Bisserbe, J.C., Lane, R.M., Flament, M.F. and the Franco-Belgian OCD Study Group (1997). A double-blind comparison of sertraline and clomipramine in outpatients with obsessive–compulsive disorder. *Eur Psychiatry*, **12**: 82–93.

Black, B. and Uhde, T.W. (1992). Acute dystonia and fluoxetine. (Letter). *J Clin Psychiatry*, **53**: 327.

Black, D.W. (1996). Compulsive buying: A review. *J Clin Psychiatry*, **57**(suppl 8): 50–4, Discussion, p. 55.

Black, D.W. and Blum, N.S. (1992a). Obsessive-compulsive disorder support groups: The Iowa model. *Compr Psychiatry*, **33**: 65–71.

Black, D.W. and Blum, N. (1992b). Trichotillomania treated with clomipramine and a topical steriod. (Letter.) *Am J Psychiatry*, **149**: 842–3.

Black, D.W., Gabel, J. and Schlosser, S. (1997). Urge to splurge. (Letter.) *Am J Psychiatry*, **154**: 1629–30.

Black, D.W., Gaffney, G., Schlosser, S. and Gabel, J. (1998a). The impact of obsessive–compulsive disorder on the family: preliminary findings. *J Nerv Ment Dis*, **186**: 440–2.

Black, D.W., Goldstein, R.B., Noyes, R. and Blum, N. (1994). Compulsive behaviors and obsessive–compulsive disorder (OCD): Lack of a relationship between OCD, eating disorders, and gambling. *Compr Psychiatry*, **35**: 145–8.

Black, D.W., Kehrberg, L.L.D., Flumerfelt, D.L. and Schlosser, S.S. (1997). Characteristics of 36 subjects reporting compulsive sexual behavior. *Am J Psychiatry*, **154**: 243–9.

Black, D.W., Noyes, R., Goldstein, R.B. and Blum, N. (1992). A family study of obsessive–compulsive disorder. *Arch Gen Psychiatry*, **49**: 362–8.

Black, D.W., Noyes, R., Pfohl, B., Goldstein, R.B. and Blum, N. (1993a). Personality disorder in obsessive–compulsive volunteers, well comparison subjects, and their first-degree relatives. *Am J Psychiatry*, **150**: 1226–32.

Black, D.W., Repertinger, S., Gaffney, G.R. and Gabel, J. (1998b). Family history and psychiatric comorbidity in persons with compulsive buying: preliminary findings. *Am J Psychiatry*, **155**: 960–3.

Black, D.W., Wesner, R. and Gabel, J. (1993b). The abrupt discontinuation of fluvoxamine in patients with panic disorder. *J Clin Psychiatry*, **54**: 146–9.

Bland, R.C., Newman, S.C. and Orn, H. (1988). Age of onset psychiatric disorders. *Acta Psychiatr Scand*, **77**(suppl 338): 43–9.

Bland, R.C., Newman, S.C., Orn, H. and Stebelsky, G. (1993). Epidemiology of pathological gambling in Edmonton. *Can J Psychiatry*, **38**: 108–12.

Blaszcynski, A. and McConaghy, N. (1994). Criminal offences in Gamblers Anonymous and hospital treated pathological gamblers. *J Gambling Studies*, **10**: 99–128.

Blaszcynski, A., McConaghy, N. and Frankova, A. (1990). Boredom proneness in pathological gambling. *Psychol Rep*, **67**: 35–42.

Blaszcynski, A. and Silove, D. (1995). Cognitive and behavioral therapies for pathological gambling. *J Gambling Stud*, **11**: 195–220.

Blaszcynski, A. and Silove, D. (1996). Pathological gambling: Forensic issues. *Aust N Z J Psychiatry*, **30**: 358–69.

Bleuler, E. (1924). *Textbook of Psychiatry*, p. 540. New York: Macmillan.

Blier, P. and Bergeron, R. (1995a). Effectiveness of pindolol with selected anti-depressant drugs in the treatment of major depression. *J Clin Psychopharmacol*, **15**: 217–22.

Blier, P. and Bergeron, R. (1995b). The safety of concomitant use of sumatriptan and antidepressant treatments. *J Clin Psychopharmacol*, **15**: 106–9.

Blier, P. and Bergeron. R. (1996). Sequential administration of augmentation strategies in treatment-resistent obsessive–compulsive disorder: Preliminary findings. *Int Clin Psychopharmacol*, **11**: 37–44.

Blumer, D. and Walker, A.E. (1967). Sexual behavior in temporal lobe epilepsy. *Arch Neurol*, **16**: 37–43.

Bodkin, J.A. and White, K. (1989). Clonazepam in the treatment of obsessive compulsive disorder associated with panic disorder in one patient. *J Clin Psychiatry*, **50**: 265–6.

Bolen, D.W. and Boyd, W.H. (1968). Gambling and the gambler. *Arch Gen Psychiatry*, **18**: 617–30.

Bolton, D., Luckie, M. and Steinberg, D. (1995). Long-term course of obsessive–compulsive disorder treated in adolescence. *Acad Child Adolesc Psychiatry*, **34**: 1441–50.

Borison, R.L., Ang, L., Chang, S., Dysken, M., Comaty, J.E. and Davis, J.M. (1992). New pharmacological approaches in the treatment of Tourette Syndrome. *Adv Neurol*, **35**: 377–82.

Bourgeois, J.A. (1996). Two cases of hair loss after sertraline use. *J Clin Psychopharmacol*, **16**: 91–2.

Bradford, J.M.W. and Gratzer, T.G. (1995). A treatment for impulse control disorders and paraphilia: A case report. *Can J Psychiatry*, **40**: 4–5.

Brawman-Mintzer, O., Lydiard, R.B., Phillips, K.A., Morton, A., Czepowicz, V., Emmanuel, N., Villareal, G., Johnson, M. and Ballenger, J.C. (1995). Anxiety disorders and body dysmorphic disorder: A comorbidity study. *Am J Psychiatry*, **152**: 1665–76.

Breiter, H.C., Rauch, S.L., Kwong, K.K., Baker, J.R., Weisskoff, R.M., Kennedy, D.N., Kendrick, A.D., Davis, T.L., Jiang, A., Cohen, M.S., Stern, C.E., Belliveau, J.W., Baer, L., O'Sullivan, R.L., Savage, C.R., Jenike, M.A. and Rosen, B.R. (1996). Functional magnetic resonance imaging of symptom provocation in obsessive–compulsive disorder. *Arch Gen Psychiatry*, **53**: 595–606.

Brickner, R.M., Rosner, A.A. and Munro, R. (1940). Physiological aspects of the obsessive state. *Psychosom Med*, **2**: 369–83.

Bridges, P. (1990). Psychosurgery revisited. *J Neuropsychiatry Clin Neurosci*, **2**: 326–30.

Brodsky, C.M. (1983). "Allergic to everything": A medical subculture. *Psychosomatics*, **24**: 731–42.

Brown, R.I.F. (1987). Pathological gambling and associated patterns of crime: Comparisons with alcohol and other drug addictions. *J Gambling Behav*, **3**: 98–114.

Brown, W.A. and Harrison, W. (1995). Are patients who are intolerant to one selective reuptake inhibitor intolerant to another? *J Clin Psychiatry*, **56**: 30–4.

Bruun, R.D. and Budman, C.L. (1993). The natural history of Gilles de la Tourette syndrome. In *Handbook of Tourette's Syndrome and Related Tic and Behavioral Disorders*, ed. R. Kurlan, pp. 27–42. New York: Marcel Dekker.

Bruun, R.D. and Budman, C.L. (1996). Risperidone as a treatment for Tourette's syndrome. *J Clin Psychiatry*, **57**: 29–31.

Buckely, P.F., Sajatovic, M. and Meltzer, H.Y. (1994). Treatment of delusional disorders with Clozapine. (Letter.) *Am J Psychiatry*, **151**: 1394–5.

Burd, L., Kerbeshian, L., Wikenheiser, M. and Fisher, W. (1986). A prevalence study of Gilles de la Tourette's syndrome in North Dakota school-age children. *J Am Acad Child Adoles Psychiatry*, **25**: 552–3.

Burka, J. and Yuen, L. (1983). *Procrastination: Why You Do It, What To Do About It.* Reading, MA: Addison-Wesley.

Burns, D.D. (1990). *The Feeling Good Handbook.* New York: Penguin Books.

Burrai, C., Bocchetta, A. and Del Zompo, M. (1991). Mania and fluvoxamine. (Letter.) *Am J Psychiatry*, **148**: 1263–4.

Burstein, A. (1992). Fluoxetine-lithium treatment for kleptomania. (Letter.) *J Clin Psychiatry*, **53**: 28–9.

Butler, G., Cullington, A., Munby, M., Amies, P. and Gelder, M. (1984). Exposure and anxiety management in the treatment of social phobia. *J Consult Clin Psychol*, **52**: 642–50.

Byrne, A. and Yatham, L.N. (1989). Pimozide in pathlogical jealousy. *Br J Psychiatry*, **155**: 249–51.

Bystritsky, A., Munford, P.R., Rosen, R.M., Marin, K.M., Vapnik, T., Gorbis, E.E. and Wolson, R.C. (1996). A preliminary study of partial hospital management of severe obsessive–compulsive disorder. *Psychiatr Serv*, **47**: 170–4.

Bystritsky, A. and Strausser, B.P. (1996). Treatment of obsessive–compulsive cutting behavior with naltrexone. (Letter.) *J Clin Psychiatry*, **57**: 423–4.

Caballero, R. (1988). Bowel obsession responsive to clomipramine (Letter.) *Am J Psychiatry*, **145**: 650–1.

Caine E.D., McBride, M.C., Chiverton, P., Bainford, K.A., Rediess, S. and Shiao, J. (1988). Tourette syndrome in Monroe county school children. *Neurology*, **38**: 472–5.

California Medical Association Scientific Board Task Force on Clinical Ecology. (1986). Clinical ecology: A critical appraisal. *West J Med*, **144**: 239–45.

Calvocoressi, L., Lewis, B., Harris, M., Trufan, S., Goodman, W., McDougle, C. and Price, L. (1995) Family accomodation in obsessive–compulsive disorder. *Am J Psychiatry*, **152**: 441–3.

Calvocoressi, L., McDougle, C.I., Wasylink, S., Goodman, W.K., Trufan, S.J. and Price, L.H. (1993). Inpatient treatment of patients with severe obsessive–compulsive disorder. *Hosp Community Psychiatry*, **44**: 1150–4.

Cameron, O.G. and Wasielewski, P. (1990). Clomipramine treatment of possible atypical obsessive–compulsive disorder. (Letter.) *J Clin Psychopharmacol*, **10**: 375–6.

Cantor, C. and Fallon, B.A. (1996). *Phantom Illness: Shattering the Myth of Hypochondria.* Boston: Houghton Mifflin Company.

Carnes, P. (1989). *Contrary to Love*, pp. 187–229. Minnesota: CompCare Publishers.

Carrion, V.G. (1995). Naltrexone for the treatment of trichotillomania: A case report. (Letter.) *J Clin Psychopharmacol*, **15**: 444–5.

Cascino, G.D. and Sutula, T.P. (1989). Thirst and compulsive water drinking in medial basal limbic epilepsy: An electroclinical and neuropathological correlation. (Letter.) *J Neurol Neurosurg Psychiatry*, **52**: 680–1.

Cassano, D., Del Buono, G. and Catapano, F. (1993). The relationship between obsessive–compulsive personality and obsessive–compulsive disorder: Data obtained by the Personality Disorder Examination. *Eur Psychiatry*, **8**: 219–21.

Castellanos, F.X., Giedd, J.N., Elia, J., Marsh, W.L., Ritchie, G.F., Hamburger, S.D. and Rapoport, J.L. (1997). Controlled stimulant treatment of ADHD and comorbid Tourette's syndrome: Effects of stimulant and dose. *J Am Acad Child Adolesc Psychiatry*, **36**: 589–96.

Chambers, C.D., Johnson K.A., Dick L.M., Felix, R.J. and Jones, K.L. (1996). Birth outcomes in pregnant women taking fluoxetine. *N Engl J Med*, **335**: 1010–15.

Chappell, P.B., Riddle, M.A., Scahill, L., Lynch, K.A., Schultz, R., Arnstein, A., Leckman, J.F. and Cohen, D.J. (1995). Guanfacine treatment of comorbid attention-deficit hyperactivity disorder and Tourette's syndrome: Preliminary clinical experience. *J Am Acad Child Adolesc Psychiatry*, **34**: 1140–6.

Chauvel, P., Kliemann, F., Vignal, J.P., Chodkiewicz, J.P., Talairach, J. and Bancaud, J. (1995). The clinical signs and symptoms of frontal lobe seizures. Phenomenology and classification. *Adv Neurol*, **66**: 115–26.

Chen, Y.W. and Dilsaver, S.C. (1995). Comorbidity for obsessive–compulsive disorder in bipolar and unipolar disorders. *Psychiatry Res*, **59**: 57–64.

Childers, M.K., Holland, D., Ryan, M.G. and Rupright, J. (1998). Obsessional disorders during recovery from severe head injury: Report of four cases. *Brain Injury* **12**: 613–16

Childers, R.T. (1958). Report of two cases of trichotillomania of long standing duration and their response to chlorpromazine. *J Clin Exp Psychopathol*, **19**: 141–4.

Chiu, H.F.K. (1995). Delusional jealousy in Chinese elderly psychiatric patients. *J Geriatr Psychiatry Neurol*, **8**: 49–51.

Chong, S.A. (1995). Fluvoxamine and mandibular dystonia. (Letter.) *Can J Psychiatry*, **40**: 430–1.

Chong, S.A. (1996). Fluvoxamine and akathisia. (Letter.) *J Clin Psychopharmacol*, **16**: 334–5.

Chong, S.A. and Low, B. L. (1996). Treatment of kleptomania with fluvoxamine. *Acta Psychiatr Scand*, **93**: 314–15.

Chouinard, G., Goodman, W., Greist, J., Jenike, M., Rasmussen, S., White, K., Hackett, E., Gaffney, M. and Bick, P.A. (1990). Results of a double-blind placebo controlled trial of a new serotonin uptake inhibitor, sertraline, in the treatment of obsessive–compulsive disorder. *Psychopharmacol Bull*, **26**: 279–84.

Christensen, R.C., Byerly, M.J. and McElroy, R.A. (1996). A case of sertraline-induced stuttering. (Letter.) *J Clin Psychopharmacol*, **16**: 92–3.

Christenson, G.A., Chernoff-Clementz, E. and Clementz, B.A. (1992a). Personality and clinical characteristics in patients with trichotillomania. *J Clin Psychiatry*, **53**: 407–13.

Christenson, G.A. and Crow, S.J. (1996). The characterization and treatment of trichotillomania. *J Clin Psychiatry*, **57**(suppl 8): 42–9.

Christenson, G.A., Crow, S.J., Mitchell, J.E., Mackenzie, T.B., Crosby, R.D. and Falls, J. (1998). Fluvoxamine in the treatment of trichotillomania: an 8-week, open-label study. *CNS Spetrums* **3**: 64–71.

Christenson, G.A., Faber, R.F., de Zwaan, M., Raymond, N.C., Specker, S.M., Ekern, M.D.,

Mackenzie, T.B., Crosby, R.D., Crow, S.J., Eckert, E.D., Mussell, M.P. and Mitchell, J.E. (1994a). Compulsive buying: Descriptive characteristics and psychiatric comorbidity. *J Clin Psychiatry*, **55**: 5–11.

Christenson, G.A., Mackenzie, T.B. and Mitchell, J.E. (1991a). Characteristics of 60 adult chronic hair pullers. *Am J Psychiatry*, **148**: 365–70.

Christenson, G.A., Mackenzie, T.B. and Mitchell, J.E. (1994b). Adult men and women with trichotillomania: A comparison of male and female characteristics. *Psychosomatics*, **35**: 142–9.

Christenson, G.A., Mackenzie, T.B., Mitchell, J.E. and Callies, A.L. (1991b). A placebo-controlled, double-blind crossover study of fluoxetine in trichotillomania. *Am J Psychiatry*, **148**: 1566–71.

Christenson, G.A., Mackenzie, T.B. and Reeve, E.A. (1992b). Familial trichotillomania. (Letter.) *Am J Psychiatry*, **149**: 283–4.

Christenson, G.A., Popkin, M.K., Mackenzie, T.B. and Realmuto, G.M. (1991c). Lithium treatment of chronic hair pulling. *J Clin Psychiatry*, **52**: 116–20.

Christenson, G.A., Pyle, R.L. and Mitchell, J.E. (1991d). Estimated lifetime prevalence of trichotillomania in college students. *J Clin Psychiatry*, **52**: 415–17.

Chua, T.P. and Vong, S.K. 1993. Hyponatremia associated with paroxetine. (Letter.) *Br Med J*, **306**: 143.

Ciarrochi, J.W. (1995). *The Doubting Disease: Help for Scrupulosity and Religious Compulsions*. New York: Paulist Press.

Ciarrocchi, J.W. and Richardson, J. (1989). Profile of compulsive gamblers in treatment: Update and comparisons. *J Gambling Stud*, **5**: 53–65.

Ciraulo, D.A., Shader, R.I., Greenblatt, D.J. and Creelman W. (Eds.). (1995). *Drug Interactions in Psychiatry*, 2nd edn. Baltimore, MD: Williams and Wilkins.

Clarkin, J.F., Pilkonis, P.A. and Magruder, K.M. (1996). Psychotherapy of depression: Implications for reform of the health care system. *Arch Gen Psychiatry*, **53**: 717–23.

The Clomipramine Collaborative Study Group. (1991). Clomipramine in the treatment of patients with obsessive–compulsive disorder. *Arch Gen Psychiatry*, 48: 730–8.

Cohen, B.J., Mahelsky, M. and Adler, L. (1990). More cases of SIADH with fluoxetine. (Letter.) *Am J Psychiatry*. **147**: 948–9.

Cohen, L.J., Stein, D.J., Simeon, D., Spadaccini, E., Rosen, J., Aronowitz, B. and Hollander, E. (1995). Clinical profile, comorbidity, and treatment history in 123 hair pullers: A survey study. *J Clin Psychiatry*, **56**: 319–26.

Cohen, L.S., Friedman, J.M., Jefferson, J.W., Johnson, E.M. and Weiner, M.L. (1994). A reevaluation of risk of in utero exposure to lithium. [Published erratum appears in JAMA (1994), **271**: 1485.] *JAMA*, **271**: 146–50.

Coleman, E. (1992). Is your patient suffering from compulsive sexual behavior? *Psychiatr Ann*, **22**: 320–5.

Comings, D.E., Himes, J.A. and Comings, B.G. (1990). An epidemiologic study of Tourette's syndrome in a single school district. *J Clin Psychiatry*, **51**: 463–9.

Committee on Safety of Medicines (1993). Dystonia and withdrawal symptoms with paroxetine (Seroxat). *Curr Prob Pharmacovigil*, **19**: 1.

Como, P.G. and Kurlan, R. (1991). An open-label trial of fluoxetine for obsessive–compulsive disorder in Gilles de la Tourette's syndrome. *Neurology*, **41**: 872–4.

Connor, K.M., Davidson, J.R.T., Potts, N.L.S., Tupler, L.A., Miner, C.M., Malik, M.L., Book, S.W.,

Colket, J.T. and Terrell, F. (1998). Discontinuation of clonazepam in the treatment of social phobia. *J Clin Psychopharmacol*, **18**: 373–8.

Corá-Locatelli, Greenberg, B.D., Martin, J.D. and Murph, D.L. (1998). Rebound psychiatric and physical symptoms after gabapentin discontinuation. (Letter.) *J Clin Psychiatry*, **59**: 131.

Coulter, D.M. and Pillans, P.I. (1995). Fluoxetine and extrapyramidal side effects. *Am J Psychiatry*, **152**: 122–5.

Coupland, N.J., Bell, C.J. and Potodar, J.P. (1996). Serotonin reuptake inhibitor withdrawal. *J Clin Psychopharmacol*, **16**: 356–62.

Crews, J.R., Potts, N.L.S., Schreiber, J. and Lipper, S. (1993). Hyponatremia in a patient treated with sertraline. (Letter.) *Am J Psychiatry*, **150**: 1564.

Crino, R.D. and Andrew, G. (1996). Personality disorder in obsessive compulsive disorder: A controlled study. *J Psychiatr Res*, **30**: 29–38.

Croisile, B., Tourniaire, D., Confavreux, C., Trillet, M. and Aimard, G. (1989). Bilateral damage to the head of the caudate nuclei. (Letter.) *Ann Neurol*, **25**: 313–14.

Cummings, J.L. (1993). Frontal-subcortical circuits and human behavior. *Arch Neurol*, **50**: 873–80.

Cummings, J.L. and Cunningham, K. (1992). Obsessive–compulsive disorder in Huntington's disease. *Biol Psychiatry*, **31**: 263–70.

Dalton, C.B. and Drossman, D.A. (1997). Diagnosis and treatment of irritable bowel syndrome. *Am Fam Physician*, **55**: 875–80, 883–5.

Damon, J.E. (1988). *Shopaholics: Serious Help for Addicted Spenders*. Los Angeles: Price Stein Sloan.

Daniele, A., Bartolomeo, P., Cassetta, E., Bentivoglio, A.R., Gainotti, G., Abanese, A. and Partolomeo, B. (1997). Obsessive–compulsive behavior and cognitive impairment in a parkinsonian patient after a left putaminal lesion. (Letter.) *J Neurol Neurosurg Psychiatry*, **62**: 288–9.

Danjou, P. and Hackett, D. (1995). Safety and tolerance profile of venlafaxine. *Int Clin Psychopharmacol*, **10**(suppl 2): 15–20.

Davidson, J.R.T. (1997). Use of benzodiazepines in panic disorder. *J Clin Psychiatry*, **58**(suppl 2): 26–8.

Davidson, J.R.T., Tupler, L.A. and Potts N.L.S. (1994). Treatment of social phobia with benzodiazepines. *J Clin Psychiatry*, **55**(suppl 6): 28–32.

Deale, A., Chalder, T., Marks, I. and Wessely, S. (1997). Cognitive behavior therapy for chronic fatigue syndrome: A randomized controlled trial. *Am J Psychiatry*, **154**: 408–14.

Degonda, M., Wyss, M. and Angst, J. (1993). The Zurich study: XVIII. Obsessive–compulsive disorders and syndromes in the general population. *Eur Arch Psychiatry Clin Neurosci*, **243**: 16–22.

Deltito, J.A. and Stam, M. (1989). Psychopharmacological treatment of avoidant personality disorder. *Compr Psychiatry*, **30**: 498–504.

den Boer, J.A. (1997). Psychopharmacology of comorbid obsessive–compulsive disorder and depression. *J Clin Psychiatry*, **58**(suppl 8): 17–19.

Denckla, M.B., Bemporad, J.R. and MacKay, M.C. (1976). Tics following methylphenidate administration: A report of 20 cases. *JAMA*, **235**: 1349–51.

DePrins, L. (Ed.) (1995). *Psychotropics 95/96*. Copenhagen: Lundbeck.

DeVane, C.L. (1996). Dr. Vane Replies. (Letter.) *J Clin Psychiatry*, **57**: 225–7.

Deveaugh-Geiss, J., Katz, R., Landau, P., Goodman, W. and Rasmussen, S. (1990). Clinical predictors of treatment response in obsessive compulsive disorder: Exploratory analyses from multicenter trials of clomipramine. *Psychopharmacol Bull*, **26**: 54–9.

Diaferia, G., Bianchi, I., Bianchi, M.L., Cavedini, P., Erzegovesi, S. and Bellodi, L. (1997). Relationship between obsessive–compulsive personality disorder and obsessive–compulsive disorder. *Compr Psychiatry*, **38**: 38–42.

Diaferia, G., Mundo, E., Bianchi, Y. and Ronchi, P. (1994). Behavioral side effects in obsessive–compulsive patients treated with fluvoxamine: A clinical description. (Letter.) *J Clin Psychopharmacol*, **14**: 78–9.

Dinan, T.G. (1993). Lithium augmentation in sertraline-resistant depression: A preliminary dose-response study. *Acta Psychiatr Scand*, **88**: 300–1.

Dodt, J.E., Byerly, M.J., Cuadros, C. and Christensen, R.C. (1997). Treatment of risperidone-induced obsessive–compulsive symptoms with sertraline. (Letter.) *Am J Psychiatry*, **154**: 582.

Dohlberg, O.T., Iancu, I., Sasson, Y. and Zohar, J. (1996). The pathogenesis and treatment of obsessive–compulsive disorder. *Clin Neuropharmacol*, **19**: 129–47.

Dolan, M. and Bishay, N. (1996). The effectiveness of cognitive therapy in the treatment of non-psychotic morbid jealousy. *Br J Psychiatry*, **168**: 588–93.

Donovan, N.J. and Barry, J.J. (1994). Compulsive symptoms associated with frontal lobe injury. (Letter.) *Am J Psychiatry*, **151**: 618.

Dorian, B.J. (1979). Monosymptomatic hypochondrial psychosis. (Letter.) *Can J Psychiatry*, **24**: 377.

Drake, W. and Gordon, G. (1994). Heart block in a patient on propranolol and fluoxetine. (Letter.) *Lancet*, **348**: 425–6.

Dreessen, L., Hoekstra, R. and Arntz, A. (1997). Personality disorders do not influence the results of cognitive and behavior therapy for obsesssive compulsive disorder. *J Anxiety Disord*, **11**: 503–21.

Drossman, D.A. (1978). Evaluation and care of medical patients with psychosocial disturbances. *Ann Int Med*, **88**: 366–72.

Drummond, L.M. and Gravestock, S. (1988). Delayed emergence of obsessive–compulsive neurosis following head injury: Case report and review of its theoretical implications. *Br J Psychiatry*, **153**: 839–42.

Dunner, D.L., ed. (1997). *Current Psychiatric Therapy*, Philadelphia: W.B. Saunders.

Dupont, R.L., Rice, D.P., Shiraki, S. and Rowland, C.R. (1995). Economic costs of obsessive–compulsive disorder. *Medical Interface*, **8**: 102–9.

Durst, R., Katz, G. and Knobler, H.Y. (1997). Buspirone augmentation of fluvoxamine in the treatment of kleptomania. (1997). *J Nerv Ment Dis*, **185**: 586–8.

Eales, M.J. and Layeni, A.O. (1994). Exacerbation of obsessive–compulsive symptoms associated with clozapine. *Br J Psychiatry*, **164**: 687–8.

Eapen, V., Trimble. R.R. and Robertson M.M. (1996). The use of fluoxetine in Gilles de la Tourette sundrome and obsessive compulsive behaviours: Preliminary clinical experience. *Prog Neuro-Psychopharmacol Biol Psychiat*, **20**: 737–43.

Egrilmez, A., Gülseren, L., Gülseren, S. and Kültür, S. (1997). Phenomenology of obsessions in a Turkish series of OCD patients. *Psychopathology*, **30**: 106–10.

Eisen, J.L., Beer, D.A., Pato, M.T., Venditto, T.A. and Rasmussen, S.A. (1997). Obsessive–compulsive disorder in patients with schizophrenia or schizoaffective disorder. *Am J Psychiatry*, **154**: 271–3.

Elliott, M.L. and Biever L.S. (1996). Head injury and sexual dysfunction. *Brain Injury*, **10**: 703–17.

Ellison, J.M., Milofsky, J.E. and Ely, E. (1990). Fluoxetine-induced bradycardia and syncope in two patients. *J Clin Psychiatry*, **51**: 385–6.

Ellison, J.M. and Stanziani, P. (1993). SSRI-associated nocturnal bruxism in four patients. *J Clin Psychiatry*, **54**: 432–4.

Emmanuel, N.P., Lydiard, R.B. and Crawford, M. (1997). Treatment of irritable bowel syndrome with fluvoxamine. (Letter.) *Am J Psychiatry*, **154**: 711–12.

Emmelkamp, P.M.G. (1982). *Phobic and Obsessive–Compulsive Disorders*. New York: Plenum Press.

England, S.L. and Gotestam, K.G. (1991). The nature and treatment of excessive gambling. *Acta Psychiatr Scand*, **84**: 113–20.

Enoch, M.D. and Trethowan, W.H. (1979). *Uncommon Psychiatric Syndromes*, 2nd edn. Bristol: J. Wright.

Erkwoh, R. (1993). FDG–PET and electroencephalographic findings in a patient suffering from musical hallucinations. *Nuklear Medizin*, **32**: 159–63.

Escalona, P.R., Adair, J.C., Roberts, B.B. and Graeber, D.A. (1997). Obsessive–compulsive disorder following bilateral globus pallidus infarction. *Biol Psychiatry*, **42**: 410–2.

Fabbri, R. and Dy, A.J. (1974). Hypnotic treatment of trichotillomania: Two cases. *Int J Clin Exp Hyp*, **22**: 210–15.

Faber, R.J. and O'Guinn, T.C. (1992). A clinical screener for compulsive buying. *J Cons Res*, **19**: 459–69.

Fallon, B.A., Campeas, R., Schneier, F.R., Hollander, E., Feerick, J., Hatterer, J., Goetz, D., Davies, S. and Liebowitz, M.R. (1992). Open trial of intravenous clomipramine in five treatment-refractory patients with obsessive–compulsive disorder. *J Neuropsychiatry Clin Neurosci*, **4**: 70–5.

Fallon, B.A., Liebowitz, M.R., Hollander, E., Schneier, F.R., Campeas, R.B., Fairbanks, J., Papp, L.A., Hatterer, J.A. and Sandberg, D. (1990). The pharmacotherapy of moral or religious scrupulosity. *J Clin Psychiatry*, **51**: 517–21.

Fallon, B.A., Liebowitz, M.R., Salman, E., Schneier, F.R., Jusino, C., Hollander, E. and Klein, D.F. (1993). Fluoxetine for hypochondriacal patients without major depression. *J Clin Psychopharmacol*, **13**: 438–41.

Fals-Stewart, W. and Lucente, S. (1993). An MCMI cluster typology of obsessive–compulsives: A measure of personality characteristics and its relationship to treatment participation, compliance and outcome in behavior therapy. *J Psychiatr Res*, **27**: 139–54.

Fava, M., Rosenbaum, J.F., McGrath, P.J., Stewart, J.W., Amsterdam, J.D. and Quitkin, F.M. (1994). Lithium and tricyclic augmentation of fluoxetine treatment for resistant major depression: A double-blind, controlled study. *Am J Psychiatry*, **151**: 1372–4.

Feder, R. (1991). Bradycardia and syncope induced by fluoxetine. (Letter.) *J Clin Psychiatry*, **52**: 139.

Feigin, A., Kurlan, R., McDermott, M.P., Beach, J., Dimitsopulos, T., Brower, C.A., Chapieski, L., Trinidad, K., Como, P. and Jankovic, J. (1996). A controlled trial of deprenyl in children with Tourette's syndrome and attention deficit hyperactivity disorder. *Neurology*, **46**: 965–8.

Fennig, S., Fennig, S.N., Pato, M. and Weitzman, A. (1994). Emergence of symptoms of Tourette's syndrome during fluvoxamine treatment of obsessive–compulsive disorder. *Br J Psychiatry*, **164**: 839–41.

Fenton, W.S. and McGlashan, T.H. (1986). The prognostic significance of obsessive–compulsive symptoms in schizophrenia. *Am J Psychiatry*, **143**: 437–41.

Figueroa, Y., Rosenberg, D.R., Birmaher, B. and Keshavan, M.S. (1998). Combination treatment with clomipramine and selective serotonin reuptake inhibitors for obsessive–compulsive disorder in children and adolescents. *J Child Adolesc Psychopharmacol* **8**: 61–7.

First, M.B., Spitzer, R.L., Gibbon, M. and Williams, J.B.W. (1995). *Structured Clinical Interview for DSM-IV Axis I Disorders – Patient Edition* (SCID-I/P, Version 2.0). New York: New York State Psychiatric Institute, Biometrics Research Department.

Fishbain, D.A. (1988). Kleptomanic behavior response to perphenazine-amitriptyline HCl combination. (Letter.) *Can J Psychiatry*, **33**: 241–2.

Flament, M.F., Whitaker, A., Rapoport, J.L., Davies, M., Berg, C.Z., Kalikow, K., Sceery, W. and Shaffer, D. (1988). Obsessive compulsive disorder in adolescence: An epidemiological study. *J Am Acad Child Adolesc Psychiatry*, **6**: 764–71.

Fleming, B. (1990). Dependent personality disorder. In *Cognitive Therapy of Personality Disorders*, ed. A.T. Beck, A. Freeman and Associates, pp. 283–308. New York: Guilford Press.

Foa, E.B. and Kozak, M.J. (1995). DSM-IV field trial: Obsessive–compulsive disorder. *Am J Psychiatry*, **152**: 90–6.

Foa, E.B. and Kozak, M.J. (1996). Psychological treatment for obsessive–compulsive disorder. In *Long-Term Treatments of Anxiety Disorders, ed. M.R. Mavissakalian and R.F. Prien*, pp. 285–309. Washington, DC: American Psychiatric Press.

Foa, E.B., Kozak, M.J., Steketee, G.S. and McCarthy, P.R. (1992). Treatment of depressive and obsessive–compulsive symptoms in OCD by imipramine and behavior therapy. *Br J Clin Psychol*, **31**: 279–92.

Foa, E.B., Steketee, G.S. and Ozarow, B.J. (1985). Behavior therapy with obsessive–compulsives: From theory to treatment. In *Obsessive-Compulsive Disorder: Psychological and Pharmacological Treatment*, ed. M. Mavissakalian, S.M. Turner and L. Michelson, pp. 59–129. New York: Plenum Press.

Fontaine, R. and Chouinard, G. (1989). Fluoxetine in the long-term maintenance treatment of obsessive compulsive disorder. *Psychiatr Ann*, **19**: 88–91.

Frankel, M., Cummings, J.L., Robertson, M.M., Trimble, M.R., Hill, M.A. and Benson, D.F. (1986). Obsessions and compulsions in Gilles de la Tourette's syndrome. *Neurology*, **36**: 378–82.

Frankenburg, F. (1984). Hoarding in anorexia nervosa. *Br J Med Psychol*, **57**: 57–60.

Freeman, C.P.L., Trimble, M.R., Dakin, J.F.W., Stokes, T.M. and Ashford, J.J. (1994). Fluvoxamine versus clomipramine in the treatment of obsessive compulsive disorder: A multicenter, randomized, double-blind, parallel group comparison. *J Clin Psychiatry*, **55**: 1–5.

Freeman, T. (1990). Psychoanalytical aspects of morbid jealousy in women. *Br J Psychiatry*, **156**: 68–72.

Freeston, M.H. and Ladouceur, R. (1997). What do patients do with their obsessive thoughts? *Behav Res Ther*, **35**: 335–48.

Freeston, M.H., Rhéaume, J. and Ladouceur, R. (1996). Correcting faulty appraisals of obsessional thoughts. *Beh Res Ther*, **34**: 433–46.

Freud, S. (1909). Notes upon a case of obsessional neurosis. In *Standard Edition of the Complete Psychological Works of Sigmund Freud*, vol. 10, ed. J. Strachey, pp.165–73. London: Hogarth Press (1955).

Freud, S. (1913). The disposition to obsessional neurosis. In *Standard Edition of the Complete Psychological Works of Sigmund Freud*, vol. 12, ed. J. Strachey, pp.311–26. London: Hogarth Press (1958).

Freud, S. (1926). Inhibitions, symptoms and anxiety. In *Standard Edition of the Complete Psychological Works of Sigmund Freud*, vol. 20, ed. J. Strachey, pp.87–178. London: Hogarth Press (1959).

Friman, P.C., Finney, J.W. and Christophersen, E.R. (1984). Behavioral treatment of trichotillomania: An evaluative review. *Behav Ther*, **15**: 249–65.

Frost, L. and Lal, S. (1995). Shock-like sensations after discontinuation of selective serotonin reuptake inhibitors. (Letter.) *Am J Psychiatry*, **152**: 810.

Frost, R.O. and Gross, R.C. (1993). The hoarding of possessions. *Behav Res Ther*, **31**: 367–81.

Frost, R.O., Hartl, T.L., Christian, R. and Williams, N. (1995). The value of possessions in compulsive hoarding: Patterns of use and attachment. *Behav Res Ther*, **33**: 897–902.

Fruensgaard, K. (1991a). Psychotherapeutic strategy and neurotic excoriations. *Int J Dermatol*, **30**: 198–203.

Fruensgaard, K. (1991b). Psychotherapy and neurotic excoriations. *Int J Dermatol*, **30**: 262–5.

Frye, P.E. and Arnold, L.E. (1981). Persistent amphetamine-induced compulsive rituals: Response to pyridoxine(B6). *Biol Psychiatry*, **16**: 583–7.

Fulcher, K.Y. and White, P.D. (1997). Randomised controlled trial of graded exercise in patients with the chronic fatigue syndrome. *Br Med J*, **314**: 1647–52.

Fux, M., Levine, J., Aviv, A. and Belmaker, R.H. (1996). Inositol treatment of obsessive–compulsive disorder. *Am J Psychiatry*, **153**: 1219–21.

Gabbard, G.O. (1994). *Psychodynamic Psychiatry in Clinical Practice: The DSM-IV Edition.* Washington, DC: American Psychiatric Press.

Gabbard, G.O. (Ed.) (1995). *Treatments of Psychiatric Disorders*, 2nd edn. vols. 1 and 2. Washington, DC: American Psychiatric Press.

Galski, T. (1981). The adjunctive use of hypnosis in the treatment of trichotillomania: A case report. *Am J Clin Hyp*, **23**: 198–201.

Gatto, E., Pikielny, R. and Micheli, F. (1994). Fluoxetine in Tourette's syndrome. (Letter.) *Am J Psychiatry*, **151**: 946–7.

Gauthier, J. and Pellerin, D. (1982). Management of compulsive shoplifting through covert sensitization. *J Beh Ther Exp Psychiatry*, **13**: 73–5.

George, M., Kellner, C. and Fossey, M. (1989). Obsessive–compulsive symptoms in a patient with multiple sclerosis. *J Nerv Ment Dis*, **177**: 304–5.

George, M.S. and Trimble, M.R. (1993). Dystonic reaction associated with fluvoxamine. (Letter.) *J Clin Psychopharmacol*, **13**: 220–1.

George, M.S., Trimble, M.R., Ring, H.A., Sallee, F.R. and Robertson, M.M. (1993a). Obsessions in obsessive–compulsive disorder with and without Gilles de la Tourette's syndrome. *Am J Psychiatry*, **150**: 93–102.

George, M.S., Trimble, M.R. and Robertson, M.M. (1993b). Fluvoxamine and sulpiride in comorbid obsessive–compulsive disorder and Gilles de la Tourette syndrome. *Human Psychopharmacol*, **8**: 327–34.

Ghaemi, S.N., Zarate, C.A., Pople, A.P., Pillay, S.S. and Cole, J.O. (1995). Is there a relationship between clozapine and obsessive–compulsive disorder? A retrospective chart review. *Compr Psychiatry*, **36**: 267–70.

Gidal, B.E., Anderson, G.D., Seaton, T.L., Miyoshi, H.R. and Wilenksy, A.J. (1993). Evaluation of the effect of fluoxetine on the formation of carbamazepine epoxide. *Ther Drug Monit*, **15**: 247–50.

Gitlin, M. (1993). Pharmacotherapy of personality disorders: Conceptual framework and clinical strategies. *J Clin Psychopharmacol*, **13**: 343–53.

Gitlin, M. (1994). Psychotropic medications and their effects on sexual function: Diagnosis, biology, and treatment approaches. *J Clin Psychiatry*, **55**: 406–13.

Gitlin, M. (1995a). Effects of depression and antidepressants on sexual functioning. *Bull Menninger Clin*, **59**: 232–48.

Gitlin, M. (1995b). Treatment of sexual side effects with dopaminergic agents. (Letter.) *J Clin Psychiatry*, **56**: 124.

Gitlin, M. (1997). Venlafaxine, monoamine oxidase inhibitors, and the serotonin syndrome. (Letter.) *J Clin Psychopharmacol,* **17**: 66–7.

Glassman, A. and Bigger, J.T. (1981). Cardiovascular effects of therapeutic doses of tricyclic antidepressants. *Arch Gen Psychiatry,* **38**: 815–20.

Glover, J.H. (1985). A case of kleptomania treated by covert sensitization. *Br J Clin Psychol,* **24**: 213–14.

Goetz, C. G., (1993). Clonidine. In *Handbook of Tourette's Syndrome and Related Tic and Behavioral Disorders,* ed. R. Kurlan, pp. 377–88. New York: Marcel Dekker.

Goetz, C.G., Tanner, C.M., Stebbins, G.T., Leipzig, G. and Carr, W.C. (1992). Adult tics in Gilles de la Tourette's syndrome: Description and risk factors. *Neurology,* **42**: 784–8.

Goetz, C.G., Tanner, C.M., Wilson, R.S., Carroll, V.S., Garron, P.G. and Shannon, K.M. (1987). Clonidine and Gilles de la Tourette's Syndrome: Double-blind study using objective rating methods. *Ann Neurol,* **21**: 307–10.

Golden, R.N. (1993). Treatment of attention deficit hyperactivity disorder. In *Handbook of Tourette's Syndrome and Related Tic and Behavioral Disorders,* ed. R. Kurlan, pp. 423–30. New York: Marcel Dekker.

Goldman, M.J. (1991). Kleptomania: Making sense of the nonsensical. *Am J Psychiatry,* **148**: 986–96.

Goldstein, D.J., Williams, M.L. and Pearson, D.K. (1991). Fluoxetine-exposed pregnancies. *Clin Res,* **39**: 768A.

Goodman, A. (1993). Diagnosis and treatment of sexual addiction. *J Sex Marital Ther,* **19**: 225–51.

Goodman, W.K., McDougle, C.J. and Price, L.H. (1992a). Pharmacotherapy of obsessive–compulsive disorder. *J Clin Psychiatry,* **53**(suppl 4): 29–37.

Goodman, W.K., McDougle, C.J. and Price, L.H. (1992b). The role of serotonin and dopamine in the pathophysiology of obsessive compulsive-disorder. *Int Clin Psychopharmacol,* **7**(suppl 1): 35–8.

Goodman, W.K., Price, L., Rasmussen, S., Mazure, C., Delgado, P., Henninger, G.R. and Charney, D.S. (1989b). The Yale-Brown Obsessive Compulsive Scale (Y-BOCS): Part II. Validity. *Arch Gen Psychiatry,* **46**: 1012–16.

Goodman, W.K., Price, L., Rasmussen, S., Mazure, C., Fleischman, R.L., Hill, C.L., Henninger, G.R. and Charney, D.S. (1989a). The Yale-Brown Obsessive Compulsive Scale (Y-BOCS): Part I. Development, use, and reliability. *Arch Gen Psychiatry,* **46**: 1006–11.

Gordon, A.G. (1994). Musical hallucinations. *Neurology,* 44: 986.

Gordon, C.T., Cotelingam, G.M., Stager, S., Ludlow, C.L., Hamburger, S.D. and Rapoport, J.L. (1995). A double-blind comparison of clomipramine and desipramine in the treatment of developmental stuttering. *J Clin Psychiatry,* **56**: 238–42.

Gorman, D.G. and Cummings J.L. (1992). Hypersexuality following septal injury. *Arch Neurol,* **49**: 308–10.

Goscinski, I., Kwiatkowski, S., Polak, J., Orlowiejska, M.J. Partyk, A. (1997). The Klüver Bucy syndrome. *J Neurol Sci,* **41**: 269–72.

Goshen, C.E. (Ed.) (1967). *Documentary History of Psychiatry: A Source Book on Historical Principles.* New York: Philosophical Library.

Gottesman, H.G. and Schubert, D.S.P. (1993). Low-dose medroxyprogesterone acetate in the management of the paraphilias. *J Clin Psychiatry,* **54**: 182–8.

Grady, T., Pigott, T.A., L'Heureux, F., Hill, J.L., Bernstein, S.E. and Murphy, D.L. (1993). Double-blind study of adjuvant buspirone for fluoxetine-treated patients with obsessive–compulsive disorder. *Am J Psychiatry*, **150**: 819–21.

Greenberg, D. (1987). Compulsive hoarding. *Am J Psychotherapy*, **41**: 409–16.

Greenberg, D. and Witztum, E. (1994). Cultural aspects of obsessive compulsive disorder. In *Current Insights in Obsessive Compulsive Disorder*, ed. E. Hollander, J. Zohar, D. Marazzitti and B. Olivier, pp. 11–21. New York: John Wiley and Sons

Greenberg, D., Witztum, E. and Levy, A. (1990). Hoarding as a psychiatric symptom. *J Clin Psychiatry* **51**: 417–21.

Greenberg, H.R. and Sarner, C.A. (1965). Trichotillomania. *Arch Gen Psychiatry*, **12**: 482–9.

Greenblatt, D.J., Miller, L.G. and Shader, R.I. (1987). Clonazepam pharmokinetics, brain uptake, and receptor interactions. *J Clin Psychiatry* **48**(suppl 10): 4–11.

Greenblatt, D.J., Preskorn, S.H., Cotreau, M.M., Horst, W.D. and Harmatz, J.S. (1992). Fluoxetine impairs clearance of alprazolam but not of clonazepam. *Clin Pharmacol Ther*, **52**: 479–86.

Greist, J., Chouinard, G., DuBoff, E., Halaris, A., Kim, S.W., Koran, L., Liebowitz, M., Lydiard, R.B., Rasmussen, S., White, K. and Sikes, C. (1995a). Double-blind parallel comparison of three doses of sertraline and placebo in outpatients with obsessive compulsive disorder. *Arch Gen Psychiatry* **52**:289–95.

Greist, J.H., Jefferson, J.W., Kobak, K.A., Chouinard, G., DuBoff, E., Halaris, A., Kim, S.W., Koran, L., Liebowitz, M.R., Lydiard, B., McElroy, S., Mendels, J., Rasmussen, S., White, K. and Flicker, C. (1995b). A 1 year double-blind placebo-controlled fixed dose study of sertraline in the treatment of obsessive–compulsive disorder. *Int Clin Psychopharmacol*, **10**: 57–65.

Greist, J.H., Jefferson, J.W., Kobak, K.A., Katzelnick, D.J. and Serlin, R.C. (1995c). Efficacy and tolerability of serotonin transport inhibitors in obsessive-compulsve disorder. *Arch Gen Psychiatry*, **52**: 53–60.

Greist, J.H., Jenike, M.A., Robinson, D. and Rasmussen, S.A. (1995d). Efficacy of fluvoxamine in obsessive–compulsive disorder: Results of a multicentre, double blind, placebo-controlled trial. *Eur J Clin Res*, **7**: 195–204.

Gross, M.D. (1991). Treatment of pathological jealousy by fluoxetine. (Letter.) *Am J Psychiatry*, **148**: 683–4.

Grossman, R. and Hollander, E. (1996). Treatment of obsessive–compulsive disorder with venlafaxine. (Letter.) *Am J Psychiatry*, **153**: 576–7.

Gruber, A.J., Hudson, J.I. and Pope, H.G. (1996). The management of treatment-resistant depression in disorders on the interface of psychiatry and medicine: Fibromyalgia, chronic fatigue syndrome, migraine, irritable bowel syndrome, atypical facial pain, and premenstrual dysphoric disorder. *Psychiatr Clin North Am*, **19**: 351–69.

Gudjonsson, G.H. (1987). The significance of depression in the mechanism of "compulsive" shoplifting. *Med Sci Law*, **27**: 171–6.

Guidry, L.S. (1969). Use of a covert punishing contingency in compulsive stealing. *J Beh Ther Exp Psychiatry*, **6**: 169.

Gupta, M.A., Gupta, A. K. and Haberman, J.F. (1986). Neurotic excoriations: A review and some new perspectives. *Compr Psychiatry*, **27**: 381–6.

Gupta, S. and Freimer, M. (1993). Trichotillomania, clomipramine, topical steroids. (Letter.) *Am J Psychiatry*, **150**: 524.

Gupta, S. and Major, L.F. (1991). Hair loss associated with fluoxetine. (Letter.) *Br J Psychiatry*, **159**: 737–8.

Guthrie, S. and Grunhaus, L. (1990). Fluoxetine-induced stuttering. (Letter.) *J Clin Psychiatry*, **51**: 85.

Guy, Y. (Ed.) (1976). *ECDEU Assessment Manual for Psychopharmacology*. Publication ADM 76-338, pp. 218–222. Washington, DC: US Department of Health, Education, and Welfare.

Haddad, P. (1997). Newer antidepressants and the discontinuation syndrome. *J Clin Psychiatry*, **58**(suppl 7): 17–22.

Hall, J.R. and McGill, J.C. (1986). Hypnobehavioral treatment of self-destructive behavior: Trichotillomania and bulimia in the same patient. *Am J Clin Hyp*, **29**:39–46.

Hall, M.J. (1994). Breast tenderness and enlargement induced by sertraline. (Letter.) *Am J Psychiatry*, **151**: 1395–6.

Hall, R.C.W. (1994). Legal precedents affecting managed care: The physician's responsibilities to patients. *Psychosomatics*, **35**: 105–17.

Haller, R. and Hinterhuber, H. (1994). Treatment of pathological gambling with carbamazepine. *Pharmacopsychiatry*, **27**: 129.

Hallopeau, M. (1889). Alopecie par grattage (trichomanie ou trichotillomanie). *Ann Dermatol Syphil*, **10**: 440–1.

Hamner, M.B. (1992). Obsessive-compulsive symptoms associated with acute intermittent porphyria. *Psychosomatics*, **33**: 329–32.

Hantouche, E.G., Lancrenon, S., Bouhassira, M., Ravily, V., and Bourgeois, M.L. (1997). Evaluation répétée de l'impulsivité dans une cohorte de 155 patients souffrant d'un trouble obsessionnel–compulsif: suivi prospectif de 12 mois. *L'Encéphale* **23**: 83–90.

Hardie, R.J., Lees, A.J. and Stern, G.M. (1984). On-off fluctuations in Parkinson's disease: A clinical and neuropharmacological study. *Brain*, **107**: 487–506.

Hassanye, F., Murray, R.B. and Rodgers, H. (1991). Adrenocortical suppression presenting with agitated depression, morbid jealousy and a dementia-like state. *Br J Psychiatry*, **159**: 870–2.

Hatch, M.L. (1997). Conceptualization and treatment of bowel obsessions: Two case reports. *Behav Res Ther*, **35**: 253–7.

Heimberg, R.G. (1993). Specific issues in the cognitive–behavioral treatment of social phobia. *J Clin Psychiatry*, **54**(suppl 12): 36–45.

Heimberg, R.G. and Juster, H.R. (1994). Treatment of social phobia in cognitive-behavioral groups. *J Clin Psychiatry*, **55**(suppl 6): 38–46.

Heimke, C., Weigmann, H., Härtter, S., Dahmen, N., Wetzel, H. and Müller, H. (1994). Elevated levels of clozapine in serum after addition of fluvoxamine. (Letter.) *J Clin Psychopharmacol*, **14**: 279–81.

Heisler, M.A., Guidry, J.R. and Arnecke, B. (1996). Serotonin syndrome induced by administration of venlafaxine and phenelzine. (Letter.) *Ann Pharmacother*, **30**: 84.

Hellings, J.A. and Warnock, J.K. (1994). Self-injurious behavior and serotonin in Prader–Willi syndrome. *Psychopharmacol Bull*, **30**: 245–50.

Helzer, J.E., Robins, L.N., McEvoy, L.T., Spitznagel, E.L., Stoltzman, R.K., Farmer, A. and Brockington, I.F. (1985). A comparison of clinical and Diagnostic Interview Schedule diagnoses. *Arch Gen Psychiatry*, **42**: 657–66.

Hendrickx, B., Van Moffaert M., Spiers R. and Von Frenckell R. (1991). The treatment of psychocutaneous disorders: A new approach. *Curr Ther Res Clin Exp*, **49**: 111–19.

Hermesh, H., Aizenberg, D. and Munitz, H. (1990). Trazodone treatment in clomipramine-resistant obsessive–compulsive disorder. *Clin Neuropharmacol*, **13**: 322–8.

Hermesh, H., Shahar, A. and Munitz, H. (1987). Obsessive-compulsive disorder and borderline personality disorder. *Am J Psychiatry*, **144**: 120–1.

Hewlett, W.A., Vinogradov, S. and Agras, W.S. (1990). Clonazepam treatment of obsessions and compulsions. *J Clin Psychiatry*, **51**: 158–61.

Hewlett, W.A., Vinogradov, S. and Agras, W.S. (1992). Clomipramine, clonazepam, and clonidine treatment of obsessive–compulsive disorder. *J Clin Psychopharmacol*, **12**: 420–30.

Hodgson, R.E., Murray, D. and Woods, M. R. (1992). Othello's syndrome and hyperthyroidism. *J Nerv Ment Dis*, **180**: 663–4.

Hoehn-Saric, R., Lipsey, J.R. and McLeod, D.R. (1990). Apathy and indifference in patients on fluvoxamine and fluoxetine. *J Clin Psychopharmacol*, **10**: 343–5.

Hollander, E. (Ed.) (1993). *Obsessive–Compulsive Related Disorders*. Washington DC: American Psychiatric Press.

Hollander, E. (1997). Gambling: Overview and new pharmacological treatments. Presented at the 150th Annual Meeting of the Amercian Psychiatric Association, San Diego, CA, May 17–22, 1997.

Hollander, E., Cohen, L.J. and Simeon, D. (1993). Body dysmorphic disorder. *Psychiatr Ann*, **23**: 359–64.

Hollander, E., DeCaria, C.M., Schneier, F.R., Schneier, H.A., Liebowitz, M. and Klein, D.F. (1990). Fenfluramine augmentation of serotonin reuptake blockade antiobsessional treatment. *J Clin Psychiatry*, **51**: 119–23.

Hollander, E., Frenkel, M., DeCaria, C., Trungold, S. and Stein, D.J. (1992a). Treatment of pathological gambling with clomipramine. *Am J Psychiatry*, **149**: 710–1.

Hollander, E. and McCarley, A. (1992). Yohimbine treatment of sexual side effects induced by serotonin reuptake blockers. *J Clin Psychiatry*, **53**: 207–9.

Hollander, E., Neville, D., Frenkel, M., Josephson, S. and Liebowitz, M.R. (1992b). Body dysmorphic disorder: Diagnostic issues and related disorders. *Psychosomatics*, **33**: 156–65.

Hollander, E. and Wong C.M. (1995). Obsessive–compulsive spectrum disorder. *J Clin Psychiatry*, **56**(suppl 4): 3–6.

Holzer, J.C., Goodman, W.K., McDougle, C., Baer, L., Boyarsky, B.K., Leckman, J.F. and Price, L.H. (1994). Obsessive–compulsive disorder with and without a chronic tic disorder: A comparison of symptoms in 70 patients. *Br J Psychiatry*, **164**: 469–73.

Hoogduin, C.A.L., Duivenvoorden, H., Schaap, C. and de Haan, E. (1989). On the outpatient treatment of obsessive compulsives: Outcome, prediction of outcome and follow-up. In *Fresh Perspectives on Anxiety Disorders*, ed. P.M.G. Emmelkamp, W.T.A.M. Everaerd, F.W. Kraaimaat and M.J.M. van Son, pp. 173–85. Amsterdam: Swets and Zeitlinger.

Humberto, N., Weissbecker, K., Mejia, J.M. and Sanchez de Camerona, M. (1993). Family study of obsessive–compulsive disorder in a Mexican population. *Arch Med Res*, **24**: 193–8.

Hunter, R. and Macalpine, I. (Ed.) (1963). *Three Hundred Years of Psychiatry 1534–1860*. London: Oxford University Press.

Husain, M.M., Lewis, S.F. and Thornton, W.L. (1993). Maintenance ECT for refractory obsessive–compulsive disorder. *Am J Psychiatry*, **150**: 1899–900.

Hwang, M.Y., Martin, A.M., Lindenmayer, J.P., Stein, D. and Hollander, E. (1993). Treatment of schizophrenia with obsessive compulsive features with serotonin reuptake inhibitors. (Letter.) *Am J Psychiatry*, **150**: 1127.

Hynes, J.V. (1982). Hypnotic treatment of five adult cases of trichotillomania. *Aust J Clin Exp Hyp*, **10**: 109–16.

Iancu, I., Kotler, M., Bleich, A. and Lepkifker, E. (1995). Clomipramine efficacy for Tourette syndrome and major depression: A case study. *Biol Psychiatry*, **38**: 407–9.

Iancu, I., Weizman, A., Kindler, S., Sasson, Y. and Zohar, J. (1996). Serotonergic drugs in trichotillomania: treatment results in 12 patients. *J Nerv Ment Dis*, **184**: 641–4.

Insel, T.R. (1992). Toward a neuroanatomy of obsessive–compulsive disorder. *Arch Gen Psychiatry*, **49**: 739–44.

Insel, T.R., Hoover, C. and Murphy, D.L. (1983). Parents of patients with obsessive–compulsive disorder. *Psychol Med*, **13**: 807–11.

Insel, T.R. and Pickar, D. (1983). Naloxone administration in obsessive–compulsive disorder: Report of two cases. *Am J Psychiatry*, **140**: 1219–20.

Irle, E., Exner, C., Thielen, K., Weniger, G. and Rüther, E. (1998). Obsessive–compulsive disorder and ventromedial frontal lesions: Clinical and neuropsychological findings. *Am J Psychiatry*, **155**: 255–63.

Iruela, L.M., Gilaberte, I., Caballero, L. and Oliveros, S.C. (1990). Pathological jealousy and pimozide. (Letter.) *Br J Psychiatry*, **156**: 749.

Jackson, C., Carson, W., Markowitz, J. and Mintzer, J. (1995). SIADH associated with fluoxetine and sertraline therapy. (Letter.) *Am J Psychiatry*, **152**: 809–10.

Jackson, S. (1986). *Melancholia and Depression From Hippocratic Times to Modern Times*. New Haven, Connecticut: Yale University Press.

Jacobsen, F.M. (1992). Fluoxetine-induced sexual dysfunction and an open trial of yohimbine. *J Clin Psychiatry*, **53**: 119–22.

Jacobsen, F.M. (1995). Risperidone in the treatment of affective illness and obsessive–compulsive disorder. *J Clin Psychiatry*, **56**: 423–9.

Jankovic, J. (1992). Diagnosis and classification of tics and Tourette syndrome. *Adv Neurol*, **58**: 7–14.

Jankovic, J. (1993). Tics in other neurological disorders. In *Handbook of Tourette's Syndrome and Related Tic and Behavioral Disorders*, ed. R. Kurlan, pp. 167–82. New York: Marcel Dekker.

Jefferson, J.W. (1995). Social phobia: A pharmacologic treatment overview. *J Clin Psychiatry*, **56**(suppl 5): 18–24.

Jefferson, J.W. (1997). Antidepressants in panic disorder. *J Clin Psychiatry*, **58**(suppl 2): 20–4.

Jefferson, J.W., Greist, J.H., Perse, T.L. and Rosenfeld, R. (1991). Fluvoxamine-associated mania/hypomania in patients with obsessive–compulsive disorder. (Letter.) *J Clin Psychopharmacol*, **11**: 391–3.

Jelliffe, S.E. (1929). Psychologic components in postencephalitic oculogyric crises: Contribution to a genetic interpretation of compulsions phenomena. *Arch Neurol Psychiatry*, **21**: 491–532.

Jelliffe, S.E. (1932). Psychopathology of forced movements in oculogyric crises. *Nerv Ment Dis Monograph Series*, **55**: 1–219.

Jenike, M.A. (1991). Severe hair loss associated with fluoxetine treatment. (Letter.) *Am J Psychiatry*, **148**: 392.

Jenike, M.A. (1992). New developments in treatment of obsessive–compulsive disorder. In *Review of Psychiatry*, vol 11, ed. A. Tasman and M.B. Riba, pp. 323–346. Washington, DC: American Psychiatric Press.

Jenike, M.A., Baer, L., Ballantine, H.T., Martuza, R.L., Tynes, S., Giriunas, I., Buttolph, M.L. and Cassem, N.H. (1991a). Cingulotomy for refractory obsessive–compulsive disorder. *Arch Gen Psychiatry*, **48**: 548–55.

Jenike, M.A., Baer, L. and Buttolph, L. (1991b). Buspirone augmentation of fluoxetine in patients with obsessive compulsive disorder. *J Clin Psychiatry*, **52**: 13–14.

Jenike, M.A., Baer, L., Minichiello, W.E., Rauch, S.L. and Buttolph, M.L. (1997). Placebo-controlled trial of fluoxetine and phenelzine for obsessive–compulsive disorder. *Am J Psychiatry*, **154**: 1261–4.

Jenike, M.A. and Rauch, S.L. (1994). Managing the patient with treatment-resistant obsessive compulsive disorder. *J Clin Psychiatry*, **55**(suppl 3): 11–17.

Jenike, M.A., Vitagliano, H.L., Rabinowitz, J., Goff, D.C. and Baer, L. (1987). Bowel obsessions responsive to tricyclic antidepressants in four patients. *Am J Psychiatry*, **144**: 1347–8.

Joffe, R.T. and Schuller, D.R. (1993). An open study of buspirone augmentation of sertonin reuptake inhibitors in refractory depression. *J Clin Psychiatry*, **54**: 269–71.

Joffe, R.T., Swinson, R.P. and Regan, J.J. (1988). Personality features of obsessive–compulsive disorder. *Am J Psychiatry*, **145**: 1127–9.

John, L., Perreault, M.M., Tao, T. and Blew, P.G. (1997). Sertonin syndrome associated with nefazodone and paroxetine. *Ann Emergency Med*, **29**: 287–9.

Judd, F.K., Chua, P., Lynch, C. and Norman, T. (1991). Fenfluramine augmentation of clomipramine treatment of obsessive compulsive disorder. *Aust N Z J Psychiatry*, **25**: 412–14.

Kafka, M.P. (1991). Successful antidepressant treatment of nonparaphilic sexual addictions and paraphilias in men. *J Clin Psychiatry*, **52**: 60–5.

Kafka, M.P. (1994). Sertraline pharmacotherapy for paraphilias and paraphilia-related disorders: An open trial. *Ann Clin Psychiatry*, **6**: 189–95.

Kafka, M.P. and Coleman, E. (1991). Serotonin and paraphilias: The convergence of mood, impulse and compulsive disorders. *J Clin Psychopharmacol*, **11**: 223–4.

Kafka, M.P. and Prentky, R. (1992). Fluoxetine treatment of nonparaphilic sexual addictions and paraphilias in men. *J Clin Psychiatry*, **53**: 351–8.

Kafka, M.P. and Prentky, R.A. (1994). Preliminary observations of DSM-III-R Axis I comorbidity in men with paraphilias and paraphilia-related disorders. *J Clin Psychiatry*, **55**: 481–7.

Kafka, M.P. and Prentky, R.A. (1997). Compulsive sexual behavior characteristics. (Letter.) *Am J Psychiatry*, **154**: 1632.

Kahne, G.J. and Wray, R.W. (1989). Clomipramine for bowel obsessions. *Am J Psychiatry*, **146**: 120–1.

Kalivas, J., Kalivas, L and Gilman, D. (1996). Sertraline in the treatment of neurotic excoriations and related disorders. (Letter.) *Arch Dermatol*, **132**: 589–90.

Kant, R., Smith-Seemiller, L. and Duffy, J.D. (1996). Obsessive compulsive disorder after closed head injury: Review of the literature and report of four cases. *Brain Injury*, **10**: 55–63.

Karno, M., Golding, J.M., Sorenson, S.B. and Burnam, A. (1988). The epidemiology of obsessive–compulsive disorder in five US communities. *Arch Gen Psychiatry*, **45**: 1094–9.

Katona, C.L., Abou-Saleh, M.T., Harrison, D.A., Nairac, B.A., Edwards, D.R., Lock, T., Burns, R.A. and Robertson, M.M. (1995). Placebo-controlled trial of lithium augmentation of fluoxetine and lofepramine. [Published erratum appears in *Br J Psychiatry* (1995); 166: 544.] [See comments.] *Br J Psychiatry*, **166**: 80–6.

Katz, R.J., Deveaugh-Geiss, J. and Landau, P. (1990). Clomipramine in obsessive–compulsive disorder. *Biol Psychiatry*, **28**: 401–14.

Katzelnick, D.J., Kobak, K.A., Greist, J.H., Jefferson, J.W., Mantle, J.M. and Serlin, R.C. (1995). Sertraline for social phobia: A double-blind, placebo-controlled crossover study. *Am J Psychiatry*, **152**: 1368–71.

Keijsers, G.P.J., Hoogduin, C. A.L. and Schaap, C.P.D.R. (1994). Predictors of treatment in the behavioural treatment of obsessive–compulsive disorder. *Br J Psychiatry*, **165**: 781–6.

Keller, M.B., Gelenberg, A.J., Hirschfeld, R.M.A. et al., (1998). A double-blind, randomized trial of sertraline or imipramine in chronic depression. *J Clin Psychiatry*. **59**: 598–607.

Kellner, R. (1985). Functional somatic symptoms and hypochondriasis: A survey of empirical studies. *Arch Gen Psychiatry*, **42**: 821–33.

Kellner, R. (1992). Diagnosis and treatments of hypochondriacal syndromes. *Psychosomatics*, **33**: 278–89.

Keuler, D.J., Altemus, M., Michelson, D., Greenberg, B. and Murphy, D.L. (1996). Behavioral effects of naloxone infusion in obsessive–compulsive disorder. *Biol Psychiatry*, **40**: 154–6.

Kenyon, F.E. (1976). Hypochondriacal states. *Br J Psychiatry*, **129**: 1–14.

Ketheun, N.J., Cyr, P., Ricciardi, J.A., Minichiello, W.E., Buttolph, M.L. and Jenike, M.A. (1994). Medication withdrawal symptoms in obsessive–compulsive disorder patients treated with paroxetine. (Letter.) *J Clin Psychopharmacol*, **14**: 206–7.

Ketheun, N.J., O'Sullivan, R.L., Hayday, C.F., Peets, K.E., Jenike, M.A. and L. Baer. (1997). The relationship of menstrual cycle and pregnancy to compulsive hairpulling. *Psychother Psychosom*, **66**: 33–7.

Ketheun, N.J., O'Sullivan, R.L., Ricciardi, J.N., Shera, D., Savage, C.R., Borgmann, A.S., Jenike, M.A. and Baer, L. (1995). The Massachusetts General Hospital (MGH) Hairpulling Scale: 1. Development and factor analyses. *Psychother Psychosom*, **64**: 141–5.

Kettl, P.A. and Marks, I.M. (1986). Neurological factors in obsessive compulsive disorder: Two case reports and a review of the literature. *Br J Psychiatry*, **149**: 315–19.

Keutzer, C. (1972). Kleptomania: A direct approach to treatment. *Br J Med Psychol*, **45**: 159–63.

Khanna, S., Kaliaperumal, V.G. and Channabasavanna, S.M. (1990). Clusters of obsessive–compulsive phenomena in obsessive–compulsive disorder. *Br J Psychiatry*, **156**: 51–4.

Kindler, S., Dannon, P.N., Iancu, I., Sasson, Y. and Zohar, J. (1997). Emergence of kleptomania during treatment for depression with serotonin selective reuptake inhibitors. *Clin Neuropharmacol*, **20**: 126–9.

Kinsey, A.C., Pomeroy, W.B. and Martin, C.E. (1948). *Sexual Behavior in the Human Male*. Philadelphia: W.B. Saunders.

Kinsey, A.C., Pomeroy, W.B., Martin, C.E. and Gebhard, P.H. (1953). *Sexual Behavior in the Human Female*. Philadelphia: W.B. Saunders.

Klerman, G.L. and Weissman, M.M. (Eds.). (1993). *New Applications of Interpersonal Psychotherapy*. Washington, DC: American Psychiatric Press.

Kline, M.D. and Koppes, S. (1994). Acidophilus for sertraline-induced diarrhea. (Letter.) *Am J Psychiatry*, **151**: 1521–2.

Kmetz, G.F., McElroy, S.L. and Collins, D.J. (1997). Response of kleptomania and mixed mania to valproate. (Letter.) *Am J Psychiatry*, **154**: 580–1.

Koizumi, H.M. (1985). Obsessive-compulsive symptoms following stimulants. *Biol Psychiatry*, **20**: 1332–7.

Kopala, L. and Honer, W. G. (1994). Risperidone, serotonergic mechanisms, and obsessive–compulsive symptoms in schizophrenia. *Am J Psychiatry*, **151**: 1714–15.

Koponen, H., Lepola, U., Leinonen, E., Jakinen, R., Penttinen, J. and Turtonen, J. (1997). Citalopram in the treatment of obsessive compulsive disorder: An open pilot study. *Acta Psychiatr Scand*, **96**: 343–6.

Koran, L.M., Cain, J.W., Dominguez, R.A., Rush, A.J. and Thiemann, S. (1996a). Are fluoxetine plasma levels related to outcome in obsessive–compulsive disorder? *Am J Psychiatry*, **153**:1450–4.

Koran, L.M., Faravelli, C. and Pallanti, S. (1994). Intravenous clomipranine for obsessive–compulsive disorder. (Letter.) *J Clin Psychopharmacol*, **14**: 216–18.

Koran, L.M., Gelenberg, A., Kornstein, S.K., Howland, R.H., Friedman, R.A., DeBattista, C., Keller, M.B., Klein, D., Kocsis, J. Schatzberg, A. and LaVange, L. (1999). Sertraline versus imipramine to prevent relapse in chronic depression. *J Clin Psychopharmacol*. (Submitted.)

Koran, L.M., McElroy, S.L., Davidson, J.R.T., Rasmussen, S.A., Hollander, E. and Jenike, M. (1996b). Fluvoxamine versus clomipramine for obsessive–compulsive disorder: A double-blind comparison. *J Clin Psychopharmacol*, **16**: 121–9.

Koran, L.M., Mueller, K. and Maloney, A. (1996c). Will pindolol augment response to an SRI in OCD? *J Clin Psychopharmacol*, **16**: 253–4.

Koran, L.M. and Pallanti, S. (1996). Intravenous pulse-loaded clomipramine in body dysmorphic disorder: Two case reports. *CNS Spectrums*, **1**: 54–7.

Koran, L.M., Pallanti, S., Paiva, R.S. and Quercioli, L. (1998). Pulse loading versus gradual dosing of intravenous clomipramine in obsessive–compulsive disorder. *Eur Neuropsychopharmacol*, **8**: 121–6.

Koran, L.M., Ringold, A. and Hewlett, W. (1992). An open clinical trial of fluoxetine for trichotillomania. *Psychopharmacol Bull*, **28**: 145–9.

Koran, L.M., Sallee, F.R. and Pallanti, S. (1997). Rapid benefit of intravenous pulse loading of clomipramine in obsessive–compulsive disorder. *Am J Psychiatry*, **154**: 396–401.

Koran, L.M., Sox, H.C., Marton, K.I., Moltzen, S., Sox, C.H., Kraemer, H.C., Imai, K., Kelsey, T.G., Rose, T.G., Levin L.C and Chandra, S. (1989). Medical evaluation of psychiatric patients: I. Results in a state mental health system. *Arch Gen Psychiatry*, **46**: 733–40.

Koran, L.M., Thienemann, M. and Davenport, R. (1996d). Quality of life in patients with obsessive compulsive disorder. *Am J Psychiatry*, **156**: 783–8.

Kornreich, C., Den Dulk, A., Verbanck, P. and Pelc, I. (1995). Fluoxetine treatment of compulsive masturbation in a schizophrenic patient. (Letter.) *J Clin Psychiatry*, **56**: 334.

Kotler, M., Iancu, I., Kindler, S., Lefkifker, E. and Zohar, J. (1994). Clomipramine-induced Tourettism in obsessive–compulsive disorder: Clinical and theoretical implications. *Clin Neuropharmacol*, **17**: 338–43.

Kotrla, K.J., Ardaman, M.F., Meyers, C.A., Novac, I.S. and Harman, L.A. (1994). Unsuspected obsessive compulsive disorder in a patient with bilateral striopallidodentate mineralizations. *Neuropsychiatry Neuropsychol Behav Neurol*, **7**: 130–5.

Kraepelin, E. (1915). *Psychiatrie*, 8th edn. pp. 408–9. Leipzig: Verlag Von Johann Ambrosius Barth.

Kreider, M.S., Bushnell, W.D., Oakes, R. and Wheadon, D.E. (1995). A double-blind, randomized study to provide safety information on switching fluoxetine-treated patients to paroxetine without an intervening washout period. *J Clin Psychiatry*, **56**: 142–5.

Krishnan, K.R.R., Davidson, J.R.T. and Guajardo, C. (1985). Trichotillomania – A review. *Compr Psychiatry*, **26**: 123–8.

Krishnan, R.R., Davidson, J. and Miller, R. (1984). MAO inhibitor therapy in trichotilomania associated with depression: Case report. *J Clin Psychiatry*, **45**: 267–8.

Kroll, L. and Drummond, L.M., (1993). Temporal lobe epilepsy and obsessive–compulsive symptoms. (Letter.) *J Nerv Ment Dis*, **181**: 457–8.

Krueger, D.W. (1988). On compulsive shopping and spending: A psychodynamic inquiry. *Am J Psychother*, **42**: 574–84.

Krüger, S., Cooke, R.G., Hasey, G.M., Jorna, T. and Persad, E. (1995). Comorbidity of obsessive compulsive disorder in bipolar disorder. *J Affect Disord*, **34**: 117–20.

Kuhn, D.R., Greiner, D. and Arseneu, L. (1998). Addressing hypersexuality in Alzheimer's disease. *J Geront Nurs*, **24**: 44–50.

Kulin, N.A., Pastuszak, A., Sage, S.R., Schick-Boschetto, B., Spivey, G., Feldkamp, M., Ormand, K., Matsui, D., Stein-Schechman, A.K. Cook, C., et al. (1998). Pregnancy outcome following maternal use of the new selective serotonin reuptake inhibitors: A prospective controlled multicenter study. *JAMA*, **279**: 609–10.

Kupfer, D.J. (1991). Long-term treatment of depression. *J Clin Psychiatry*, **52**(suppl 5): 28–34.

Kupfer, D.J., Frank, E., Perel, J.M., Cornes, C., Mallinger, A.G., Thase, M.E., McEachran, A.B. and Grochocinski, V.J. (1992). Five-year outcome for maintenance therapies in recurrent depression. *Arch Gen Psychiatry*, **49**: 769–73.

Kurlan, R., Como, P.G., Deeley, C., McDermot, M. and McDermot, M.P. (1993). A pilot controlled study of fluoxetine for obsessive compulsive symptoms in children with Tourette syndrome. *Clin Neuropharmacol*, **16**: 167–72.

Kurlan, R. and Trinidad, K.S. (1995) Treatment of tics. In *Treatment of Movement Disorders*, ed. R. Kurlan, pp. 365–406. Philadelphia: J.B. Lippincott

Kushner, H.I. and Kiessling, L.S. (1996). The controversy over the classification of Gilles de la Tourette's syndrome, 1800–1995. *Perspect Biol Med*, **39**: 409–35.

Labbate, L.A. and Pollack, M.H. (1994). Treatment of Fluoxetine-induced sexual dysfunction with buproprion: A case report. *Ann Clin Psychiatry*, **6**: 13–15.

Ladouceur, R. (1991). Prevalence estimates of pathological gambling in Quebec. *Can J Psychiatry*, **36**: 732–4.

Laegreid, L., Hagberg, G. and Lundberg, A. (1992). Neurodevelopment in late infancy after prenatal exposure to benzodiazepines – A prospective study. *Neuroped*, **23**: 60–7.

Lane, R. and Baldwin, D. (1997). Selective serotonin reuptake inhibitor-induced serotonin syndrome: Review. *J Clin Psychopharmacol*, **17**: 208–21.

Lane, R.D. (1990). Successful fluoxetine treatment of pathologic jealousy. *J Clin Psychiatry*, **51**: 345–6

Laplane, D., Levasseur, M., Pillon, B., Dubois, B., Baulac, M., Mazoyer, B., Dinh, S.T., Sette, G., Danze, F. and Baron, J.C. (1989). Obsessive–compulsive and other behavioural changes with bilateral basal ganglia lesions. *Brain*, **112**: 699–725.

LaPorta, L.D. (1993). Sertraline-induced akathisia. (Letter.) *J Clin Psychopharmacol*, **13**: 219–20.

Leckman, J.F., Goodman, W.K., North, W.G., Chappell, P.B., Price, L.H., Pauls, D.L., Anderson, G.M., Riddle, M.A., McSwiggan-Hardin M., McDouble, C.J, Barr, L.C. and Cohen D.J. (1994a). Elevated cerbrospinal fluid levels of oxytocin in obsessive–compulsive disorder: Comparison with Tourette's syndrome and healthy controls. *Arch Gen Psychiatry*, **51**: 782–92.

Leckman, J.F., Grice, D.E., Barr, L.C., de Vries, A.L.C., Martin, C., Cohen, D.J., McDougle, C.J., Goodman, W.K. and Rasmussen, S.A. (1995). Tic-related vs. non-tic-related obsessive compulsive disorder. *Anxiety*, **1**: 208–15.

Leckman, J.F., Grice, D.E., Boardman, J., Zhang, H., Vitale, A., Bondi, C., Alsobrook, J., Peterson, B.S., Cohen, D.J., Rasmussen, S.A., et al. (1997a). Symptoms of obsessive–compulsive disorder. *Am J Psychiatry*, **154**: 911–17.

Leckman, J.F., Hardin, M.T., Riddle, M.A., Stevenson, J., Ort, S.I. and Cohen, D.J. (1991). Clonidine treatment of Gilles de la Tourette's syndrome. *Arch Gen Psychiatry*, **48**: 324–8.

Leckman, J.F., Peterson, D.S., Anderson, G.M., Arnstein, A.F.T., Pauls, D.I. and Cohen, D.J. (1997b). Pathogenesis of Tourette's syndrome. *J Child Psychol Psychiatry*, **38**: 119–42.

Leckman, J.F., Riddle, M.A., Hardin, M.T., Ort, S.I., Swartz, K.L., Stevenson, J. and Cohen, D.J. (1989). The Yale Global Tic Severity Scale: Initial testing of a clinician-rated scale of tic severity. *J Am Acad Child Adolesc Psychiatry*, 28: 566–73.

Leckman, J.F., Walker, D.E., Goodman, W.K., Pauls, D.L. and Cohen, D.J. (1994b). Just right perceptions associated with compulsive behavior in Tourette's syndrome. *Am J Psychiatry*, **151**: 675–80.

Legarda, J.J., Babio, R. and Abreu, J.M. (1992). Prevalence estimates of pathological gambling in Seville (Spain). *Br J Addict*, **87**: 767–70.

Lejoyeux, M. and Adès, J. (1994). Les Achats Pathologiques: Une addiction comportementale. *Neuro-Psy*, **9**: 25–32.

Lejoyeux, M. and Adès, J. (1997). Antidepressant discontinuation: A review of the literature. *J Clin Psychiatry*, **58**(suppl 7): 11–16.

Lejoyeux, M., Adès, J., Tassain, V. and Solomon J. (1996). Phenomenology and psychophathology of uncontrolled buying. *Am J Psychiatry*, **153**: 1524–9.

Lejoyeux, M., Hourtané, M. and Adès, J. (1995). Compulsive buying and antidepressants. (Letter.) *J Clin Psychiatry*, **56**: 38.

Lelliott, P.T., Noshirvani, H.F., Basoglu, M., Marks. I.M. and Monteiro, W.O. (1988). Obsessive–compulsive beliefs and treatment outcome. *Psychol Med*, **18**: 697–702.

Lenane, M.C., Swedo, S.E., Rapoport, J.L., Leonard, H., Sceery, W. and Guroff, J.J. (1992). Rates of obsessive compulsive disorder in first degree relatives of patients with trichotillomania: A research note. *J Child Psychol Psychiatry*, **33**: 925–33.

Lensi, P., Cassano, G.B., Correddu, G., Ravagli, S., Kunovac, J.L. and Akiskal, H.S. (1996). Obsessive–compulsive disorder: Familial-developmental history, symptomatology, comorbidity and course with special reference to gender-related differences. *Br J Psychiatry*, **169**: 101–7.

Leon, A.C., Olfson, M., Broadhead, W.E., Barrett, J.E., Blacklow, R.S., Keller, M.B., Higgins, E.S. and Weissman, M.M. (1995). Prevalence of mental disorders in primary care: Implications for screening. *Arch Fam Med*, **4**: 857–61.

Leon, A.C., Portera, L. and Weissman, M.M. (1995). The social costs of anxiety disorders. *Br J Psychiatry*, **166**(suppl 27): 19–22.

Leonard, H.L., Lenane, M.C., Swedo, S.E., Rettew, D.C., Rapoport, J.L. (1991). A double-blind comparison of clomipramine and desipramine treatmemt of severe onychophagia (nail biting). *Arch Gen Psychiatry*, **48**: 821–7.

Leonard, H.L., Swedo, S.E., Lenane, M.C., Rettew, D.C., Hamburger, S.D., Bartko, J.J., and Rapoport, J.L. (1993). A 2- to 7-year follow-up study of 54 obsessive–compulsive children and adolescents. *Arch Gen Psychiatry* **50**: 429–39.

Leonard, H.L., Topal, D., Bukstein, O., Hindmarsh, D., Allen, A.J. and Swedo, S.E. (1994). Clonazepam as an augmenting agent in the treatment of childhood-onset obsessive–compulsive disorder. *J Am Acad Child Adolesc Psychiatry*, **33**: 792–4.

Lepola, U.M., Wade, A.G., Leinonen, E.V., Koponen, H.J., Frazer, J., Sjödin, I., Perittinen, J.T., Pederson, T. and Lehto, H.J. (1998). A controlled, prospective, 1-year trial of citalopram in the treatment of panic disorder. *J Clin Psychiatry*, **59**: 528–34.

Lepold, U., Koponow, H. and Leinonen, E. (1994). Citalopram in the treatment of social phobia: a report of three cases. *Pharmacopsychiatry*, **27**: 181–8.

Lesieur, H.R. (1984). *The Chase: Career of the Compulsive Gambler*. Cambridge, MA: Schenkman Books.

Lesieur, H.R. and Blume, S.B. (1987). The South Oaks Gambling Screen (SOGS): A new instrument for the identification of pathological gamblers. *Am J Psychiatry*, **144**: 1184–8.

Lesieur, H.R. and Blume, S.B. (1991). Evaluation of patients treated for pathological gambling in a combined alcohol, substance abuse and pathological gambling treatment unit using the Addiction Severity Index. *Br J Addict*, **86**: 1017–28.

Lesieur, H.R. and Rosenthal, R.J. (1991). Pathological gambling: A review of the literature (prepared for the American Psychiatric Association Task Force of DSM-IV Committee on Disorders of Impulse Control Not Elsewhere Classified). *J Gambling Studies*, **7**: 5–39.

Lester, B.M., Cucca, J., Andreozzi, L., Flanagan, P. and Oh, W. (1993). Possible association between fluoxetine hydrochloride and colic in an infant. *J Am Acad Child Adolesc Psychiatry*, **32**: 1253–5.

Leung, A.K.C and Robson, L.M. (1990). Nail biting. *Clin Ped*, **29**: 690–2.

Levin, B. and Duchowny, M. (1991). Childhood obsessive–compulsive disorder and cingulate epilepsy. *Biol Psychiatry*, **30**: 1049–55.

Levine, M.P. and Troiden, R.R. (1988). The myth of sexual compulsivity. *J Sex Res*, **25**: 347–63.

Liebowitz, M.R. (1987). Social phobia. In *Modern Problems in Pharmacopsychiatry: Anxiety*, vol. 22, ed. D.F. Klein, pp. 141–73. Basel: S. Krager.

Liebowitz, M.R., Schneier, F., Campeas, R., Hollancder, E., Hatterer, J., Fyer, A., Gorman, J., Papp, L., Davies, S., Gully, R. and Klein D.F. (1992). Phenelzine vs atenolol in social phobia: A placebo-controlled comparison. *Arch Gen Psychiatry*, **49**: 290–300.

Linden, R.D., Pope, H.G. Jr. and Jonas, J.M. (1986). Pathological gambling and major affective disorder: Preliminary findings. *J Clin Psychiatry*, **47**: 201–3.

Lindenmayer, J.P., Vakharia, M. and Kanofsky, D. (1990). Fluoxetine in chronic schizophrenia. (Letter.) *J Clin Psychopharmacol*, **10**: 76.

Lindhout, D., Meinardi, H. and Meijer, J. (1992). Antiepileptic drugs and teratogenesis in two consecutive cohorts: changes in prescription policy paralleled by changes in pattern of malformations. *Neurology*, **42**(suppl 5): 94–110.

Linehan, M.M. (1993). *Cognitive Behavioral Treatment of Borderline Personality Disorder*. New York: Guilford Press.

Lipinski, J.F., Mallya, G., Zimmerman, P. and Pope, H.G. (1989). Fluoxetine-induced akathisia: Clinical and theoretical implications. *J Clin Psychiatry*, **50**: 339–42.

Lombroso, P.J., Scahill, L., King, R.A., Lynch, K.A., Chappell, P.B., Peterson, B.S., McDougle, C.J. and Leckman, J.F. (1995). Risperidone treatment of children and adolescents with chronic tic disorders: A preliminary report. *J Am Acad Child Adolesc Psychiatry*, **34**: 1147–52.

Lopez, O.L., Berthier, M.L., Backer, J.T. and Boller, F. (1997). Creutzfeldt-Jakob disease with features of obsessive–compulsive disorder and anorexia nervosa: The role of cortical–subcortical systems. *Neuropsychiatry Neuropsychol Behav Neurol*, **10**: 120–4.

López-Ibor Jr., J.J., Saiz, J., Cottraux, J., Note, I., Viñas, R., Bourgeois, M., Hernández, M. and Gómez-Pérez, J.C. (1996). Double-blind comparison of fluoxetine versus clomipramine in the treatment of obsessive compulsive disorder. *Eur Neuropsychopharmacol*, **6**: 111–18.

Lopez-Villegas, D., Kulisevsky, J., Deus, J., Junque, C., Pujol, J., Guardia, E. and Grau, J.M. (1996). Neuropsychological alterations in patients with computed tomography-detected basal ganglia calcification. *Arch Neurol*, **53**: 251–6.

LoPiccolo, J. and Van Male, L.M. (1997). Paraphilias. In *Current Psychiatric Therapy*, 2nd edn., ed. D.L. Dunner, pp. 377–85. Philadelphia: W.B. Saunders

Louie, A.K., Lannon, R.A. and Ajari, L.J. (1994). Withdrawal reactions after sertraline discontinuation. (Letter.) *Am J Psychiatry*, **151**: 450–1.

Lowe, T.L., Cohen, D.J., Detlar, J., Kraemenitzer, M.W. and Shaywitz, B.A. (1982). Stimulant medications precipitate Tourette's Syndrome. *JAMA*, **247**: 1168–9.

Luchins, D.J., Goldman, M.B., Lieb, M. and Hanrahan, P. (1992). Repetitive behaviors in chronically institutionalized schizophrenic patients. *Schizophrenia Res*, **8**: 119–23.

Lyketsos, C.G. (1992). Successful treatment of bowel obsessions with nortriptyline. (Letter.) *Am J Psychiatry*, **149**: 573.

Magliana, L., Tosini, P., Guarneri, M., Marasco, C. and Catapano, F. (1996). Burden on the families of patients with obsessive–compulsive disorder: A pilot study. *Eur Psychiatry*, **11**: 192–7.

Mahendran, R. (1998). Obsessional symptoms associated with risperidone treatment. *Aust NZ J Psychiatry*, **32**: 299–301.

Mahgoub, O.M. and Abdel-Hafeiz, H.B. (1991). Pattern of obsessive–compulsive disorder in Eastern Saudi Arabia. *Br J Psychiatry*, **158**: 840–2.

Mahr, G. (1990). Isotretinoin and trichotillomania (Letter.) *Psychosomatics*, **31**: 235.

Makela, E.H., Sullivan, P. and Taylor, M. (1994). Sertraline and speech blockage. (Letter.) *J Clin Psychopharmacol*, **14**: 432–3.

Mallya, G., White, K. and Gunderson, C. (1993). Is there a serotoninergic withdrawal syndrome? (Letter.) *Biol Psychiatry*, **33**: 851–2.

Mallya, G., White, K., Waternaux, C., Quay, S. (1992). Short- and long-term treatment of obsessive–compulsive disorder with fluvoxamine. *Ann Clin Psychiatry*, **4**: 77–80.

Mammen, O.K., Perel, J.M., Rudolph, G., Foglia, J.P. and Wheeler, S.B. (1997). Sertraline and norsertraline levels in three breastfed infants. *J Clin Psychiatry*, **58**: 100–3.

Mannino, F.V. and Delgado, R.A. (1969). Trichotillomania in children: A review. *Am J Psychiatry*, **126**: 505–11.

March, J.S., Frances, A., Carpenter, D. and Kahn, D.A. (Eds.) (1997). The Expert Consensus Guideline Series: Treatment of Obsessive–Compulsive Disorder. *J Clin Psychiatry*, **58**(suppl 4): 1–72.

Markovitz, P.J., Stagno, S.J. and Calabrese, J.R. (1990). Buspirone augmentation of fluoxetine in obsessive–compulsive disorder. *Am J Psychiatry*, **147**: 798–800.

Markowitz, J.C. (1994). Religiosity and psychopathology. (Letter.) *J Clin Psychiatry*, **55**: 414–15.

Marks, I. (1992). *Fears, Phobias and Rituals.* Oxford: Oxford University Press.

Marshall, J.R. (1997). Alcohol and substance abuse in panic disorder. [Discussion: Treating the substance-abusing patient.] *J Clin Psychiatry*, **58**:(suppl 2): 46–49, 49–50.

Marshall, R.D., Schneier, F.R., Fallon, B.A., Ferrick, J. and Liebowitz, M.R. (1994). Medication therapy for social phobia. *J Clin Psychiatry*, **55**(suppl 6): 33–7.

Mavissakalian, M., Hamann, M., Haidar, S.A. and de Groot, C.M. (1993). DSM-III personality disorder in generalized anxiety, panic/agoraphobia, and obsessive–compulsive disorders. *Compr Psychiatry*, **34**: 243–8.

Mavissakalian, M., Hamann, M.S. and Jones, B. (1990a). Correlates of DSM-III personality disorder in obsessive–compulsive disorder. *Compr Psychiatry*, **31**: 481–9.

Mavissakalian, M., Hamann, M.S. and Jones, B. (1990b). DSM-III personality disorders in obsessive–compulsive disorder: Changes with treatment. *Compr Psychiatry*, **31**: 432–7.

Mavissakalian, M., Jones, B., Olson, S. and Perel, J.M. (1990c). Clomipramine in obsessive–compulsive disorder: Clinical response and plasma levels. *J Clin Psychopharmacol*, **10**: 261–8.

Mavissakalian, M.R. and Perel, J.M. (1989). Imipramine dose-response relationship in panic disorder with agoraphobia. *Arch Gen Psychiatry*, **46**: 127–31.

Mavissakalian, M.R. and Perel, J.M. (1992). Protective effects of imipramine maintenance treatment in panic disorder with agoraphobia. *J Am Psychiatry*, **194**: 1053–7.

May, W.S. and Terpenning, M.S. (1991). Delusional parsitosis in geriatric patients. *Psychosomatics*, **32**: 88–93.

Mayou, R., Bryant, B., Forfar, C. and Clark, D. (1994). Non-cardiac chest pain and benign palpitations in the cardiac clinic. *Br Heart J*, **72**: 548–53.

Mazzi, E. (1977). Possible neonatal diazepam withdrawal: A case report. *Am J Obstet Gynecol*, **129**: 586–7.

McCain, G.A. (1996). A cost-effective approach to the diagnosis and treatment of fibromyalgia. *Rheum Dis Clin North Am*, **22**: 323–49.

McCall, W.V. (1994). Sertraline-induced stuttering. (Letter.) *J Clin Psychiatry*, **55**: 316.

McConaghy, N., Armstrong, M.S. and Blaszczynski, A. (1985). Expectancy, covert sensitization and imaginal desensitization in compulsive sexuality. *Acta Psychiatr Scand*, **72**: 176–87.

McConaghy, N., Armstrong, M.S., Blaszcynski, A. and Allcock, C. (1983). Controlled comparison of aversive therapy and imaginal desensitization in compulsive gambling. *Br J Psychiatry*, **142**: 366–72.

McConaghy, N. and Blaszczynski, A. (1988). Imaginal desensitization: A cost-effective treatment in two shop-lifters and a binge-eater resistant to previous therapy. *Aust N Z J Psychiatry*, **22**: 78–82

McConaghy, N., Blaszczynski, A. and Frankova, A. (1991). Comparison of imaginal desensitization with other behavioural treatments of pathological gambling: A two- to nine-year follow-up. *Br J Psychiatry*, **159**: 390–3.

McCormick, R.A., Russo, A.M., Ramirez, L.F. and Taber, J.I. (1984). Affective disorders among pathological gamblers seeking treatment. *Am J Psychiatry*, **141**: 215–18.

McCormick, S., Olin, J. and Brotman, A.W. (1990). Reversal of fluoxetine-induced anorgasmia by cyproheptadine in two patients. (Letter.) *J Clin Psychiatry*, **51**: 383–4.

McDaniel, J.S. and Johnson, K.M. (1995). Obsessive-compulsive disorder in HIV disease. *Psychosomatics*, **36**: 147–50.

McDougle, C.J., Barr, L.C., Goodman, W.K., Pelton, G.H., Aronson, S.C., Anand, A. and Price, L.H. (1995a). Lack of efficacy of clozapine monotherapy in refractory obsessive–compulsive disorder. *Am J Psychiatry*, **152**: 1812–14.

McDougle, C.J., Fleischmann, R.L., Epperson, C.N., Wasylink, S., Leckman, J.F. and Price, L.H. (1995b). Risperidone addition in fluvoxamine-refractory obsessive–compulsive disorder: Three cases. *J Clin Psychiatry*, **56**: 526–8.

McDougle, C.J., Goodman, W.K., Leckman, J.F., Barr, L.C., Heninger, G.R. and Price, L.H. (1993a). The efficacy of fluvoxamine in obsessive compulsive disorder: Effects of comorbid chronic tic disorder. *J Clin Psychopharmacol*, **13**: 354–8.

McDougle, C.J., Goodman, W.K., Leckman, J.F., Holzer, J.C., Barr, L.C., McCance-Katz, E., Heninger, G.R. and Price, L.H. (1993b). Limited therapeutic effect of addition of buspirone in fluvoxamine refractory obsessive–compulsive disorder. *Am J Psychiatry*, **150**: 647–9.

McDougle, C.J., Goodman, W.K., Leckman, J.F., Lee, N.C., Heninger, G.R. and Price, L.H. (1994a). Haloperidol addition in fluvoxamine-refractory obsessive–compulsive disorder. *Arch Gen Psychiatry*, **51**: 302–8.

McDougle, C.J., Goodman, W.K. and Price, L.H. (1994b). Dopamine antagonists in tic-related and psychotic spectrum obsessive compulsive disorder. *J Clin Psychiatry*, **55**(suppl 3): 24–31.

McDougle, C.J., Goodman, W.K., Price, L.H., Delgado, P.L., Krystal, J.H. and Charney, D.S. (1990). Neuroleptic addition in fluvoxamine-refractory obsessive–compulsive disorder. *Am J Psychiatry*, **147**: 652–4.

McDougle C.J., Kresch, L.E., Goodman, W.K., Naylor, S.T., Volkmar, F.R., Cohen, D.J. and Price, L.H. (1995c). A case-controlled study of repetitive thoughts and behavior in adults with autistic disorder and obsessive-compulsive disorder. *Am J Psychiatry*, **152**: 772–7.

McDougle, C.J., Price, L.H., Goodman, W.K., Charney, D.S. and Heninger, G.R. (1991). A controlled trial of lithium augmentation in fluvoxamine-refractory obsessive–compulsive disorder: Lack of efficacy. *J Clin Psychopharmacol*, **11**: 175–84.

McElhatton, P.R. (1992). The use of phenothiazines during prgnancy and lactation. *Reprod Toxicol*, **6**: 475–90.

McElhatton, P.R. (1994). The effects of benzodiazepine use during pregnancy and lactation. *Reprod Toxicol*, **8**: 461–75.

McElroy, S.L., Hudson J.I., Phillips, K.A., Keck, P.E. and Pope, H.G. (1993). Clinical and theoretical implications of a possible link between obsessive–compulsive and impulse control disorders. *Depression*, **1**: 121–32.

McElroy, S.L., Hudson, J.I., Pope, H.G. and Keck, P.E. (1991a). Kleptomania: Clinical characteristics and associated psychopathology. *Psychol Med*, **21**: 93–108.

McElroy, S.L., Hudson, J.I., Pope, H.G., Keck, P.E. and Aizley, H.G. (1992). The DSM-III-R Impulse Control Disorders Not Elsewhere Classified: Clinical characteristics and relationship to other psychiatric disorders. *Am J Psychiatry*, **149**: 318–27.

McElroy, S.L. and Keck, P.E. (1995). Antiepileptic Drugs. In *American Psychiatric Press Textbook of Psychopharmacology*, ed. A.F. Schatzberg and C.B. Nemeroff, pp. 351–75. Washington, DC: American Psychiatric Press.

McElroy, S.L., Keck, P.E. and Friedman, L.M. (1995). Minimizing and managing antidepressant side effects. *J Clin Psychiatry*, **56**(suppl 2): 49–55.

McElroy, S.L., Keck, P.E., Pope, H.G. and Hudson, J.I. (1989). Pharmacological treatment of kleptomania and bulimia nervosa. *J Clin Psychopharmacol*, **9**: 358–60.

McElroy, S., Keck, P.E., Pope, H.G., Smith, J.M.R. and Strakowski, S.M. (1994a). Compulsive buying: A report of 20 cases. *J Clin Psychiatry*, **55**: 242–8.

McElroy S.L., Phillips, K.A. and Keck, P.E. (1994b). Obsessive compulsive spectrum disorder. *J Clin Psychiatry*, **55**(suppl 10): 33–51.

McElroy, S.L., Pope, H.G., Hudson, J.I., Keck, P.E. and White, K.L. (1991b). Kleptomania: A report of 20 cases. *Am J Psychiatry*, **148**: 652–7.

McGuire, P.K., Bench, C.J., Frith, C.D., Marks, I.M., Frackowiak, R.S.J. and Dolan, R.J. (1994). Functional anatomy of obsessive–compulsive phenomena. *Br J Psychiatry*, **164**: 459–68.

McKay, D., Todaro, J., Neziroglu, F., Campisi, T., Moritz, E.K. and Yaryura-Tobias, J.A. (1997). Body dysmorphic disorder: A preliminary evaluation of treatment and maintenance using exposure with response prevention. *Behav Res Ther*, **35**: 67–70.

McKeon, J., McGuffin, P. and Robinson, P. (1984). Obsessive–compulsive neurosis following head injury: A report of four cases. *Br J Psychiatry*, **144**: 190–2.

McLean, J.D., Forsythe, R.G. and Kapkin, I.A. (1983). Unusual side effects of clomipramine associated with yawning. *Can J Psychiatry*, **28**: 569–70.

McNamara, P. and Durso, R. (1991). Reversible pathologic jealousy (Othello syndrome) associated with amantadine. *J Geriatr Psychiatry Neurol*, **4**: 157–9.

Medical Economics Company, Inc. (1998). *Physicians' Desk Reference*, 52nd edn., Montvale: Medical Economics Company.

Medical Letter. (1992). Drugs that cause sexual dysfunction: An update. **34**: 73–8.

Megens, J. and Vandereycken, W. (1988). Hospitalization of obsessive–compulsive patients: The forgotten factor in the behavior therapy literature. *Compr Psychiatry*, **30**: 161–9.

Mehregan, A.H. (1970). Trichotillomania: A clinicopathologic study. *Arch Dermatol*, **102**: 129–33.

Mena, I., Marin, O., Fuenzalida, S. and Cotzias, G.C. (1967). Chronic manganese poisoning: Clinical picture and manganese turnover. *Neurology*, **17**: 128–36.

Michael, A., Mirza, K.A.H., Mirza, V.S., Babu, V.S. and Vithayathil, E. (1995). Morbid jealousy in alcoholism. *Br J Psychiatry*, **167**: 668–72.

Miguel, E.C., Baer, L., Coffey, B.J., Rauch, S.L., Savage, C.R., O'Sullivan, R.L., Phillips, K., Moretti, C., Leckman, J.F. and Jenike, M.A. (1997). Phenomenological differences appearing with repetitive behaviours in obsessive–compulsive disorder and Gilles de la Tourette's syndrome. *Br J Psychiatry*, **170**: 140–5.

Miguel, E.C., Stein, M.C., Rauch, S.L., O'Sullivan, R.L., Stern, T.A. and Jenike, M.A. (1995). Obsessive–compulsive disorder in patients with multiple sclerosis. *J Neuropsychiatry Clin Neurosci*, 7: 507–10.

Milanfranchi, A., Ravigli, S., Lensi, P., Marazziti, D. and Cassano, G.B. (1997). A double-blind study of fluvoxamine and clomipramine in the treatment of obsessive–compulsive disorder. *Int Clin Psychiapharmacol*, 12: 131–6.

Mindham, R.H.S., Scadding, J.G. and Cawley, R.H. (1992). Diagnoses are not diseases. *Br J Psychiatry*, 161: 686–91.

Mindus, P. and Jenike M.A. (1992). Neurosurgical treatment of malignant obsessive compulsive disorder. *Psychiatr Clin North Am*, 15: 921–38.

Minichiello, W.E., O'Sullivan, R.L., Osgood-Hynes, D. and Baer, L. (1994). Trichotillomania: Clinical aspects and treatment strategies. *Harvard Rev Psychiatry*, 1: 336–44.

Mirow, S. (1991). Cognitive dysfunction associated with fluoxetine. (Letter.) *Am J Psychiatry*, 148: 948–9.

Misri, S. and Sivertz, K. (1991). Tricyclic drugs in pregnancy and lactation: A preliminary report. *Int J Psychiatry Med*, 21: 157–71.

Modell, J.G. (1989). Repeated observations of yawning, clitoral engorgement, and orgasm associated with fluoxetine administration. (Letter.) *J Clin Psychopharmacol*, 9: 63–5.

Modell, J.G., Mountz, J.M., Curtis, G.C. and Greden, J.F. (1989). Neurophysiologic dysfunction in basal banglia/limbic striatal and thalamocortical circuits as a pathogenetic mechanism of obsessive–compulsive disorder. *J Neuropsychiatry Clin Neurosci*, 1: 27–36.

Monahan, P., Black, D.W. and Gabel, J. (1996). Reliability and validity of a scale to measure change in persons with compulsive buying. *Psychiatry Res*, 64: 59–67.

Monga, T.N., Monga, M., Raina, M.S., Hardjasudarma, M. (1986). Hypersexuality in stroke. *Arch Phys Med Rehabil*, 67: 415–17.

Monroe, J.T. and Abse, D.W. (1963). The psychopathology of trichotillomania and trichophagy. *Psychiatry*, 26: 95–103.

Monteiro, W.O., Noshirvani, H.F., Marks, I.M. and Lelliott, P.T. (1987). Anorgasmia from clomipramine in obsessive–compulsive disorder. *Br J Psychiatry*, 151: 107–12.

Montgomery, S. (1998). Citalopram treatment of obsessive compulsive disorder: Results from a double-blind, placebo-controlled trial. Abstract presented at the *37th American College of Neuropsychopharmacology Annual Meeting*, December 14–18, 1998, Puerto Rico, USA.

Montgomery, S.A. and Åsberg, M. (1979). A new depression scale designed to be sensitive to change. *Br J Psychiatry*, 134: 382–9.

Montgomery, S.A., McIntyre, A., Osterheider, M., Sarteschi, P., Zitterl, W., Zohar, J., Birkett, M., Wood, A.J. and The Lilly European OCD Study Group. (1993). A double-blind, placebo-controlled study of fluoxetine in patients with DSM-III-R obsessive–compulsive disorder. *Eur Neuropsychopharmacol*, 3: 143–52.

Moore, D.P. (1996). Neuropsychiatric aspects of Sydenham's Chorea: A comprehensive review. *J Clin Psychiatry*, 57: 407–14.

Moran, E. (1970). Varieties of pathological gambling. *Br J Psychiatry*, 116: 593–7.

Moriarty, J., Trimble, M. and Hayward, R. (1993). Obsessive–compulsive disorder onset after removal of a brain tumor. *J Nerv Ment Dis*, 181: 331.

Mulder, D.S. (1953). Paroxysmal psychiatric symptoms observed in epilepsy. *Staff Meetings Mayo Clin*, 28: 31–5.

Muldoon, C. (1996). The safety and tolerability of citalopram. *Int Clin Psychopharmacol*, 11(suppl 1): 35–40.

Mullen, P.E. (1991). Jealousy: The pathology of passion. *Br J Psychiatry*, **158**: 593–601.

Mullen, P.E. and Martin, J. (1994). Jealousy: A community study. *Br J Psychiatry*, **164**: 35–43.

Muller, S.A. (1987). Trichotillomania. *Dermatol Clin*, **5**: 595–601.

Muller, S.A. (1990). Trichotillomania: A histopathologic study in sixty-six patients. *J Am Acad Dermatol*, **23**: 56–62.

Mundo, E., Bareggi, S.R., Pirola, R., Bellodi, L. and Smeraldi, E. (1997). Long-term pharmaco-therapy of obsessive–compulsive disorder: A double-blind controlled study. *J Clin Psychopharmacol*, **17**: 4–10.

Mundo, E., Bianchi, L. and Bellodi, L. (1997). Efficacy of fluvoxamine, paroxetine, and citalo-pram in the treatment of obsessive–compulsive disorder: A single-blind study. *J Clin Psychopharmacol*, **17**: 267–71.

Munro, A. (1984). Excellent response of pathologic jealousy to pimozide. *Can Med Assoc J*, **131**: 852–3.

Munro, A. (1988). Monosymptomatic hypochondriacal psychosis. *Br J Psychiatry*, **153**(suppl 2): 37–40.

Munro, A. and Chmara, J. (1982). Monosymptomatic hypochondriacal psychosis: A diagnostic checklist based on 50 cases of the disorder. *Can J Psychiatry*, **27**: 374–6.

Murphy T.K., Goodman, W.K., Fudge, M.W., Williams, R.C., Ayoub, E.M., Dalal, M., Lewis, M.H. and Zabriskie, J.B. (1997). B lymphocyte antigen D8/17: A peripheral marker for childhood-onset obsessive–compulsive disorder and Tourette's syndrome? *Am J Psychiatry*, **154**: 402–7.

Murray, J.B. (1992). Kleptomania: A review of the research. *J Psychology*, **126**: 131–8.

Murray, J.B. (1993). Review of research on pathological gambling. *Psychological Rep*, **72**: 791–810.

Nelson, E.B., Keck, P.E. and McElroy, S.L. (1997). Resolution of fluoxetine-induced sexual dysfunction with the 5-HT$_3$ antagonist granisetron. (Letter.) *J Clin Psychiatry*, **58**: 496–7.

Nelson, E. and Rice, J. (1997). Stability of diagnosis of obsessive–compulsive disorder in the epi-demiologic catchment area study. *Am J Psychiatry*, **154**: 826–31.

Nemeroff, C.B., DeVane, L. and Pollock, B.G. (1996). Newer antidepressants and the cytochrome P450 system. *Am J Psychiatry*, **153**: 311–20.

Nestadt, G., Romanoski, A.J., Brown, C.H, Chahal, R., Merchant, A., Folstein M.F., Gruenberg, E.M. and McHugh, P.R. (1991). DSM-III compulsive personality disorder: An epidemiolog-ical survey. *Psychol Med*, **21**: 461–71.

Nestadt, G., Samuels, J.F., Romanoski, A.J., Folstein M.F. and McHugh, P.R. (1994). Obsessions and compulsions in the community. *Acta Psychiatr Scand*, **89**: 219–24.

Nierenberg, A.A. and Amsterdam, J.D. (1990). Treatment-resistant depression: Definition and treatment approaches. *J Clin Psychiatry*, **51**(suppl 6): 39–47.

Nierenberg, D.W. and Semprebon, M. (1993). The central nervous system serotonin syndrome. *Clin Pharmacol Ther*, **53**: 84–8.

Ninan, P. T., Rothbaum, B.O., Stipetic, M., Lewine, R.J. and Risch, S.C. (1992). CSF 5–HIAA as a predictor of treatment response in trichotillomania. *Psychopharmacol Bull*, **28**: 451–5.

Noble, S. and Benfield, P. (1997). Citalopram: A review of its pharmacology, clinical efficacy and tolerability in the treatment of depression. *CNS Drugs*, **8**: 410–31.

Norden, M.J. (1994). Buspirone treatment of sexual dysfunction associated with selective sero-tonin re-uptake inhibitors. *Depression*, **2**: 109–12.

Noshirvani, H.F., Kasvikis, Y., Marks, I.M., Tsakiris, F. and Monteiro, W.O. (1991). Gender-diver-gent aetiological factors in obsessive–compulsive disorder. *Br J Psychiatry*, **158**: 260–3.

Noyes, R., Kathol, R.G., Fisher, M.M., Phillips, B.M., Suelzer, M.T. and Holt, C.S. (1993). The validity of DSM-III-R hypochondriasis. *Arch Gen Psychiatry*, **50**: 961–70.

Noyes, R., Kathol, R.G., Fisher, M.M., Phillips B.M., Suelzer, M.T. and Woodman, C.L. (1994). One-year follow-up of medical outpatients with hypochondriasis. *Psychosomatics*, **35**: 533–45.

Nulman, I., Rovet, J., Stewart, D.E., Wolpin J., Gardner, H.A., Theis, J.G.W., Kulin, N. and Koren, G. (1997). Neurodevelopment of children exposed in utero to antidepressant drugs. *N Engl J Med*, **336**: 258–63.

Ogilvie, A.D. (1993). Hair loss during fluoxetine treatment. (Letter.) *Lancet*, **342**: 1423.

Okasha, A., Saad, A., Khalil, A.H., Seif El Dawla, A. and Yehia, N. (1994). Phenomenology of obsessive–compulsive disorder: A transcultural study. *Comp Psychiatry*, **35**: 191–7.

Oldham, J.M., Skodol, A.E., Kellman, H.D., Hyler, W.E., Doidge, N., Rosnick, L. and Gallaher, P.E. (1995). Comorbidity of Axis I and Axis II disorders. *Am J Psychiatry*, **152**: 571–8.

Orford, J. (1978). Hypersexuality: Implications for a theory of dependence. *Br J Addict*, **73**: 299–310.

O'Sullivan, R.L., Keuthen, N.J., Christenson, G.A., Mansueto, C.S., Stein, D.J. and Swedo, S.E. (1997). Trichotillomania: Behavioral symptom or clinical syndrome? *Am J Psychiatry*, **154**: 1442–9.

O'Sullivan, R.L., Keuthen, N.J., Hayday, C.F., Ricciardi, J.N., Buttolph, M.L., Jenike, M.A. and Baer, L. (1995). The Massachusetts General Hospital (MGH) Hiarpulling Scale: 2. Reliability and validity. *Psychother Psychosom*, **64**: 146–8.

O'Sullivan, R.L, Keuthen, N.J., Jenike, M.A. and Gumley, G. (1996). Trichotillomania and carpal tunnel syndrome. (Letter.) *J Clin Psychiatry*, **57**: 174.

O'Sullivan, R.L., Keuthen, N.J., Rodriguez, D., Goodchild, P., Christenson, G.A., Rauch, S.L., Jenike, M.A. amd Baer, L. (1998). Venlafaxine treatment of trichotillomania: An open series of ten cases. *CNS Spectrums*, **3**: 56–63.

Ottervanger J.P., Stricker, B.H.C.H., Huls, J. and Weeda, J.N. (1994). Bleeding attributed to the intake of paroxetine. (Letter.) *Am J Psychiatry*, **151**: 781–2.

Otto, M.W. (1992). Normal and abnormal information processing: A neuropsychological perspective on obsessive–compulsive disorder. *Psychiatr Clin North Am*, **15**: 825–48.

Pacella, B.L., Polatin, P. and Nagler, S.H. (1944). Clinical and EEG studies in obsessive–compulsive states. *Am J Psychiatry*, **100**: 830–5.

Pallanti, S. and Koran, L.M. (1996). Intravenous, pulse-loaded clomipramine in body dysmorphic disorder: Two case resports. *CNS Spectrums*, **1**: 54–7.

Pallanti, S., Quercioli, L., Paiva, R.S. and Koran, L.M. (1998). Citalopram plus clomipramine for treatment resistant obsessive–compulsive disorder. *European Psychiatry*. **8**: 121–6

Papp, L.A., Schneier, F.R., Fyer, A.J., Liebowitz, M.R., Gorman, J.M., Coplan, J.D., Campeas, R., Fallon, B.A. and Klein D.F. (1997). Clomipramine treatment of panic disoder: Pros and cons. *J Clin Psychiatry* **58**: 423–5.

Paradis, C.M., Friedman, S. and Hatch, M. (1992). Obsessive–compulsive disorder onset after removal of a brain tumor. *J Nerv Ment Dis*, **180**: 535–6.

Parameshwar, E. (1996). Hair loss with fluvoxamine use. (Letter.) *Am J Psychiatry*, **153**: 581–2.

Pastuszak, A., Schick-Boschetto, B., Zuber, C., Feldkamp, M., Pinelli, M., Sihn, S., Donnenfeld, A., McCormack, M., Leen-Mitchell, M., Woodland, C., Gardner, A., Horn, M. and Koren, G. (1993). Pregnancy outcome following first-trimester exposure to fluoxetine (Prozac). *JAMA*, **269**: 2246–8.

Patil, V.J. (1992). Development of transient obsessive–compulsive symptoms during treatment with clozapine. (Letter.) *Am J Psychiatry*, **149**: 272.

Pato, M.T., Hill, J.L. and Murphy, D.L. (1990). A clomipramine dosage reduction study in the course of long-term treatment of obsessive–compulsive disorder patients. *Psychopharmacol Bull*, **26**: 211–14.

Pato, M.T. and Pato, C.N. (1991). Psychometrics in obsessive–compulsive disorder. In *The Psychobiology of Obsessive-Compulsive Disorder*, eds. J. Zohar, T. Insel and S. Rasmussen, pp. 44–88. New York: Springer.

Pato, M.T., Zohar-Kadouch, R., Zohar, J. and Murphy, D.L. (1988). Return of symptoms after discontinuation of clomipramine in patients with obsessive–compulsive disorder. *Am J Psychiatry*, **145**: 1521–2.

Patterson, W.M. (1993). Fluoxetine-induced sexual dysfunction. (Letter.) *J Clin Psychiatry*, **54**: 71.

Pauls, D.L. (1992). The genetics of obsessive–compulsive disorder and Gilles de la Tourette's syndrome. *Psychiatr Clin North Am*, **15**: 759–66.

Pauls, D.L., Alsobrook II, J.P., Phil, M., Goodman, W., Rasmussen, S. and Leckman, J.F. (1995). A family study of obsessive–compulsive disorder. *Am J Psychiatry*, **151**: 76–84.

Pauls, D.L., Raymond, C.L., Stevenson, J.M. and Leckman, J.F. (1991). A family study of Tourette's syndrome. *Am J Hum Genet*, **48**: 154–63.

Pauls, D.L., Towbin, K.E., Leckman, J.F., Zahner, G.E.P. and Cohen, D.J. (1986). Gilles de la Tourette's syndrome and obsessive–compulsive disorder. *Arch Gen Psychiatry*, **43**: 1180–2.

Penfield, W. and Jasper, H. (1954). *Epilepsy and the Functional Anatomy of the Brain*, pp. 468–9. London: Churchill.

Perciaccante, M. and Perciaccante, R.G. (1993). Progestin treatment for obsessive–compulsive disorder. *Psychosomatics*, **34**: 284–5.

Perry, J.C. (1992). Problems and considerations in the valid assessment of personality disorders. *Am J Psychiatry*, **149**: 1645–53.

Perry, J.C. (1995). Dependent personality disorder. In G.O. Gabbard ed., *Treatments of Psychiatric Disorders*, 2nd edn., vol. 2, pp. 2356–66. Washington, DC: American Psychiatric Press.

Perugi, G., Akiskal, H.S., Giannotti, D., Frare, F., Di Vaio, S. and Cassano, G.B. (1997a). Gender-related differences in body dysmorphic disorder (dysmorphophobia). *J Nerv Ment Dis*, **185**: 578–82.

Perugi, G., Akiskal, H.S., Pfanner, C., Presta, S., Gemignani, A., Milanfranchi, A., Lensi, P., Ravagli, S. and Cassano, G.B. (1997b). The clinical impact of bipolar and unipolar affective comorbidity on obsessive–compulsive disorder. *J Affect Disord*, **46**: 15–23.

Peterson, B. S. (1996). Considerations of natural history and pathophysiology in the psychopharmacology of Tourette's syndrome. *J Clin Psychiatry*, **57**(suppl 9): 24–34.

Peterson, B.S. and Cohen, D.J. (1998). The treatment of Tourette's syndrome: Multimodal, developmental intervention. *J Clin Psychiatry*, **59**(suppl 1): 62–72.

Petter, T., Richter, M.A. and Sandor, P. (1998). Clinical features distinguishing patients with Tourette's syndrome and obsessive–compulsive disorder from patients with obsessive–compulsive disorder without tics. *J Clin Psychiatry* **59**: 456–9

Phillippopoulos, G.S. (1961). A case of trichotillomania. *Acta Psychother*, **9**: 304–12.

Phillippopoulos, G.S. (1979). The analysis of a case of dysmorfophobia. *Can J Psychiatry*, **24**: 397–401.

Phillips, K.A. (1991). Body dysmorphic disorder: The distress of imagined ugliness. *Am J Psychiatry*, **148**: 1138–49.

Phillips, K.A. (1995). Body dysmorphic disorder: Clinical features and drug treatment. *CNS Drugs*, **3**: 30–40.

Phillips, K.A. (1996a). An open study of buspirone augmentation of serotonin-reuptake inhibitors in body dysmorphic disorder. *Psychopharmacol Bull*, **32**: 175–80.

Phillips, K.A. (1996b). Body dysmorphic disorder: Diagnosis and treatment of imaged ugliness. *J Clin Psychiatry*, **57**(suppl 8): 61–5.

Phillips, K.A. (1996c). Pharmacologic treatment of body dysmorphic disorder. *Psychopharmacol Bull*, **32**: 597–605.

Phillips, K.A. (1996d). *The Broken Mirror: Understanding and Treating Body Dysmorphic Disorder*. New York: Oxford University Press.

Phillips, K.A. and Diaz, S.F. (1997). Gender differences in body dysmorphic disorder. *J Nerv Ment Dis*, **185**: 570–7.

Phillips, K.A., Dwight, M.M. and McElroy, S.L. (1998). Efficacy and safety of fluvoxamine in body dysmorphic disorder. *J Clin Psychiatry*, **59**: 165–71.

Phillips, K.A., Hollander, E., Rasmussen, S.A., Aronowitz, B.R., DeCaria, C. and Goodman, S.K. (1997a). A severity rating scale for body dysmorphic disorder: Development, reliability, and validity of a modified version of the Yale–Brown Obsessive Compulsive Scale. *Psychopharmacol Bull*, **33**: 17–22.

Phillips, K.A., McElroy, S.L., Hudson, J.I. and Pope, H.C. (1995). Body dysmorphic disorder: An obsessive–compulsive spectrum disorder, a form of affective spectrum disorder, or both? *J Clin Psychiatry*, **56**(suppl 4): 41–51.

Phillips, K.A., McElroy S.L., Keck, P.E., Hudson, J.I. and Pope, H.G. (1994). A comparison of delusional and nondelusional body dysmorphic disorder in 100 cases. *Psychopharmacol Bull*, **30**: 179–86.

Phillips, K.A., McElroy, S.L., Keck, P.E., Pope, H.G. and Hudson, J.I. (1993). Body dysmorphic disorder: 30 cases of imagined ugliness. *Am J Psychiatry*, **150**: 302–8.

Phillips, K.A. and Nierenberg, A.A. (1994). The assessment and treatment of refractory depression. *J Clin Psychiatry*, **55**(suppl 2): 20–6.

Phillips, K.A., O'Sullivan, R.L. and Pope, H.G. (1997b). Muscle dsymorphia. (Letter.) *J Clin Psychiatry*, **58**: 361.

Phillips, K.A. and Taub, B.A. (1995). Skin picking as a symptom of body dysmorphic disorder. *Psychopharm Bull*, **31**: 279–88.

Phillips, K.A., Van Noppen, B.L. and Shapiro, L. (1997c). *Learning to Live With Body Dysmorphic Disorder*. Milford, CT: The Obsessive-Compulsive Foundation.

Piccinelli, M., Pini, S., Bellantuono, C. and Wilkinson, G. (1995). Efficacy of drug treatment in obsessive–compulsive disorder: A meta-analytic review. *Br J Psychiatry*, **166**: 424–43.

Pigott, T., Altemus, M., Rubentein, C., Hill, J., Bihari, K., L'Heureux, F., Bernstein, S. and Murphy, D. (1991a). Symptoms of eating disorders in patients with obsessive–compulsive disorder. *Am J Psychiatry*, **148**: 1552–7.

Pigott, T., L'Heureux, F., Hill, J.L., Bihari, K., Bernstein, S.E. and Murphy, D.L. (1992a). A double-blind study of adjuvant buspirone hydrochloride in clomipramine-treated patients with obsessive–compulsive disorder. *J Clin Psychopharmacol*, **12**: 11–18.

Pigott, T., L'Heureux, F., Rubenstein, C.S., Bernstein, S.E., Hill, J.L. and Murphy, D.L. (1992b). A double-blind, placebo controlled study of trazodone in patients with obsessive–compulsive disorder. *J Clin Psychopharmacol*, **12**: 156–62.

Pigott, T., Pato, M.T., Bernstein, S.E., Grover, G.N., Hill, J.L., Tolliver, T.J. and Murphy, D.L. (1990). Controlled comparisons of clomipramine and fluoxetine in the treatment of obsessive compulsive disorder. *Arch Gen Psychiatry*, **47**: 926–32.

Pigott, T., Pato, M.T., L'Heureux, F., Hill, J.L., Grover, G.N., Bernstein, S.E. and Murphy, D.L. (1991b). A controlled comparison of adjuvant lithium carbonate or thyroid hormone in clomipramine treated patients with obsessive–compulsive disorder. *J Clin Psychopharmacol*, **11**: 242–8.

Pilowsky, I. (1967). Dimensions of hypochondriasis. *Br J Psychiatry*, **113**: 89–93.

Pincu, L. (1989). Sexual compulsivity in gay men: Controversy and treatment. *J Counsel Devel*, **68**: 63–8.

Pitman, R.K. (1987). Pierre Janet on obsessive–compulsive disorder (1903). *Arch Gen Psychiatry*, **44**: 226–32.

Pitman, R.K., Green, R.C., Jenike, M.A. and Mesulam, M.M. (1987). Clinical comparison of Tourette's disorder and obsessive–compulsive disorder. *Am J Psychiatry*, **144**: 1166–71.

Pollack, J. (1987). Relationship of obsessive–compulsive personality to obsessive–compulsive disorder: A review of the literature. *J Psychology*, **121**: 137–48.

Pollack, M.H. and Otto, M.W. (1997). Long-term course and outcome of panic disorder. *J Clin Psychiatry*, **58**(suppl 2): 57–60.

Pollack, M.H., Otto, M.W., Tesar, G.E., Cohen, L.S., Meltzer-Brody, S. and Rosenbaum, J.F. (1993). Long-term outcome after acute treatment with alprazolam or clonazepam for panic disorder. *J Clin Psychopharmacol*, **13**: 257–63.

Pollack, M.H., Otto, M.W., Worthington, J.J., Manfro, G.G. and Wolfow, R. (1998). Sertraline in the treatment of panic disorder: a flexible-dose multicenter trial. *Arch Gen Psychiatry*, **55**: 1010–16.

Pollack, M.H. and Rosenbaum, J.F. (1987). Management of antidepressant-induced side effects: A practical guide for the clinician. *J Clin Psychiatry*, **48**: 3–8.

Pollard, C.A., Ibe, I.O., Krojanker, D.N., Kitchen, A.D., Bronson, S.S. and Flynn, T.M. (1991). Clomipramine treatment of trichotillomania: A follow-up report on four cases. *J Clin Psychiatry*, **52**: 128–30.

Pollock, B.G. (1982). Successful treatment of pathological jealousy with pimozide. (Letter.) *Can J Psychiatry*, **27**: 86–7.

Popper, C.W. (1997). Antidepressants in the treatment of attention-deficit/hyperactivity disorder. *J Clin Psychiatry*, **58**(suppl 14): 14–29.

Porto, L., Bermanzohn, P.C., Pollack, S., Morrissey, R. and Siris, S.G. (1997). A profile of obsessive–compulsive symptoms in schizophrenia. *CNS Spectrums*, **2**: 21–5.

Powers, R. (1993). Fibromyalgia: An age-old malady begging for respect. *J Gen Intern Med*, **8**: 93–103.

Preskorn, S.H. (1989). Tricyclic antidepressants: The whys and hows of therapeutic drug monitoring. *J Clin Psychiatry*, **50**(suppl 7): 34–42.

Preskorn, S.H. (1993). Pharmacokinetics of antidepressants: Why and how are they relevant to treatment. *J Clin Psychiatry*, **54**(suppl 9): 14–34.

Preskorn, S.H. (1995). What is the message in the alphabet soup of cytochrome P450 enzymes? *J Prac Psychiatry Behav Health*, **1**: 237–40.

Preskorn, S.H. (1996a). *Clinical Pharmacology of Selective Serotonin Reuptake Inhibitors.* 1st edn. Caddo, OK: Professional Communications, Inc.

Preskorn, S.H. (1996b). Drug-drug interactions. *J Clin Psychiatry*, **57**: 223–5.

Preskorn, S.H. and Magnus, R.D. (1994). Inhibition of hepatic P-450 isoenzymes by serotonin selective reuptake inhibitors: In vitro and in vivo findings and their implications for patient care. *Psychopharmacol Bull*, **30**: 251–9.

Price, R.A., Kidd, K.K., Cohen, D.J., Pauls, D.L. and Leckman, J.F. (1985). A twin study of Tourette syndrome. *Arch Gen Psychiatry*, **42**: 815–20.

Pulst, S-M., Walshe, T.M. and Romero, J.A. (1983). Carbon monoxide poisoning with features of Gilles de la Tourette's syndrome. *Arch Neurol*, **40**: 443–4.

Pupko, H. (1997). I've got the music in me: A look at intrusive music and OCD. *OCD Newsletter*, **11**: 2–3.

Quadland, M.C. (1985). Compulsive sexual behavior: Definition of a problem and an approach to treatment. *J Sex Marital Ther*, **11**: 121–32.

Quadland, M.C. and Shattls, W.D. (1987). AIDS, sexuality and sexual control. *J Homosex*, **14**: 277–98.

The Quality Assurance Project. (1991). Treatment outlines for avoidant, dependent and passive–aggressive personality disorders. *Aust N Z J Psychiatry*, **25**: 404–11.

Rahman, M.A. and Gregory, R. (1995). Trichotillomania associated with HIV infection and response to sertraline. *Psychosomatics*, **36**: 417–18.

Ramchandani, D. (1990). Trazodone for bowel obsession.(Letter.) *Am J Psychiatry*, **147**: 124.

Rasmussen, S.A. (1984). Lithium and tryptophan augmentation in clomipramine-resistant obsessive–compulsive disorder. *Am J Psychiatry*, **141**: 1283–5.

Rasmussen, S.A. (1994). Commentary: Obsessive compulsive spectrum disorders. *J Clin Psychiatry*, **55**: 89–91.

Rasmussen, S.A. and Eisen, J.L. (1988). Clinical and epidemiologic findings of significance to neuropharmacologic trials in OCD. *Psychopharmacol Bull*, **24**: 466–70.

Rasmussen, S.A. and Eisen, J.L. (1992a). The epidemiology and clinical features of obsessive–compulsive disorder. *Psychiatr Clin North Am*, **15**: 743–58.

Rasmussen, S.A. and Eisen, J.L. (1992b). The epidemiology and differential diagnosis of obsessive–compulsive disorder. *J Clin Psychiatry*, **53**(Suppl 10): 4–10.

Rasmussen, S.A. and Eisen, J.L. (1997). Treatment strategies for refractory obsessive–compulsive disorder. *J Clin Psychiatry*, **58**(suppl 13): 9–13.

Rasmussen, S.A., Eisen, J.L. and Pato, M.T. (1993). Current issues in the pharmacologic management of obsessive–compulsive disorder. *J Clin Psychiatry*, **54**: 4–9.

Rasmussen, S., Hackett, E., Duboff, E., Greist, J., Halaris, A., Koran, L.M., Liebowitz, M., Lydiard, R.B., McElroy, S., Mendels, J. et al. (1997). A 2–year study of sertraline in the treatment of obsessive–compulsive disorder. *Int Clin Psychopharmacol*, **12**: 309–16.

Ratzoni, G., Hermesh, H., Brandt, N., Lauffer, M. and Munitz, H. (1990). Clomipramine efficacy for tics, obsessions, and compulsions in Tourette's syndrome and obsessive–compulsive disorder: A case study. *Biol Psychiatry*, **27**: 95–8.

Rauch, S.L., O'Sullivan, R.L. and Jenike, M.A. (1996). Open treatment of obsessive compulsive disorder with venlafaxine: A series of ten cases. (Letter.) *J Clin Psychopharmacol*, **16**: 81–3.

Ravizza, L., Barzega, G., Bellino S., Bogetto, F. and Maina G. (1995). Predictors of drug treatment response in obsessive–compulsive disorder. *J Clin Psychiatry*, **56**: 368–73.

Ravizza, L., Barzega, G., Bellino S., Bogetto, F. and Maina G. (1996a). Drug treatment of obsessive–compulsive disorder (OCD): Long-term trial with clomipramine and selective serotonin reuptake inhibitors (SSRIs). *Psychopharmacol Bull*, **32**: 167–73.

Ravizza, L., Barzega, G., Bellino S., Bogetto, F. and Maina G. (1996b). Therapeutic effect and safety of adjunctive risperidone in refractory obsessive–compulsive disorder (OCD). *Psychopharmacol Bull*, **32**: 677–82.

Reeve, E.A., Bernstein, G.A. and Christenson, G.A. (1992). Clinical characteristics and psychiatric comorbidity in children with trichotillomania. *J Am Acad Child Adolesc Psychiatry*, **31**: 132–8.

Reeves, R. (1995). Serotonin syndrome produced by paroxetine and low-dose trazodone. *Psychosomatics*, **36**: 159–60.

Reid, T.L. (1992). Treatment of generalized anxiety disorder and trichotillomania with buspirone. (Letter.) *Am J Psychiatry*, **149**: 573–4.

Reimherr, F.W., Amsterdam, J.D., Quitkin, F.M. et al. (1998). Optimal length of continuation therapy in depression: A prospective assessment during long-term fluoxetine tratment. *Am J Psychiatry*, **155**: 1247–53.

Reisenman, C. (1995). Antidepressant drug interactions and the cytochrome P450 system: A critical appraisal. *Pharmacotherapy*, **15**(6 Pt 2): 84S–99S.

Remillard, G.M., Andermann, F., Gloor, P., Olivier, A. and Martin, J.B. (1981). Water-drinking as ictal behaviour in complex partial seizures. *Neurology*, **31**: 117–24.

Remington, G. and Adams, M. (1994). Risperidone and obsessive–compulsive symptoms. (Letter.) *J Clin Psychopharmacol*, **14**: 358–9.

Reynolds, R.D. (1997). Sertraline-induced anorgasmia treated with intermittent nefazodone. (Letter.) *J Clin Psychiatry*, **58**: 89.

Reznik, I. and Sirota, P. (1996). Combined fluvoxamine and neuroleptic therapy for schizophrenic patients with obsessive compulsive disorder. *Israel J Psychiatry*, **33**: 269–70.

Ricciardi, J.N., Baer, L., Jenike, M.A., Fischer, S.C., Sholtz, D. and Buttolph, M.L. (1992). Changes in DSM-III-R Axis II diagnoses following treatment of obsessive–compulsive disorder. *Am J Psychiatry*, **149**: 829–31.

Riddle, M.A., Hardin, M.T., King, R., Scahill, L. and Woolston, J.L. (1990). Fluoxetine treatment of children and adolescents with Tourette's and obsessive-compulsive disorders: Preliminary clinical experience. *J Am Acad Child Adolesc Psychiatry*, **29**: 45–8.

Riggs, D.S. and Foa, E.G. (1993). Obsessive compulsive disorder. In *Clinical Handbook of Psychological Disorders*, 2nd edn., ed. D.H. Barlow, pp. 189–239. New York: Guilford Press.

Robert, E. (1996). Treating depression in pregnancy. *N Engl J Med*, **335**: 1056–8.

Robertson, M.M. (1989). The Gilles de la Tourette syndrome: The current status. *Br J Psychiatry*, **154**: 147–69.

Robertson, M.M. (1994). Annotation: Gilles de la Tourette syndrome – An update. *J Child Psychol Psychiatry*, **35**: 597–611.

Robertson, M.M and Gourdie, A. (1990). Familial Tourette's syndrome in a large British pedigree. Associated psychopathology, severity, and potential for linkage analysis. *Br J Psychiatry*, **156**: 515–21.

Robertson, M.M and Yakeley, J.W. (1993). Obsessive–compulsive disorder and self-injurious behavior. In *Handbook of Tourette's Syndrome and Related Tic and Behavioral Disorders*, ed. R. Kurlan, pp. 45–87. New York: Marcel Dekker.

Rogers, M.P. and Mendoza, A.Y. (1994). Development of obsessive–compulsive disorder after brain tumor surgery and radiation. *Psychosomatics*, **35**: 402–6.

Rosa, F. (1994). Medicaid antidepressant pregnancy exposure outcomes. *Reprod Toxicol*, **8**: 444.

Rosen, J.C. and Reiter, J. (1996). Development of the body dysmorphic disorder examination. *Behav Res Ther*, **34**: 755–66.

Rosenbaum, M.S. and Ayllon, T. (1981). The habit reversal technique in treating trichotillomania. *Behav Ther*, **12**: 473–81.

Rosenfeld, R., Dar, R., Anderson, D., Kobak, K.A. and Greist, J.H. (1992). A computer-assisted version of the Yale–Brown Obsessive–Compulsive Scale. *Psychol Assessment*, **4**: 329–32.

Rosenthal, R.J. and Lorenz, V.C. (1992). The pathological gambler as criminal offender. *Clin Forensic Psychiatry*, **15**: 647–60.

Roth, A.S., Ostroff, R.B. and Hoffman, R.E. (1996). Naltrexone as a treatment for repetitive self-injurious behavior: An open-label trial. *J Clin Psychiatry*, **57**: 233–7.

Rothbaum, B.O., Shaw, L., Morris, R. and Ninan, P.T. (1993). Prevalence of trichotillomania in a college freshman population. (Letter.) *J Clin Psychiatry*, **54**: 71.

Rothenberg, A. (1990). Adolescence and eating disorder: The obsessive–compulsive syndrome. *Psychiatr Clin North Am*, **13**: 469–88.

Rothschild, A.J. (1995). SSRI-induced sexual dysfunction: Efficacy of a drug holiday. *Am J Psychiatry*, **152**: 1514–16.

Rowen, R. (1981). Hypnotic age regression in the treatment of a self-destructive habit: Trichotillomania. *Am J Clin Hyp*, **23**: 195–7.

Rubenstein, C.S., Pigott, T.A., L'Heureux, F., Hill, J.H. and Murphy, D.L. (1992). A preliminary investigation of the lifetime prevalence of anorexia and bulimia nervosa in patients with obsessive–compulsive disorder. *J Clin Psychiatry*, **53**: 309–14.

Rubey, R., Brady, K.T. and Norris, G.T. (1993). Clomipramine treatment of sexual preoccupation. (Letter.) *J Clin Psychopharmacol*, **13**: 158–9.

Ruegg, R.G., Evans, D.L., Comer, W.S. and Golden, R.N. (1992). Lithium augments fluoxetine treatment of obsessive compulsive disorder. *Lithium*, **3**: 69–76.

Ruiz, F. (1994). Fluoxetine and the serotonin syndrome. *Ann Emerg Med*, **24**: 983–5.

Russell, J.L. (1996). Relatively low doses of cisapride in the treatment of nausea in patients treated with venlafaxine for treatment-refractory depression. *J Clin Psychopharmacol*, **16**: 35–7.

Russo, A.M., Taber, J.I., McCormick, R.A. and Ramirez, L.F. (1984). An outcome study of an inpatient treatment program for pathological gamblers. *Hosp Community Psychiatry*, **35**: 823–47.

Rylander, G. (1969). Clinical and medicocriminological aspects of addictions to central stimulating drugs. In *Abuse of Central Stimulants*, ed. E. Sjoquiste and M. Tottie, pp. 251–73. New York: Raven Press.

Sachdeva, J.S. and Sidhu, B.S. (1987). Trichotillomania associated with depression. *J Indian Med Assoc*, **85**: 151–2.

Sacks, O.W., Messeloff, C., Schartz, W., Goldfarb, A. and Kohl, M. (1970). Effects of l-dopa in patients with dementia. *Lancet*, **1**: 1231.

Sadovnick, D. and Kurlan, R. (1997). The increasingly complex genetics of Tourette's syndrome. *Neurology*, **48**: 801–2.

Salzberg, A.D. and Swedo, S.E. (1992). Oxytocin and vasopressin in obsessive–compulsive disorder. (Letter.) *Am J Psychiatry*, **149**: 713–14.

Salzman, L. (1980). *Treatment of the Obsessive Personality*. New York: Jason Aronson.

Salzman, L. (1983). Psychoanalytic therapy of the obsessional patient. *Curr Psychiatr Ther*, **22**: 53–9.

Sandler, N.H. (1996). Tardive dyskinesia associated with fluoxetine. (Letter.) *J Clin Psychiatry*, **57**: 91.

Sandor, P. (1993). Gilles de la Tourette syndrome: A neuropsychiatric disorder. *J Psychosom Research*, **37**: 211–26.

Sandor, P., Musisi, S., Moldofsky, H. and Lang, A. (1990). Tourette syndrome: A follow-up study. *J Clin Psychopharmacol*, **10**: 197–9.

Saper, B. (1971). A report on behavior therapy with outpatient clinic patients. *Psychiatr Q*, **45**: 209–15.

Sasson, Y., Bermanzohn, P.C. and Zohar, J. (1997). Treatment of obsessive–compulsive syndromes in schizophrenia. *CNS Spectrums*, **2**: 34–6, 45.

Savard, R. and Walker, E. (1965). Changes in social functioning after surgical treatment for temporal lobe epilepsy. *Soc Work* **10**: 87–95.

Saxena, S., Wang, D., Bystritsky, A. and Baxter, L.R. (1996). Risperidone augmentation of SRI treatment for refractory obsessive–compulsive disorder. *J Clin Psychiatry*, **57**: 303–6.

Scahill, L., Riddle, M.A., King, R.A., Hardin, M.T., Rasmusson, A., Makuch, R.W. and Leckman, J.F. (1997). Fluoxetine has no marked effect on tic symptoms in patients with Tourette's syndrome: a double-blind placebo-controlled study. *J Child Adolesc Psychopharmacol*, **7**: 75–85.

Schacter, M (1961). Trichotillomania in children. *Prax Kinderpsychol Kinderpsychiatry*, **10**: 120–4.

Schatzberg, A.F., Cole, J.O. and DeBattista, C. (1997). *Manual of Clinical Psychopharmacology*, 3rd edn. Washington, DC: American Psychiatric Press, Inc.

Schilder, P. (1938). The organic background of obsessions and compulsions. *Am J Psychiatry*, **94**: 1397–416.

Schlosser, S., Black, D.W., Blum, N. and Goldstein, R.B. (1994a). The demography, phenomenology, and family history of 22 persons with compulsive hair pulling. *Ann Clin Psychiatry*, **6**: 147–52.

Schlosser, S., Black, D.W., Repertinger, S. and Freet, D. (1994b). Compulsive buying: Demography, phenomenology, and comorbidity in 46 subjects. *Gen Hosp Psychiatry*, **16**: 205–12.

Schneier, F.R., Johnson, J., Hornig, C.D., Liebowitz, M.R. and Weissman, M.M. (1992). Social phobia: Comorbidity and morbidity in an epidemiologic sample. *Arch Gen Psychiatry*, **49**: 282–8.

Schneier, F.R., Saoud, J.B., Campeas, R., Fallon, B.F., Hollander, E., Coplan, J. and Liebowitz, M.R. (1993). Buspirone in social phobia. *J Clin Psychopharmacol*, **13**: 251–6.

Schneier, F.R., Spitzer, R.L., Gibbon, M., Fyer, A.T. and Liebowitz, M.R. (1991). The relationship of social phobia subtypes and avoidant personality disorder. *Comp Psychiatry*, **32**: 496–502.

Schou, M. (1976). What happened later to the lithium babies? A follow-up study of children born without malformations. *Acta Psychiatr Scand*, **54**: 193–7.

Schou, M. (1990). Lithium treatment during pregnancy, delivery, and lactation: An update. *J Clin Psychiatry*, **51**: 410–13.

Schuckit, M.A. and Hesslbrock, V. (1994). Alcohol dependence and anxiety disorders: What is the relationship? *Am J Psychiatry*, **151**: 1723–34.

Schulberg, H.C., Saul, M., McClelland, M. Ganfuli, M., Christy, W. and Frank, R. (1985). Assessing depression in primary medical and psychiatry practices. *Arch Gen Psychiatry*, **42**: 1164–70.

Schwartz, J.H. (1992). Psychoanalytic psychotherapy for a woman with diagnoses of kleptomania and bulimia. *Hosp Community Psychiatry*, **43**: 109–10.

Schwartz, J.M. (1996). *Brain Lock*. New York: Harper Collins.

Schwartz, J.M., Stoessel, P.W., Baxter, L.R., Martin, K.R. and Phelps, M.E. (1996). Systematic changes in cerebral glucose metabolic rate after successful behavior modification treatment of obsessive–compulsive disorder. *Arch Gen Psychiatry*, **53**: 109–13.

Schwartz, M.F. (1992). Sexual compulsivity as post-traumatic stress disorder: Treatment perspectives. *Psychiatr Ann*, **22**: 333–8

Schwartz, M.F. and Brasted, W.S. (1985). Sexual addiction: Self-hatred, guilt, and passive rage contribute to this deviant behavior. *Med Aspects Hum Sex*, **19**: 103–7.

Schwarz, J. and Lindner, A. (1992). Inpatient treatment of male pathological gamblers in Germany. *J Gambling Stud*, **8**: 93–109.

Schweitzer, I., Tuckwell, V. and Johnson, G. (1997). A review of the use of augmentation therapy for the treatment of resistant depression: Implications for the clinician. *Aust NZ J Psychiatry,* **31**: 340–52.

Schweizer, E., Pohl, R., Balon, R., Fox, I., Rickels, K. and Yeragani, V.K. (1990). Lorazepam vs. alprazolam in the treatment of panic disorder. *Pharmacopsychiatry,* **23**: 90–3.

Scolnik, D., Nulman, I. Rovet, J., Gladstone, D., Czuchta, D., Gardner, H.A., Gladstone, R., Ashby, P, Weksberg, R., Emerson, T., et al. (1994). Neurodevelopment of children exposed in utero to phenytoin and carbamazepine monotherapy. [Erratum, (1994). *JAMA,* **271**: 1745.] *JAMA,* **271**: 767–70.

Sebit, M.B., Acuda, W. and Chibanda, D. (1996). A case of the frontal lobe syndrome following head injury in Harare, Zimbabwe. *Central African J Med,* **42**: 51–3.

Seeman, M.V. (1979). Pathological jealousy. *Psychiatry,* **42**: 351–61.

Seibyl, J.P., Krystal, J.H., Goodman, W.K. and Price, L.H. (1989). Obsessive–compulsive symptoms in a patient with a right frontal lobe lesion: Respose to lithium augmentation of tranylcypromine. *Neuropsychiatry Neuropsychol Behav Neurol,* **1**: 295–9.

Seidman, S.N. and Rieder, R.O. (1994). A review of sexual behavior in the United States. *Am J Psychiatry,* **151**: 330–41.

Seitz, P.F.D. (1953). Dynamically-oriented brief psychotherapy: Psychocutaneous excoriation syndromes. *Psychosom Med,* **15**: 200–13.

Sexson, W.R. and Barak, Y. (1989). Withdrawal emergent syndrome in an infant associated with maternal haloperidol therapy. *J Perinatol,* **9**: 170–2.

Shapiro E., Shapiro, A.K., Fulop, G., Hubbard, M., Mandeli, J., Nordlie, J. and Phillips, R.A. (1989). Controlled study of haloperidol, pimozide, and placebo for the treatment of Gilles de la Tourette's syndrome. *Arch Gen Psychiatry,* **46**: 722–30.

Sharma, V. (1991). Bowel obsessions and clomipramine. (Letter.) *Can J Psychiatry,* **36**: 233–4.

Sharpe, M. (1996). Chronic fatigue syndrome. *Psychiatr Clin North Am.* **19**: 549–73.

Sharpe, M., Hawton, K., Simkin, S., Surawy, C., Hackmann, A., Klimes, I., Peto, T., Warrell, D. and Seagroatt, V. (1996). Cognitive behaviour therapy for the chronic fatigue syndrome: A randomised controlled trial. *Br Med J,* **312**: 22–6.

Sharpe, M., Peveler, R. and Mayou R. (1992). The psychological treatment of patients with functional somatic symptoms: A practical guide. *J Psychosom Res,* **36**: 515–29.

Shear, M.K., Pilkonis, P.A., Cloitre, M. and Leon, A.C. (1994). Cognitive behavioral treatment compared with nonprescriptive treatment of panic disorder. *Arch Gen Psychiatry,* **51**: 395–401.

Shear, M.K. and Weiner, K. (1997). Psychotherapy for panic disroder. *J Clin Pychiatry,* **58** (suppl. 2): 38–42.

Sheehan, D.V. (1983). *The Anxiety Disease,* p. 151. New York: Charles Scribner and Sons.

Sheehan, D.V., Harnett-Sheehan, K. and Raj, B.A. (1996). The measurement of disability. *Int Clin Psychopharmacol,* **11**(suppl 3): 89–95.

Sheehan, D.V., Raj, A.B., Harnett-Sheehan, K., Soto, S. and Knapp, E. (1993). The relative efficacy of high dose buspirone and alprazolam in the treatment of panic disorder: A double-blind placebo-controlled study. *Acta Psychiatr Scand,* **88**: 1–11.

Shooka, A., al-Haddad, M.K. and Raees, A. (1998). OCD in Bahrain: a phenomenological profile. *Internat J Soc Psychiatry,* **44**: 147–54.

Shrivastava, R.K., Shrivastava, S., Overweg, N. and Schmitt, M. (1995). Amantadine in the treatment of sexual dysfunction associated with selective serotonin reuptake inhibitors. (Letter.) *J Clin Psychopharmacol,* **15**: 83–4.

Silber, K.P. and Haynes, C.E. (1992). Treating nailbiting: A comparative analysis of mild aversion and competing response therapies. *Behav Res Ther*, **30**: 15–22.

Silva, R.R., Muñoz, D.M., Daniel, W., Barickman J. and Friedhoff, A.J. (1996). Causes of haloperidol discontinuation in patients with Tourette's Disorder: Managment and alternatives. *J Clin Psychiatry*, **57**: 129–35.

Silver, P.A. (ed.) (1994). *Psychotropic Drug Use in the Medically Ill*. Basel: Karger

Simeon, D., Cohen, L.J., Stein, D.J., Schmeidler, J., Spadaccini, E. and Hollander, E. (1997a). Comorbid self-injurious behaviors in 71 female hair-pullers: A survey study. *J Nerv Ment Dis*, **185**: 117–19.

Simeon, D., Stein D.J., Gross, S., Islam, N., Schmeidler, J. and Hollander, E. (1997b). A double-blind trial of fluoxetine in pathologic skin picking. *J Clin Psychiatry*, **58**: 341–7.

Simon, G.E., Katon W.J. and Sparks, P.J. (1990). Allergic to life: Psychological factors in environmental illness. *Am J Psychiatry*, **147**: 901–6.

Simon K.M. and Myer J. (1990). Obsessive-compulsive personality disorder. In *Cognitive Therapy of Personality Disorders*, ed. A.T. Beck, A. Freeman and Associates, pp. 309–32. New York: Guilford Press.

Singer, H.S. and Walkup, J.T. (1991). Tourette Syndrome and other tic disorders. Diagnosis, pathophysiology, and treatment. *Medicine*, **70**: 15–32.

Singer, S., Brown, J., Quaskey, S., Rosenberg, L., Mellits, E. and Denckla, M. (1995). The treatment of attention-deficit hyperactivity disorder in Tourette's syndrome: A double-blind placebo controlled study with clonidine and desipramine. *Pediatrics*, **95**: 74–81.

Singh, A.N. and Maguire, J. (1989). Trichotillomania and incest. *Br J Psychiatry*, **155**: 108–10.

Skop, B.P. and Brown T.M. (1996). Potential vascular and bleeding complications of treatment with selective serotonin reuptake inhibitors. *Psychosomatics*, **37**: 12–16

Smith, K.C. and Pittkow, M.R. (1989). Naltrexone for neurotic excoriations. *J Am Acad Dermatol*, **20**: 860–1.

Snyder, S. (1980). Trichotillomania treated with amitriptyline. *J Nerv Ment Dis*, **168**: 505–7.

Sofuoglu, M. and DeBattista, C. (1996). Development of obsesssive symptoms during nefazodone treatment. (Letter.) *Am J Psychiatry*, **153**: 577–8.

Soriano, J.L., O'Sullivan, R.L., Baer, L., Phillips, K.A., McNally, R.J. and Jenike, M.A. (1996). Trichotillomania and self-esteem: A survey of 62 female hair pullers. *J Clin Psychiatry*, **57**: 77–82.

Soyka, M., Naber, G. and Völcker, A. (1991). Prevalence of delusional jealousy in different psychiatric disorders: An analysis of 93 cases. *Br J Psychiatry*, **158**: 549–53.

Spencer, T., Biederman, J., Kerman, K., Steingard, R. and Wilens, T. (1993a). Desipramine treatment of children with attention-deficit hyperactivity disorder and tic disorder or Tourette's syndrome. *J Am Acad Child Adolesc Psychiatry*, **32**: 354–60.

Spencer, T., Biederman, J., Steingard, R. and Wilens, T. (1993b). Bupropion exacerbates tics in children with attention-deficit hyperactivity disorder and Tourette's syndrome. *J Am Acad Child Adolesc Psychiatry*, **32**: 211–14.

Spencer, T., Biederman, J., Wilens, T., Steingard, R. and Geist, D. (1993c). Nortriptyline treatment of children with attention-deficit hyperactivity disorder and tic disorder or Tourette's syndrome. *J Am Acad Child Adolesc Psychiatry*, **32**: 205–10.

Spencer, T., Wilens, T., Biederman, J., Faraone, S.V., Ablon, J.S. and Lapey, K. (1995). A double-blind, crossover comparison of methylphenidate and placebo in adults with childhood-onset attention-deficit hyperactivity disorder. *Arch Gen Psychiatry*, **52**: 434–43.

Spier, S.A. (1992). Capgras' syndrome and the delusions of misidentification. *Psychiatric Ann*, **22**: 279–85.

Spitzer, R.L., Williams, J.B.W., Gibbon, M. and First, M.B. (1990). Structured Clinical Interview for DSM-III-R – Patient Edition (SCID-P, Version 1.0). Washington, DC: American Psychiatric Press.

Staab, J.P., Yerkes, S.A., Cheney, E.M. and Clayton, A.H. (1990). Transient SIADH associated with fluoxetine. (Letter.) *Am J Psychiatry*, **147**: 1569.

Staley, D., Wand, R. and Shady, G. (1997). Tourette disorder: A cross-cultural review. *Comp Psychiatry*, **38**: 6–16.

Stanley, M.A., Bowers, T., Swann, A.C. and Taylor, D.J. (1991). Treatment of trichotillomania with fluoxetine. (Letter.) *J Clin Psychiatry*, **52**: 282.

Stanley, M.A., Breckenridge, J.K., Swann, A.C., Freeman, E.B. and Reich, L. (1997). Fluvoxamine treatment of trichotillomania. *J Clin Psychopharmacol*, **17**: 278–83.

Stanley, M.A., Prather, R.C., Wagner, A.L., Davis, M.L. and Swann, A.C. (1993). Can the Yale–Brown Obsessive–Compulsive Scale be used to assess trichotillomania? A preliminary report. *Beh Res Ther*, **31**: 171–7.

Stanley, M.A., Swann, A.C., Bowers, T.C., Davis, M.L. and Taylor, D.J. (1992). A comparison of clinical features in trichotillomania and obsessive–compulsive disorder. *Behav Res Ther*, **30**: 39–44.

Stanley, M.A., Turner, S.M. and Borden, J.W. (1990). Schizotypal features in obsessive–compulsive disorder. *Compr Psychiatry*, **31**: 511–18.

Staudenmayer, H. (1996). Clinical consequences of the EI/MCS "diagnosis": Two paths. *Regul Toxicol Pharmacol*, **24**(1 Pt 2): S96–110.

Stein, D.J., Bouwer, C., Hawkridge, S. and Emsley, R.A. (1997a). Risperidone augmentation of serotonin reuptake inhibitors in obsessive–compulsive and related disorders. *J Clin Psychiatry*, **58**: 119–22.

Stein, D.J., Bouwer, C. and Maud, C.M. (1997b). Use of the selective serotonin reuptake inhibitor citalopram in treatment of trichotillomania. *Eur Arch Psychiatry Clin Neurosci*, **247**: 254–6.

Stein, D.J., Bruun, R.D., Josephson, S.C. and Hollander, E. (1991). Obsessional severity in Tourette's syndrome. (Letter.) *J Clin Psychiatry*, **52**: 388.

Stein, D.J. and Hollander, E. (1992). Low-dose pimozide augmentation of serotonin reuptake blockers in the treatment of trichotillomania. *J Clin Psychiatry*, **53**: 123–6.

Stein, D.J., Hollander, E., Anthony, D.T., Schneier, F.R., Fallon, B.A., Liebowitz, M.R. and Klein, D.F. (1992). Sertonergic medications for sexual obsessions, sexual addictions, and paraphilias. *J Clin Psychiatry*, **53**: 267–71.

Stein, D.J., Hollander, E., and Josephson, S.C. (1994a). Serotonin reuptake blockers for the treatment of obsessional jealousy. *J Clin Psychiatry*, **55**: 30–3.

Stein, D.J., Hutt, C.S., Spitz, J.L. and Hollander, E. (1993). Compulsive picking and obsessive–compulsive disorder. *Psychosomatics*, **34**: 177–80.

Stein, D.J., Keating, J., Zar, H.J. and Hollander, E. (1994b). A survey of the phenomenology and pharmacotheraoy of compulsive and impulsive-aggressive symptoms in Prader-Willi syndrome. *J Neuropsychiatry Clin Neurosci*, **6**: 23–9.

Stein, D.J., Wessels, C., Carr J., Hawkridge, S., Bouwer, C. and Kalis, N. (1997c). Hair pulling in a patient with Sydenham's chorea. (Letter.) *Am J Psychiatry*, **154**: 1320.

Stein, M.B., Forde, D.R., Anderson, G. and Walker, J.R. (1997d). Obsessive–compulsive disorder in the community: An epdemiolgic survey with clinical reappraisal. *Am J Psychiatry*, **154**: 1120–6.

Steiner, W. (1991). Fluoxetine-induced mania in a patient with obsessive–compulsive disorder. *Am J Psychiatry*, **148**: 1403–4.

Steiner, W. and Fontaine, R. (1986). Toxic reaction following the combined administration of fluoxetine and l-tryptophan: Five case reports. *Biol Psychiatry*, **21**: 1067–71.

Steingard, R., Biederman, J., Spencer, T., Wilens, T. and Gonzalez. A. (1993). Comparison of clonidine response in the treatment of attention deficit hyperactivity disorder with and without comorbid tic disorders. *J Am Acad Child Adolesc Psychiatry*, **32**: 350–3.

Stern, R.S. and Cobb, J.P. (1978). Phenomenology of obsessive–compulsive neurosis. *Br J Psychiatry*, **132**: 233–9.

Sternbach, H. (1991). The serotonin syndrome. *Am J Psychiatry*, **148**: 705–13.

Sternlicht, H.C. (1993). Obsessive–compulsive disorder, fluoxetine, and buspirone. (Letter.) *Am J Psychiatry*, **150**: 526.

Stewart, A.L., Hays, R.D. and Ware, J.E. (1988). The MOS Short-Form General Health Survey. *Med Care*, **26**: 724–32.

Stewart, R.M. and Brown, R.I.F. (1988). An outcome study of Gamblers Anonymous. *Br J Psychiatry*, **152**: 284–8.

Stone, M.H. (1990). Toward a comprehensive typology of personality. *J Person Disord*, **4**: 416–21.

Stone, M.H. (1993). Long-term outcome in personality disorders. *Br J Psychiatry*, **162**: 299–313.

Stout, R.J. (1990). Fluoxetine for the treatment of compulsive facial picking. (Letter.) *Am J Psychiatry*, **147**: 370.

Stowe, Z.N. and Nemeroff, C.B. (1995). Psychopharmacology during pregnancy and lactation. In *The American Psychiatric Press Textbook of Psychopharmacology*, eds. A.F. Schatzberg and C.B. Nemeroff, pp. 823–37. Washington DC: American Psychiatric Press.

Stowe, Z.N., Owen, M.J., Landry, J.C., Kilts, C.D., Ely, T., Llewellyn, A. and Nemeroff, C.B. (1997). Sertraline and desmethylsertraline in human breast milk and nursing infants. *Am J Psychiatry*, **154**: 1255–60.

Stravynski, A., Belisle, M., Marcouillier, M., Lavallee, Y.J. and Elie, R. (1994). The treatment of avoidant personality disorder by social skills training in the clinic or in real-life settings. *Can J Psychiatry*, **39**: 377–83.

Streichenwein, S.M. and Thornby, J.I. (1995). A long-term, double-blind, placebo-controlled crossover trial of the efficacy of fluoxetine for trichotillomania. *Am J Psychiatry*, **152**: 1192–6.

Sullivan, C. (1989). Trichotillomania (Letter.) *Br J Psychiatry*, **155**: 869.

Sunkureddi, K. and Markovitz, P. (1993). Trazodone treatment of obsessive–compulsive disorder and trichotillomania. *Am J Psychiatry*, **150**: 523–4.

Suppes, T. and Rush, A.J. (1996). Medication optimization during clozapine treatment. (Letter.) *J Clin Psychiatry*, **57**: 307–8.

Sverd, J., Gadow, K.D., Nolan, E.E., Sprafkin, J and Ezor, S.N. (1992). Methylphenidate in hyperactive boys with comorbid tic disorder: I. Clinic evaluations. *Adv Neurol*, **58**: 271–81.

Swedo, S.E. (1994). Sydenham's chorea: A model for childhood autoimmune neuropsychiatric disorder. *JAMA*, **272**: 1788–91.

Swedo, S.E., Lenane, M.C. and Leonard, H.L. (1993). Long-term treatment of trichotillomania (hair pulling). (Letter.) *N Engl J Med*, **329**: 141–2.

Swedo, S.E. and Leonard, H.L. (1992). Trichotillomania: An obsessive compulsive spectrum disorder? *Psychiatr Clin North Am*, **15**: 777–90.

Swedo, S.E., Leonard, H.L., Garvey, M., Mittleman, B., Allen, A.J., Perlmutter, S., Dow, S., Zamkoff, J., Dubbert, B.K., Lougee, L. (1998). Pediatric autoimmune neuropsychiatric disorders associated with streptococcal infections: Clinical description of the first 50 cases. *Am J Psychiatry*, **155**: 264–71.

Swedo, S.E., Leonard, H.L. and Kiessling, L.S. (1994). Speculations on antineuronal antibody-mediated neuropsychiatric disorders of childhood. *Pediatrics*, **93**: 323–6.

Swedo, S.E., Leonard, H.L., Mittleman, B.B., Allen, A.J., Rapoport, J.L., Dow, S.P., Kanter, M.E., Chapman, F. and Zabriskie, J. (1997). Identification of children with pediatric autoimmune neuropsychiatric disorders associated with streptococcal infections by a marker associated with rheumatic fever. *Am J Psychiatry*, **154**: 110–12.

Swedo, S.E., Leonard, H.L., Rapoport, J.L., Lenane, M.C., Goldberger, E.L. and Cheslow, D.L. (1989a). A double-blind comparison of clomipramine and desipramine in the treatment of trichotillomania (hair pulling). *N Engl J Med*, **321**: 497–501.

Swedo, S.E., Rapoport, J.L., Leonard, H.L., Lenane, M. and Cheslow, D. (1989b). Obsessive–compulsive disorder in children and adolescents. *Arch Gen Psychiatry*, **46**: 335–41.

Swedo, S.E., Rapoport, J.L., Leonard, H.L., Schapiro, M.B., Rapoport, S.I. and Grady, C.L. (1991). Regional cerebral glucose metabolism of women with trichotillomania. *Arch Gen Psychiatry*, **48**: 828–33.

Swims, M.P. (1993). Potential terfenadine-fluoxetine interaction. (Letter.) *Ann Pharmacother*, **27**: 1404–5.

Swoboda, K.J. and Jenike, M.A. (1995). Frontal abnormalities in a patient with obsessive–compulsive disorder: The role of structural lesions in obsessive–compulsive behavior. *Neurology*, **45**: 2130–4.

Szegedi, A., Wetzel, H., Leal, M., Härtter, S. and Hiemke, C. (1996). Combination treatment with clomipramine and fluvoxamine: Drug monitoring, safety, and tolerability data. *J Clin Psychiatry*, **57**: 257–64.

Taber, J. and Chaplin, M. (1988). Group psychotherapy with pathological gamblers. *J Gambl Beh*, **4**: 183–96.

Taber, J., McCormick, R.A., Russo, A., Adkins, B.J. and Ramirez, L.F. (1987). Follow-up of pathological gamblers after treatment. *Am J Psychiatry*, **144**: 757–61.

Takeuchi, T., Nakagawa, A., Harai, H., Nakatani, E., Fujikawa, S., Yoshizato, C. and Yamagami, T. (1997). Primary obsessional slowness: Long-term findings. *Beh Res Ther*, **35**: 445–9.

Tarnowski, K.J., Rosen, L.A., McGrath, M.L. and Drabman, R.S. (1987). A modified habit reversal procedure in a recalcitrant case of trichotillomania. *J Behav Ther Exp Psychiatry*, **18**: 157–63.

Tarrier, N., Beckett, R., Harwood S. and Bishay, N. (1990). Morbid jealousy: A review and cognitive–behavioural formulation. *Br J Psychiatry*, **157**: 319–26.

Tejera, C.A., Mayerhoff, D.I. and Ramos-Lorenzi, J. (1993). Clomipramine for obsessive–compulsive symptoms in schizophrenia. (Letter.) *J Clin Psychopharmacol*, **13**: 290–1.

Thase, M.E. and Rush, A.J. (1997). When at first you don't succeed: Sequential strategies for antidepressant nonresponders. *J Clin Psychiatry*, **58**(suppl 13): 23–9.

Theil, A., Broocks, A., Olhmeier, M., Jacoby, G.E. and Schubler, G. (1995). Obsessive–compulsive disorder among patients with anorexia nervosa and bulimia nervosa. *Am J Psychiatry*, **151**: 72–5.

Thompson, J.W., Ware, M.R. and Blashfield, R.K. (1990). Psychotropic medication and priapism: A comprehensive review. *J Clin Psychiatry*, **51**: 430–3.

Thomsen, P.H. (1997). Child and adolescent obsessive–compulsive disorder treated with citalopram: Findings from an open trial of 23 cases. *J Child Adolesc Psychopharmacol*, **7**: 157–66.

Thomsen, P.H. and Mikkelsen, H.U. (1993). Development of personality disorders in children and adolescents with obsessive–compulsive disorder: A 6– to 22–year follow-up study. *Acta Psychiatr Scand*, **87**: 456–62.

Thomsen, P.H. and Mikkelsen, H.U. (1995). Course of obsessive–compulsive disorder in children and adolescents: A prospective follow-up study of 23 Danish cases. *J Am Acad Child Adolesc Psychiatry*, **34**: 1432–40.

Thornton, S.L. and Resch, D.S. (1995). SIADH associated with sertraline therapy. (Letter.) *Am J Psychiatry*, **152**: 809.

Tielens, J.A.E. (1997). Vitamin C for paroxetine- and fluvoxamine-associated bleeding. (Letter.) *Am J Psychiatry*, **153**: 883–4.

Tollefson, G.D. (1985). Alprazolam in the treatment of obsessive symptoms. *J Clin Psychopharmacol*, **5**: 39–42.

Tollefson, G.D., Birkett, M., Koran, L. and Genduso, L. (1994a). Continuation treatment of OCD: Double-blind and open-label experience with fluoxetine. *J Clin Psychiatry*, **55**(suppl 10): 69–76.

Tollefson, G.D., Rampey, A.H., Potvin, J.H., Jenike, M.A., Rush, A.J., Dominguez, R.A., Koran, L.M., Shear, K., Goodman, W. and Genduso, L.A. (1994b). A multicenter investigation of fixed-dose fluoxetine in the treatment of obsessive–compulsive disorder. *Arch Gen Psychiatry*, **51**: 559–67.

Tolstoy, L.N. (1985). *Kreutzer Sonata and Other Stories*. New York: Penguin.

Tonkonogy, J. (1993). OCD and Pick's Disease: Clinical and neuropathological correlation. (Abstract). *J Neuropsychiatry Clin Neurosci*, **5**: 447.

Tonkonogy, J. and Barreira, P. (1989). Obsessive–compulsive disorder and caudate-frontal lesion. *Neuropsychiatry Neuropsychol Behav Neurol*, **2**: 203–9.

Torres, A. R. and Del Porto, J.A. (1995). Comorbidity of obsessive–compulsive disorder and personality disorders: A Brazilian controlled study. *Psychopathology*, **28**: 322–9.

Towbin, K.E. and Riddle, M.A. (1993). Attention deficit hyperactivity disorder. In *Handbook of Tourette's Syndrome and Related Tic and Behavioral Disorders*, ed. R. Kurlan, pp. 89–109. New York: Marcel Dekker

Trivedi, M.H. (1996). Functional neuroanatomy of obsessive–compulsive disorder. *J Clin Psychiatry*, **57**(suppl 8): 26–36.

Troyer, W.A., Pereira, G.R., Lannon, R.A., Belik, J. and Yoder, M.C. (1993). Association of maternal lithium exposure and premature delivery. *J Perinatol*, **13**: 123–7.

Uitti, R.J., Ranner, C.M., Rajput, A.H., Goetz, C.G., Klawans, H.L., Thiessen, B. (1989). Hypersexuality with antiparkinsonian therapy. *Clin Neuropharmacol*, **12**: 375–83.

Vallejo, J., Olivares, J., Marcos, T., Bulbena, A. and Menchon, J.M. (1992). Clomipramine versus phenelzine in obsessive–compulsive disorder: A controlled trial. *Br J Psychiatry*, **161**: 665–70.

Van Ameringen, M.A. and Mancini, C.L. (1996). Haloperidol in the treatment of trichotillomania. *Annual Meeting New Research Program and Abstracts*, p. 261. Washington DC: American Psychiatric Association.

Van der Burght, M. (1994). *Citalopram Product Monograph*. Denmark: Lundbeck A/S.

Van der Kolk, B.A. and Van der Hart, O. (1989). Pierre Janet and the breakdown of adaptation in psychological trauma. *Am J Psychiatry*, **146**: 1530–40.

van der Pol, M.C., Hadders-Algra, M., Huisjes, H.J. and Touwen, B.C. (1991). Antiepileptic medication in pregnancy: Late effects on the children's central nervous system development. *Am J Obstet Gynecol*, **164**: 121–8.

Van Moffaert, M. (1992). Psychodermatology: An overview. *Psychother Psychosom*, **58**: 125–36.

Van Oppen, P. and Arntz, A. (1994). Cognitive therapy for obsessive–compulsive disorder. *Behav Res Ther*, **32**: 79–87.

Van Vliet, I.M., den Boer, J.A. and Westerberg, H.G.M. (1994). Psychopharmacological treatment of social phobia; A double blind placebo controlled study with fluvoxamine. *Psychopharmacol*, **115**: 128–34.

Veale, D. (1993). Classification and treatment of obsessional slowness. *Br J Psychiatry*, **162**: 198–203.

Veale, D., Boocock, A., Gournay, K., Dryden, W., Shah, F., Willson, R. and Walburn, J. (1996a). Body dysmorphic disorder: A survey of fifty cases. *Br J Psychiatry*, **169**: 196–201.

Veale, D., Gournay K., Dryden, W., Boocock, A., Shah, F., Willson R. and Walburn, J. (1996b). Body dysmorphic disorder: A cognitive behavioural model and pilot randomised controlled trial. *Behav Res Ther*, **34**: 717–29.

Veith, R.C., Friedel, R.O., Bloom, V. and Bielski, R. (1980). Electrocardiogram changes and plasma desipramine levels during treatment of depression. *Clin Pharmacol Ther*, **27**: 796–802.

Vieta, E. and Bernardo, M. (1992). Antidepressant-induced mania in obsessive–compulsive disorder. (Letter.) *Am J Psychiatry*, **149**: 1282–3.

Viggedal, G., Hagberg, B.S., Laegreid, L. and Aronsson, M. (1993). Mental development in late infancy after prenatal exposure to benzodiazepines – A prospective study. *J Child Psychol Psychiatry*, **32**: 295–305.

Viswanathan, R. and Paradis, C. (1991). Treatment of cancer phobia with fluoxetine. (Letter.) *Am J Psychiatry*, **148**: 1090.

Volberg, R.A. (1994). The prevalence and demographics of pathological gamblers: Implications for public health. *Am J Pub Health*, **84**: 237–41.

Volberg, R.A. and Banks, S.M. (1990). A review of two measures of pathological gambling in the United States. *J Gambling Studies*, **6**: 153–63.

Volberg, R.A. and Steadman, H.J (1988). Refining prevalence estimates of pathological gambling. *Am J Psychiatry*, **145**: 502–5.

Wade, A.G., Lepola, U., Koponen, H.J., Pederson, V. and Pederson, T. (1997). The effect of citalopram in panic disorder. *Br J Psychiatry*, **170**: 549–53.

Wagstaff, G.F. and Royce, C. (1994). Hypnosis and the treatment of nail biting: A preliminary trial. *Contemp Hypnosis*, **11**: 9–13.

Walker, E.A., Roy-Byrne, P.P. and Katon, W.J. (1990). Irritable bowel syndrome and psychiatric illness. *Am J Psychiatry*, **147**: 565–72.

Walkup, J.T., Leckman, J.F., R. Price, A., Hardin, M., Ort, S.I. and Cohen, D.J. (1988). The relationship between obsessive–compulsive disorder and Tourette's syndrome: A twin study. *Psychopharmacol Bull*, **24**: 375–9.

Walkup, J.T., Rosenberg, L.A., Brown, J. and Singer, H.S. (1992). The validity of instruments measuring tic severity in Tourette's syndrome. *J Am Acad Child Psychiatry*, **31**: 472–7.

Wallace, D.J. (1997). The fibromyalgia syndrome. *Ann Med*, **29**: 9–21.

Walley, T., Pirmohamed, M., Proudlove, C. and Maxwell, D. (1993). Interaction of metoprolol and fluoxetine (Letter.) *Lancet*, **341**: 967–8.

Ward, C.D. (1988). Transient feelings of compulsion caused by hemispheric lesions: Three cases. *J Neurol Neurosurg Psychiatry*, **51**: 266–8.

Ware, J.E., Snow, K.K, Kosinski, M., Gandek, B. (1993). *SF-36 Health Survey Manual and Interpretation Guide*, pp. B19–B24. Boston: Health Institute, New England Medical Center.

Warneke, L.B. (1984). The use of intravenous chlorimipramine in the treatment of obsessive compulsive disorder. *Can J Psychiatry*, **29**: 135–41.

Warneke, L.B. (1985). Intravenous chlorimipramine in the treatment of obsessional disorder in adolescence: case report. *J Clin Psychiatry*, **46**: 100–3.

Warneke, L.B. (1989). Intravenous chlorimipramine therapy in obsessive–compulsive disorder. *Can J Psychiatry*, **34**: 853–9.

Warneke, L. (1997). A possible new treatment approach to obsessive–compulsive disorder. *Can J Psychiatry*, **42**: 667–8.

Warnock, J.K. and Kestenbaum, T. (1992). Pharmacologic treatment of severe skin-picking behavoirs in Prader-Willi syndrome. *Arch Dermatol*, **128**: 1623–5.

Warwick, H.C. and Marks, I.M. (1988). Behavioural treatment of illness phobia and hypochondriasis: A pilot study of 17 cases. *Brit J Psychiatry*, **152**: 239–41.

Warwick, H.M.C., Clark, D.M., Cobb, A.M. and Salkovskis, P.M. (1996). A controlled trial of cognitive-behavioral treatment of hypochondriasis. *Br J Psychiatry*, **169**: 189–95.

Weaver, Y.M. (1996). Medical management of the multiple chemical sensitivity patient. *Reg Toxicol Pharmacol*, **24**: S111–5.

Weilburg, J.B., Mesulam, M.-M., Weintraub, S., Buonanno, F., Jenike, M. and Stakes, J.W. (1989a). Focal striatal abnormalities in a patient with obsessive–compulsive disorder. *Arch Neurol*, **46**: 233–5.

Weilburg, J.B., Rosenbaum, J.F., Biederman, J., Sachs, G.S., Pollack, M.H. and Kelly, K. (1989b). Fluoxetine added to non-MAOI antidepressants converts nonresponders to responders: A preliminary report. *J Clin Psychiatry*, **50**: 447–9.

Weilburg, J.B., Rosenbaum, J.F., Meltzer-Brody, S. and Shustari, B.S. (1991). Tricyclic augmentation of fluoxetine. *Ann Clin Psychiatry*, **3**: 209–13.

Weissman, M.M., Bland, R.C., Canino, G.J., Greenwald, S., Hwu, H.G., Lee, C.K., Newman, S.C., Oakley-Browne, M.A., Rubio- Stipec, M.R., Wickramarante, P.J., Wihchen, H.U. and Yeh, E.K. (1994). The cross national epidemiology of obsessive compulsive disorder. *J Clin Psychiatry*, **55**(Suppl 3): 5–10.

Wesner, R.B. and Noyes, R. (1991). Imipramine an effective treatment for illness phobia. *J Affect Disord*, **22**: 43–8.

Wesson, C. (1990). *Women Who Shop too Much: Overcoming the Urge to Splurge*. New York: St. Martin's Press.

Westphal, J.R. and Rush, J. (1996). Pathological gambling in Louisiana: An epidemiological perspective. *J La State Med Soc*, **148**: 353–8.

Wetzel, H., Anghelescu, I., Szegedi, A., Wiesner, J., Weigman, H., Hartter, S. and Hiemke, C. (1998). Pharmacokinetic interactions of clozapine with selective serotonin reuptake inhibitors: Differential effects of fluvoxamine and paroxetine in a prospective study. *J Clin Psychopharmacol*, **18**: 2–9.

Wexberg, E. (1937). Remarks on the psychopathology of oculogyric crises in epidemic encephalitis. *J Nerv Ment Dis*, **85**: 56–69.

Wheadon, D.E., Bushnell, W.D. and Steiner, M. (1993). A fixed dose comparison of 20, 40, or 60 mg paroxetine to placebo in the treatment of obsessive compulsive disorder. *Abstracts of Panels and Posters, 32nd Annual Meeting, Honolulu Hawaii*, p. 194. Nashville, TN: American College of Neuropsychopharmacology.

Whitelaw, A.G., Cummings A.J. and McFadyen I.R. (1981). Effect of maternal lorazepam on the neonate. *Br Med J*, **282**: 1106–8.

Wilens, T.E., Biederman, J., Prince, J., Spencer, T.J., Faraone, S.V., Warbutton, R., Schleifer, D., Harding M., Linehan, C. and Geller, D. (1996). Six-week, double-blind, placebo-controlled study of desipramine for adult attention deficit hyperactivity disorder. *Am J Psychiatry*, **153**: 1147–53.

Wilens, T.E., Biederman, J., Spencer, T.J. and Prince, J. (1995). Pharmcotherapy of adult attention deficit/hyperactivity disorder: A review. *J Clin Psychopharmacol*, **15**: 270–9.

Williams, A.C., Owen, C. and Heath, D.A. (1988). Compulsive movement disorder with cavitation of caudate nucleus. (Letter.) *J Neurol Neurosurg Psychiatry*, **51**: 447–8.

Williams, K.E. and Koran, L.M. (1997). Obsessive compulsive disorder in pregnancy, the puerperium and the premenstruum. *J Clin Psychiatry*, **58**: 330–4.

Winchel, R.M., Jones, J.S., Molcho, A., Parsons, B., Stanley, B. and Stanley, M. (1992a). Rating the severity of trichotillomania: Methods and problems. *Psychopharmcol Bull*, **28**: 457–62.

Winchel, R.M., Jones, J.S., Molcho, A., Parsons, B., Stanley, B. and Stanley, M. (1992b). The Psychiatric Institute Trichotillomania Scale (PITS). *Psychopharmacol Bull*, **28**: 463–76.

Winchel, R.M., Jones, J.S., Stanley, B., Molcho, A. and Stanley, M. (1992c). Clinical characteristics of trichotillomania and its response to fluoxetine. *J Clin Psychiatry*, **53**: 304–8.

Winsberg, M.E., Cassic, K.S. and Koran, L.M. (1999). Hoarding in obsessive–compulsive disorder: A report of 20 cases. *J Clin Psychiatry*. (In press.)

Wisner, K.L., Perel, J.M. and Findling, R.L. (1996). Antidepressant treatment during breast-feeding. *Am J Psychiatry*, **153**: 1132–7.

Wisner, K.L., Perel, J.M. and Wheeler, S. B. (1993). Tricyclic dose requirements across pregnancy. *Am J Psychiatry*, **150**: 1541–2.

Wolfe, F., Smythe, H.A., Yunus, M.B., Bennett, A.M., Bombardier, C., Goldenberg, D.L., Tugwell, P., Campbell, S.M., Abeles, M., Clark, P. et al. (1990). The American College of Rheumatology 1990 criteria for the classification of fibromyalgia: Report of the multicenter criteria committee. *Arthritis Rheum.*, **33**: 160–72.

World Health Organization. (1992). *The ICD-10 Classification of Mental and Behavioral Disorders: Clinical Descriptions and Diagnostic Guidelines.* Geneva: World Health Organization.

Wright, S. (1994). Familial obsessive–compulsive disorder presenting as pathological jealousy successfully treated with fluoxetine. (Letter.) *Arch Gen Psychiatry*, **51**: 430–1.

Wyszynski, B., Meriam, A., Medalia, A. and Lawrence, C. (1989). Choreoacanthocytosis: Report of a case with psychiatric features. *Neuropsychiatry Neuropsychol Behav Neurol*, **2**: 137–44.

Yaryura-Tobias, J.A. and Bhagavan, H.N. (1977). L-tryptophan in obsessive–compulsive disorders. *Am J Psychiatry*, **134**: 1298–9.

Yaryura-Tobias, J.A. and Neziroglu, F.A. (1996). Venlafaxine in obsessive compulsive disorder. *Arch Gen Psychiatry*, **53**: 653–4.

Yaryura-Tobias, J.A., Kirschen, H., Ninan, P. and Mosberg, H.J. (1991). Fluoxetine and bleeding in obsessive–compulsive disorder. (Letter.) *Am J Psychiatry*, **148**: 949.

Zajecka, J., Tracy, K.A. and Mitchell, S. (1997). Discontinuation symptoms after treatment with serotonin reuptake inhibitors: Literature review. *J Clin Psychiatry*, **58**: 291–7.

Zajecka, J.M., Fawcett, J. and Guy, C. (1990). Coexisting major depression and obsessive–compulsive disorder treated with venlafaxine. *J Clin Psychopharmacol*, **10**: 152–3.

Zajecka, J.M., Jeffriess, H. and Fawcett, J. (1995). The efficacy of fluoxetine combined with a heterocyclic antidepressant in treatment-resistant depression: A retrospective analysis. *J Clin Psychiatry*, **56**: 338–43.

Zanardi, R., Artigas, F., Franchini, L., Sforzini, L., Gasperini, M., Smeraldi, E. and Perez, J. (1997). How long should pindolol be associated with paroxetine to improve the antidepressant response: *J Clin Psychopharmacol*, **17**: 446–50.

Zilboorg, G. (1967). *A History of Medical Psychology*. New York: W.W. Norton.

Zitzow, D. (1996). Comparative study of problematic gambling behaviors between Americn Indian and non-Indian adults in a Northern Plains reservation. *Am Indian Alsk Native Ment Health Res*, **7**: 27–41.

Zohar, J., Judge, R. and the OCD Paroxetine Study Investigators. (1996). Paroxetine versus clomipramine in the treatment of obsessive–compulsive disorder. *Br J Psychiatry*, **169**: 468–74.

Zohar, J., Kaplan, Z. and Benjamin, J. (1994). Clomipramine treatment of obsessive–compulsive symptomology in schizophrenic patients. *J Clin Psychiatry*, **54**: 385–8.

Index

Note: OCD = obsessive–compulsive disorder

acute intermittent porphyria 129–30
adrenocortical insufficiency 180
advocacy organizations 256–68
affective disorder 179
agoraphobia 21, 26
alcoholism in OCD 40, 51, 53
  advocacy and information 256
  Internet resources 270
  nonparaphilic sexual disorders and 241
  panic disorder and 23
  pathological gambling and 232–3
  pathological jealousy and 180, 181
alopecia 186
  see also trichotillomania
alprazolam
  panic disorder treatment 25
  pharmacokinetics 88
  social phobia treatment 19
  trademark drug names 304
amantadine 180
  trademark drug names 311–12
amitriptyline
  fibromyalgia treatment 166
  kleptomania treatment 224
  major depression treatment 14
  trichotillomania treatment 197
d-amphetamine, attention deficit hyperactivity disorder
    treatment 147–8
anorexia nervosa
  advocacy and information 256
  body dysmorphic disorder and 152
  kleptomania and 222
  OCD and 40, 51–2
antidepressants
  drug interactions 100–2
  pharmacokinetic comparison 86–7
  pregnancy/breast-feeding and 110–11
  see also individual drugs; tricyclic antidepressants
anxiety disorders and OCD 39, 50–1, 53
  advocacy and information 256
  generalized anxiety disorder 39, 50, 169, 241
  Internet resources 270–1
anxiolytics
  pharmacokinetic comparison 88
  pregnancy/breast-feeding and 111
  see also individual drugs
Asperger's syndrome 137

assertiveness training, body dysmorphic disorder and 160
athetoid movements 137
attention deficit hyperactivity disorder (ADHD) 142
  advocacy and information 256
  Internet resources 271
  treatment 146–9
aversive conditioning
  kleptomania treatment 225
  pathological gambling treatment 235
avoidant personality disorder 17, 27–9
  comorbidity 156
  diagnostic criteria 27
  differential diagnosis 152–3
  pharmacotherapy 27–8
  psychotherapy 28–9
awareness training, trichotillomania treatment 196

BDD-YBOCS scale 155, 161
Beck Anxiety Inventory 161
Beck Depression Inventory 161
behavior therapy
  body dysmorphic disorder 160–2
  hypochondriasis 170–2
  kleptomania 224–6
  major depression 17
  nail biting 209–10
  OCD 73–8
  panic disorder 25–6
  pathological gambling 234–6
  social phobia 19–21
  trichotillomania 193–6
  see also cognitive-behavioral therapy
benzodiazepines
  drug interactions 101
  obsessive–compulsive personality disorder treatment
    255
  panic disorder treatment 23–5
  pathological gambling treatment 236–7
  pharmacokinetics 88
  pregnancy/breast-feeding and 111
  serotonin syndrome management 106
  social phobia 19
  see also individual drugs
bipolar mood disorder
  advocacy and information 257
  Internet resources 271
  kleptomania and 221, 223
  OCD and 50, 51
  pathological gambling and 232, 233

body dysmorphic disorder 40, 51, 151–62
  assessment instruments 154–5
  clinical picture 153–4
  comorbidity 155–6
  diagnostic criteria 151–2
  differential diagnosis 152–3
  prevalence 155
  skin picking and 204, 206
  treatment 156 62; cognitive behavioral therapy
    160–2; combining psychotherapy with medication
    160; pharmacotherapy 156–9; treatment planning
    guidelines 162
Body Dysmorphic Disorder Examination 155
book resources for patients 268–9
bowel obsessions, management of 72
brain lock approach 79
brain tumours 125–6
breast-feeding
  antidepressants and 111
  anxiolytics and 111
  mood stabilizing drugs and 111–12
  neuroleptic drugs and 111
  serotonin reuptake inhibitors and 109–10
breathing retraining 26
brofaromine, social phobia treatment 19
bulimia nervosa
  kleptomania and 222, 224
  OCD and 40, 51–2
bupropion
  attention deficit hyperactivity disorder treatment 147
  major depression treatment 15, 16, 157
  pharmacokinetics 87
  side effects 15
buspirone
  augmentation of OCD treatment 62–3
  body dysmorphic disorder treatment 158
  kleptomania treatment 223–4
  major depression treatment 14, 15
  obsessive–compulsive personality disorder treatment
    255
  pharmacokinetics 88
  side effects 19, 63, 85
  social phobia treatment 19, 157
  SSRI sexual side effects treatment 107
  trademark drug names 305
  trichotillomania treatment 197
buying, compulsive *see* compulsive buying

carbamazepine
  pathological gambling treatment 236–7
  pregnancy and 112
  trademark drug names 306
carbon monoxide poisoning and OCD 130–1
case history elements 7–8
cerebrovascular accidents and OCD 127
cetirizine, trademark drug names 312
changing the internal monologue, trichotillomania
  treatment 194
chlorpromazine 106
choreiform movements 137
  Sydenham's chorea 123
chronic fatigue syndrome 166, 167

citalopram
  drug interactions 103
  OCD treatment 56
  panic disorder treatment 23
  pharmacokinetics 86
  side effects 85
  social phobia treatment 19
  trademark drug names 306
clinical assessment of patients 7–9
Clinical Global Impressions scale 297
clomipramine (CMI)
  body dysmorphic disorder treatment 156, 158–9
  breast-feeding and 109–10
  compulsive buying treatment 218
  major depression treatment 14
  nail biting treatment 210–11
  nonparaphilic sexual disorder treatment 246
  OCD treatment 54, 55, 60–2; augmentation of SSRI
    treatment 66–7; comparison studies 57–8;
    intravenous treatment of refractory cases 68–9;
    serotonin hypothesis and 47; with schizophrenia
    117; with Tourette's disorder 149
  panic disorder treatment 25
  pathological gambling treatment 236
  pathological jealousy treatment 183
  plasma levels 14, 66–7
  pregnancy and 108, 109
  side effects 25, 60, 89–91; cardiovascular system
    89–90, 118; digestive system 90; musculoskeletal
    system 90; nervous system 91; respiratory system
    91; sexual side effects 106; urogenital system 91
  skin picking treatment 206
  trichotillomania treatment 196–200
  withdrawal symptoms 113
clonazepam
  augmentation of OCD treatment 62–3
  panic disorder treatment 25
  pharmacokinetics 88
  side effects 19, 63
  social phobia treatment 19, 157
  trademark drug names 304
clonidine
  side effects 144
  Tourette's disorder treatment 143–4, 150; comorbid
    attention deficit hyperactivity disorder 148, 149
  trademark drug names 312
clozapine
  inducing OCD symptoms 115–16
  OCD treatment 69; with comorbid schizophrenia 118
  pregnancy and 111
  schizophrenia and 115–16
  trademark drug names 309
codeine 69
cognitive–behavioral therapy
  avoidant personality disorder 28
  body dysmorphic disorder 157, 160–2
  dependent personality disorder 30
  hypochondriasis 171–3
  major depression 17
  nail biting 210
  nonparaphilic sexual disorders 244
  obsessive–compulsive personality disorder 251–3

cognitive–behavioral therapy (*cont.*)
  OCD 73–5
  panic disorder 25–7
  pathological gambling 234–6
  pathological jealousy 182
  social phobia 19–21
  trichotillomania 193–6
  see also behavior therapy
competing response
  nail biting treatment 210
  trichotillomania treatment 196
compulsions 35–6, 37–9, 41, 119
  differential diagnosis 40, 119–21, 138
  frequency of various compulsive behaviors 42
  see also obsessive–compulsive disorder (OCD);
    schizophrenia
compulsive buying 40, 213–18
  assessment instruments 215–16
  clinical picture 214–15
  comorbidity 216
  diagnosis 213–14; differential diagnosis 215
  prevalence 214
  treatment 216–18; pharmacotherapy 217;
    psychotherapy 217–18; treatment planning
    guidelines 218
Compulsive Buying Scale 216
coping strategies, trichotillomania treatment 194
counselling, pregnancy and 112
couple therapy, nonparaphilic sexual disorders 244–5
covert sensitization
  kleptomania treatment 224–5
  nonparaphilic sexual disorder treatment 244
Creutzfeldt–Jakob disease 128
cultural influences 43
cyproheptadine
  and SSRI sexual side effects 106–7
  trademark drug names 312
cytochrome P450 isoenzymes 98–9, 100–2

dantrolene 106
delusions of parasitosis 159, 166, 203
dementia
  OCD and 40, 128
  pathological jealousy and 179
dependent personality disorder 29–31
  diagnostic criteria 30
L-deprenyl
  attention deficit hyperactivity disorder treatment 148
  trademark drug names 308
depression 39
  see major depression
dermatitis artefacta 203
desipramine
  major depression treatment 13, 14, 16, 157
  nail biting treatment 210–11
  OCD treatment 69–70; comorbid attention deficit
    hyperactivity disorder 147, 148, 149
  pregnancy/breast-feeding and 111
  side effects 147
  trademark drug names 307
  trichotillomania treatment 199
diabetes insipidus and OCD 130

diagnosis, definition of 5
diazepam, trademark drug names 304
disease, definition of 5
disorder, definition of 5
drug abuse
  see substance abuse
Dysfunctional Thought Record and obsessive–compulsive
  personality disorder 251, 252–3
dysmorfophobia 151
  see also body dysmorphic disorder
dysthymia
  hypochondriasis and 169
  obsessive–compulsive personality disorder and 241
  trichotillomania and 187, 197
dystonic movements 137

eating disorders
  see anorexia nervosa; bulimia nervosa
elderly patients, dosing regimes and 59–60
encephalitis lethargica and OCD 121–2
environmental illness 165
epilepsy
  OCD and 121, 124–5
  pathological jealousy and 180
exposure and response prevention (ERP)
  body dysmorphic disorder treatment 161
  bowel obsessions management 72
  compulsive buying treatment 216–18
  hoarding behavior management 73–4
  hypochondriasis treatment 171, 172
  kleptomania treatment 224
  obsessional slowness management 75
  OCD treatment 53, 75–8; acute treatment 76–8;
    enhancing long-term outcome 78

family studies
  OCD 47–8
  Tourette's disorder 141
  trichotillomania 190, 191
fenfluramine, augmentation of OCD treatment 63–4
fibromyalgia 166–7
fluocinolone, trichotillomania treatment 200
fluoxetine
  body dysmorphic disorder treatment 156, 158
  breast-feeding and 109–10
  drug interactions 100, 102, 103
  hypochondriasis treatment 173
  kleptomania and 221, 223, 224
  major depression treatment 11, 12, 14, 15
  nail biting treatment 211
  nonparaphilic sexual disorder treatment 245–6
  OCD treatment 54, 55, 57, 58, 60–1, 66; with
    comorbid Tourette's disorder 149
  panic disorder treatment 23
  pathological jealousy treatment 182–3
  pharmacokinetics 86
  pregnancy and 108–9
  side effects 91–4; cardiovascular system 91; digestive
    system 92; endocrine system 92; hemic and
    lymphatic system 92; nervous system 93–4;
    respiratory system 94; skin and appendages 94;
    urogenital system 94

skin picking treatment 205
social phobia treatment 19
trademark drug names 307
trichotillomania treatment 197, 199
withdrawal symptoms 113, 114
fluphenazine 111
  Tourette's disorder treatment 145
  trademark drug names 309
fluvoxamine
  body dysmorphic disorder treatment 156, 157–8, 159
  compulsive buying treatment 217
  drug interactions 100, 101, 102, 103–4
  irritable bowel syndrome treatment 166
  kleptomania and 221, 223–4
  major depression treatment 14
  obsessive–compulsive personality disorder treatment 254
  OCD treatment 55, 61, 67; with schizophrenia 117–18; with Tourette's disorder 149
  panic disorder treatment 23
  pathological gambling treatment 236
  pharmacokinetics 86
  pregnancy and 109
  side effects 94–5
  skin picking treatment 205
  social phobia treatment 19
  trademark drug names 307
  trichotillomania treatment 198
  withdrawal symptoms 113
forced thinking 124, 125
frontal lobe seizures 125

gabapentin
  augmentation of OCD treatment 64
  trichotillomania treatment 200
gambling, pathological see pathological gambling
gender identity disorder 152
generalized anxiety disorder 39, 50, 169, 241
genetic factors in OCD 47–8
graded exposure
  see exposure and response prevention
Grand Mal seizures 125
Group A β-hemolytic streptococcal (GABHS) infections 122, 123, 135
group psychotherapy
  nonparaphilic sexual disorders 245
  pathological gambling 236
guanfacine, attention deficit hyperactivity treatment 148, 149, 150

habit reversal treatment
  nail biting 210
  skin picking 207
  trichotillomania 193–4
hair pulling see trichotillomania
haloperidol in OCD 58
  pregnancy and 111
  side effects 144
  Tourette's disorder treatment 144; comorbid OCD 149
  trademark drug names 309–10
  trichotillomania treatment 197–9
head injury 126–7

hemiballismic movements 137
hoarding behavior
  compulsive buying and 215
  differential diagnosis 72
  frequency in OCD 41, 42
  management of 73–4
Hopkins Motor–Vocal Tic Scale 140
human immunodeficiency virus (HIV) 122
Huntington's disease and OCD 128, 137
hypergraphia versus compulsion 124–5
hypersexuality 238
  see also nonparaphilic sexual disorders
hyperthyroidism and pathological jealousy 180
hypnotic treatment, trichotillomania 200
hypochondriasis 40, 51, 163–77
  assessment instruments 168–9; Whiteley Index 168, 293–4
  clinical picture 167–8
  comorbidity 169–70
  course 169
  diagnostic criteria 163–4
  differential diagnosis 164–7
  prevalence 169
  treatment 170–7; in primary care 174–7; pharmacotherapy 173–4; psychotherapy 170–3; treatment planning guidelines 174
hypoparathyroidism 129

illness, definition of 5
imaginal desensitization
  kleptomania treatment 225
  nonparaphilic sexual disorder treatment 244
  pathological gambling treatment 234
imaginal flooding 78
imipramine
  drug interactions 100, 101, 102
  hypochondriasis treatment 173
  kleptomania treatment 223
  major depression treatment 14
  panic disorder treatment 23, 25
  side effects 25
  trademark drug names 307
  trichotillomania treatment 197
impulse control disorders 185, 202, 208, 213, 219, 227, 238, 240, 241
  see also individual disorders
informational organizations for patients 256–68
inheritance
  Huntington's disease 128
  neuroacanthocytosis 129
  OCD 47–8
  Sydenham's chorea 123
  Tourette's disorder 141
inositol
  augmentation of OCD treatment 64–5
  side effects 64
intermittent explosive disorder 216
Internet resources 269–74
  Usenet groups 273–4
interpersonal therapy
  body dysmorphic disorder 160
  major depression 17

intravenous clomipramine treatment
  body dysmorphic disorder 159
  OCD 14, 68–9
intrusive music in OCD, management of 74–5
irritable bowel syndrome 166
isocarboxazid, trichotillomania treatment 197

jealousy, pathological *see* pathological jealousy

kleptomania 40, 216, 219–26
  assessment 222
  clinical picture 221
  comorbidity 221–2
  diagnosis 219–20; differential diagnosis 220–1
  treatment 223–6; pharmacotherapy 223–4;
    psychotherapy 224–6; treatment planning guidelines
    226

levodopa 127–8
Liebowitz Social Anxiety Scale 18, 160, 295
lithium
  augmentation of OCD treatment 65
  kleptomania treatment 221, 222, 223
  major depression treatment 12, 15–16
  pregnancy/breast-feeding and 111–12
  side effects 15–16
  trichotillomania treatment 200
lorazepam
  panic disorder treatment 25
  trademark drug names 304–5

major depression 9–17, 50–1
  advocacy and information 257
  comorbidity; body dysmorphic disorder 155, 157;
    compulsive buying 216; hypochondriasis 169;
    nonparaphilic sexual disorders 241; OCD 50–1, 53;
    pathological gambling 232–3; trichotillomania 187,
    190–1
  diagnostic criteria 10
  differential diagnosis 11, 153
  Internet resources 271
  treatment 9–17; pharmacotherapy 12–16, 157;
    psychotherapy 17
malingering 203
manganese poisoning and OCD 131
Massachusetts General Hairpulling Scale 189
meclobemide, social phobia treatment 19
medical conditions associated with OCD 120
  see also individual conditions
melancholia hypochondriaca 163
methylphenidate
  attention deficit hyperactivity disorder treatment
    147–8, 149
  SSRI sexual side effect treatment 107
  trademark drug names 311
mirtazapine 16
  drug interactions 104–5
  for SSRI sexual side effects 108
  pharmacokinetics 87
  side effects 95
  trichotillomania treatment 199
monoamine oxidase inhibitors (MAOIs)
  body dysmorphic disorder treatment 158

depression treatment 12
drug interactions 99–103
OCD treatment 68
panic disorder treatment 23, 25
social phobia treatment 19
see also individual drugs
Montgomery–Åsberg Depression Rating Scale 161, 276–9
moral scrupulosity, management of 72
morphine, OCD treatment 69
MOS 36–item short-form health survey 298–302
motivation enhancement
  nail biting treatment 210
  trichotillomania treatment 194
multiple chemical sensitivity 165
multiple sclerosis 129, 164
muscle dysmorphia 153
myasthenia gravis 164
myoclonic jerks 137

nail biting 208–12
  clinical picture 208–9
  prevalence 208
  treatment 209–12; pharmacotherapy 210–12;
    psychological and behavioral treatments 209–10;
    treatment planning guidelines 212
naloxone 69
naltrexone
  nail biting treatment 211–12
  side effects 211
  skin picking treatment 206–7
  trademark drug names 312
  trichotillomania treatment 199
nefazodone 16
  for SSRI sexual side effects 108
  OCD as a side effect 131
  pharmacokinetics 87
  trademark drug names 307
neurasthenia 36
neuroacanthocytosis 129, 137
neuroleptics
  for refractory OCD 58, 67–8, 69
  pregnancy/breast-feeding and 111
  Tourette's disorder treatment 144–6, 150
  see also individual drugs
neuronal loop hypothesis 46–7
NIMH Trichotillomania Questionnaire 189
nonparaphilic sexual disorders 238–47
  advocacy and information 258
  assessment 242
  comorbidity 240–2, 243
  diagnosis 238–40
  Internet resources 271
  prevalence 240
  treatment 243–7; couple therapy 244–5; group
    psychotherapy 245; pharmacotherapy 245–7;
    psychotherapy 243–5; treatment planning guidelines
    246
nortriptyline
  attention deficit hyperactivity disorder treatment 147,
    149
  drug interactions 100
  kleptomania treatment 223
  major depression treatment 13, 14, 16, 157

pathological gambling treatment 237
pregnancy/breast-feeding and 111
side effects 147
trademark drug names 308

obsessional slowness, management of 75
obsessions
    differential diagnosis 4, 119, 152
    frequency of obsessional themes 41
    frequency in OCD 37–9
    history of the concept 35–6
    in Tourette's patients 141–2
    treatment of 78–80
    see also obsessive–compulsive disorder (OCD);
        schizophrenia
obsessive–compulsive disorder (OCD)
    advocacy and information 257
    assessment instruments 48–9
    associated medical conditions 119–32
    biological models 45–8; autoimmune disease
        (Sydenham's chorea) 122–4; functional
        neuroanatomy 45–7; genetic contributions 47–8;
        serotonin and other neurotransmitters 47
    clinical picture 41–5; age at onset 43–4; course and
        prognosis 44–5; cultural influences 43; morbid
        themes 41, 42; quality of life 45; symptom clusters
        42–3
    comorbidity 50–2; effective on treatment outcome
        53–4, 58, 149–50; obsessive–compulsive personality
        disorder 250; schizophrenia 115–16; Tourette's
        disorder 141–2
    diagnostic criteria 37–9
    differential diagnosis 39–40, 165–6
    history of 35–7
    international advocacy and information 258–62
    Internet resources 271–2
    OCD spectrum concept 3–5
    prevalence 49–50
    prognosis 44–5
    rating scales; see assessment instruments
    treatment 52–80; behavior therapy 73–4, 75–8; bowel
        obsessions 72; cognitive therapy 78–80; comparison
        studies 57–8; dosing regimes 58–60; efficacy studies
        55–7; exposure and response prevention; see
        behavior therapy; hoarding 72–4; inpatient
        treatment and partial hospitalization 71;
        maintenance treatment and discontinuation 61–2;
        neurosurgical interventions 70–1; obsessional
        slowness 75; patients with obsessions only 78–80;
        pharmacological augmentation strategies 62–7;
        pharmacotherapy 54–70; predictors of outcome
        53–4, 58; psychotherapy 75–80; refractory cases
        67–70; scrupulosity 72; special symptom
        management 72–5; treatment planning guidelines
        79
    trichotillomania relationship 191–3
obsessive–compulsive personality disorder (OCPD)
    comorbidity 52, 250
    diagnostic criteria 248–9
    differential diagnosis 40
    prevalence 249–50
    procrastination in 250, 251, 253–4
    treatment 250–5; pharmacotherapy 254–5;

psychotherapy 251–3; treatment planning guidelines
        255
obsessive–compulsive spectrum disorders 3–5
    see also individual disorders
olanzapine 58
    pathological jealousy treatment 183
    pregnancy and 111
olfactory reference syndrome 159, 166
oniomania 213
    see also compulsive buying
onychophagia see nail biting
oxytocin and OCD 130

panic attacks 21
    diagnostic criteria 22
    panic control treatment 26
panic disorder 21–7
    advocacy and information 256
    comorbidity 50, 170, 241
    diagnostic criteria 21, 22
    pharmacotherapy 23–5, 60
    psychotherapy 25–7
parasitosis, delusions of 159, 166, 203
Parkinson's disease 127–8, 180
    post-encephalitic Parkinson's disease 121
paroxetine
    body dysmorphic disorder treatment 156
    drug interactions 100, 105
    OCD treatment 55, 57
    panic disorder treatment 23
    pharmacokinetics 86
    pregnancy and 109
    side effects 96
    social phobia treatment 19
    trademark drug names 308
    withdrawal symptoms 113–14
partial complex seizures 124–5
pathological gambling 227–37
    advocacy and information 257
    assessment instruments 231
    clinical picture 229–31
    comorbidity 216, 232–3
    diagnostic criteria 227–9
    differential diagnosis 229
    Internet resources 272
    pharmacotherapy 236–7
    prevalence 231–2
    treatment 233–7; psychotherapeutic and multimodal
        approaches 234–6; treatment planning guidelines
        237
pathological jealousy 178–84
    clinical picture 180–1
    comorbidity 181
    diagnostic criteria 178–9
    differential diagnosis 179–80
    prevalence 180
    treatment 181–4; pharmacotherapy 182–4;
        psychotherapy 181–2; treatment planning guidelines
        183
pemoline
    attention deficit hyperactivity disorder treatment
        147–8
    side effects 148

pemoline (*cont.*)
  trademark drug names 311
perphenazine 111
  kleptomania treatment 224
personality disorders (PDs)
  comorbidity 156, 191, 192, 203, 241; body dysmorphic
    disorder 156; nonparaphilic sexual disorders 241;
    OCD 52, 54, 58, 250; skin picking 203; tricho-
    tillomania 191, 192
  pathological gambling and 231, 232–3
  treatment 58
  validity of diagnosis 248
  see also avoidant personality disorder; dependent
    personality disorder; obsessive–compulsive
    personality disorder
phenelzine
  avoidant personality disorder treatment 28
  OCD treatment 68
  panic disorder treatment 25
  social phobia treatment 19
  trademark drug names 308
Pick's disease and OCD 128–9
pimozide
  body dysmorphic disorder treatment 158
  OCD and 58
  parasitosis, delusions of, treatment 159
  pathological jealousy treatment 182, 183
  side effects 145
  Tourette's disorder treatment 144–5; comorbid OCD
    149
  trademark drug names 310
  trichotillomania treatment 197, 199
pindolol
  major depression treatment 14–15
  OCD treatment 65–6
  side effects 15
porphyria and OCD 129–30
post-encephalitic Parkinson's disease and OCD 121
post-traumatic stress disorder 39
postponement of obsessions 79
Prader-Willi syndrome and OCD 203
pregnancy
  antidepressant drug use 110–11
  anxiolytic drug use 111
  counselling 112
  mood stabilizing drug use 111–12
  neuroleptic drug use 111
  serotonin reuptake inhibitor use 108–9
procrastination, psychotherapy for 253–4
propranolol
  drug interactions 100, 102
  for tremor treatment 91
  serotonin syndrome and 106
  trademark drug names 312–13
Psychiatric Institute Trichotillomania Scale 189
psychodynamic therapy
  avoidant personality disorder 29
  body dysmorphic disorder 160
  dependent personality disorder 31
  major depression 17
  obsessive–compulsive personality disorder 251
  skin picking 207

rating scales 276–302
relaxation training
  kleptomania treatment 225
  nail biting treatment 210
  trichotillomania treatment 196
religious scrupulosity, management of 72
rheumatic fever 122–3, 135–6
risperidone
  drug interactions 100
  OCD treatment 58, 67–8
  pathological jealousy treatment 183
  pregnancy and 111
  schizophrenia and 116
  side effects 67–8
  Tourette's disorder treatment 145
  trademark drug names 310
  trichotillomania treatment 197, 199

satiation treatment for obsessions 78
schizophrenia
  obsessive–compulsive symptoms 72, 115–18; clinical
    picture 115–16; jealous delusions and 179;
    prevalence 50, 116; treatment 117–18
secondary hypochondriasis 165
seizure disorders and OCD 124–5
  frontal lobe seizures 125
  partial complex seizures 124–5
  tonic-clonic (Grand Mal) seizures 125
selective serotonin reuptake inhibitors (SSRIs) *see*
    serotonin reuptake inhibitors (SRIs)
selegiline
  attention deficit hyperactivity disorder treatment
    148
  trademark drug names 308
self-monitoring
  nail biting treatment 210
  trichotillomania treatment 194
serotonin hypothesis of OCD 47
serotonin reuptake inhibitors (SRIs) 81–114
  body dysmorphic disorder treatment 156–9
  breast-feeding and 109–10
  compulsive buying treatment 217
  drug interactions 98–105; individual drugs 103–5
  hypochondriasis treatment 173
  kleptomania and 221
  major depression treatment 11, 12–16
  nail biting treatment 211–12
  nonparaphilic sexual disorder treatment 243, 245–7
  obsessive–compulsive personality disorder treatment
    254–5
  OCD symptoms in schizophrenia and 117–18
  OCD treatment; augmentation strategies 62–7;
    clomipramine augmentation 66–7; comparison
    studies 57; dosing 58–60; efficacy studies 54, 55–6;
    maintenance treatment and discontinuation 61–2;
    predictors of outcome 53–4, 58; with exposure and
    response prevention 53, 61; with Tourette's disorder
    149
  panic disorder treatment 23–5
  pathological gambling treatment 236–7
  pathological jealousy treatment 182–4
  pharmacokinetic comparison 86

pregnancy and 108–9
side effects 60, 81; general principles of management
    81–2; individual drugs 82–98; serotonin syndrome
    105–6, 114; sexual side effects 106–8
skin picking treatment 205–6
trichotillomania treatment 192
withdrawal symptoms 113–14
see also individual drugs
serotonin syndrome 66, 105–6, 114
sertraline
    body dysmorphic disorder treatment 156
    breast-feeding and 109, 110
    drug interactions 102, 105
    major depression treatment 12, 14
    nonparaphilic sexual disorder treatment 246
    OCD treatment 56, 57, 61
    panic disorder treatment 23
    pathological jealousy treatment 183
    pharmacokinetics 86
    pregnancy and 109
    side effects 96–7
    skin picking treatment 205
    social phobia treatment 19
    trademark drug names 308
    trichotillomania treatment 197
    withdrawal symptoms 114
sexual disorders *see* nonparaphilic sexual disorders
Sexual Outlet Inventory 242
sexual side effects, management of 106–8
Shapiro Tourette Syndrome Severity Scale 139
Sheehan Disability Scale 18, 23, 296
shoplifting *see* kleptomania
side effects *see individual drugs*
skin picking 202–7
    clinical picture 202–3
    comorbidity 204
    diagnosis 202; differential diagnosis 203–4
    prevalence 204
    treatment 205–7; pharmacotherapy 205–7;
        psychotherapy 207; treatment guidelines 207
social costs of OCD 45
social phobia 17–21
    comorbidity 155–6, 157, 241
    diagnostic criteria 18
    differential diagnosis 152–3
    Internet resources 272
    treatment planning 19–21, 157; pharmacotherapy 19,
        20; psychotherapy 19–21
social skills training
    avoidant personality disorder treatment 28
    dependent personality disorder treatment 31
somatization disorder 165, 170
South Oaks Gambling Screen (SOGS) 231
strokes and OCD 127
substance abuse
    advocacy and information 256
    attention deficit hyperactivity disorder and 146
    Internet resources 270
    nonparaphilic sexual disorders and 241
    OCD and 40, 50, 51, 132
    pathological gambling and 232–3
    see also alcoholism

suicide risk
    body dysmorphic disorder 154
    major depression and 11
    pathological gambling and 232–3, 237
sulpiride
    Tourette's disorder treatment 145
    trademark drug names 310–11
Sydenham's chorea
    diagnosis 137
    OCD and 121, 122–4
    Tourette's disorder and 135
sykninesias 137

Taijin-phobia 153
tardive dyskinesia 138
thought stopping for obsessions 78–9
tic disorders
    and OCD treatment outcome 58
    differential diagnosis 137
    distinguished from compulsions 40
    Yale Global Tic Severity Scale 140, 290–2
    see also Tourette's disorder
tonic-clonic (Grand Mal) seizures 125
total allergy syndrome 165
Tourette Syndrome Global Scale 139–40
Tourette's disorder 135–50
    advocacy and information 258
    assessment instruments 139–40
    autoimmunity and 123, 136
    clinical picture 138–9
    comorbidity 52, 141–2
    diagnosis 136–7; differential diagnosis 40, 137–8
    genetics 141
    history of 135–6
    international contacts 262–8
    Internet resources 272–3
    prevalence 140
    prognosis 139
    treatment 142–50; comorbid attention deficit
        hyperactivity disorder 146–9; comorbid OCD
        149–50; pharmacotherapy 143–6; treatment
        planning guidelines 150
Tourette's Syndrome–Clinical Global Impression Scale
    140
transient hypochondriasis 165
tranylcypromine, avoidant personality disorder treatment
    28
trazodone
    kleptomania treatment 223, 224
    OCD treatment 70
    trademark drug names 309
    trichotillomania treatment 197
trichobezoar 188
trichotillomania 52, 185–201
    advocacy and information 258
    assessment instruments 188–9
    clinical picture 187–8
    comorbidity 190–1
    diagnostic criteria 185–6
    differential diagnosis 186–7
    Internet resources 272
    prevalence 189–90

trichotillomania (*cont.*)
  relationship to OCD 191–3
  treatment 193–201; behavior therapy 193–6; hypnotic
    treatments 200; pharmacotherapy 196–200;
    treatment planning guidelines 201
tricyclic antidepressants
  attention deficit hyperactivity disorder treatment
    146–7
  drug interactions 100, 101, 102
  hypochondriasis treatment 173–4
  irritable bowel syndrome treatment 166
  kleptomania treatment 223
  major depression treatment 13–16, 157
  panic disorder treatment 23–5
  pregnancy/breast-feeding and 110–11
  side effects 13–14
  see also individual drugs
trifluoperazine 111
  Tourette's disorder treatment 145
triiodothyronine (T$_3$)
  major depression treatment 16
  side effects 16
tryptophan
  augmentation of OCD treatment 65–6
  trademark drug names 313
twin studies
  OCD 47
  Tourette's disorder 141

Usenet groups 273–4

valproate
  combining with an SSRI 13

kleptomania treatment 222, 223
pregnancy and 112
trademark drug names 306
trichotillomania treatment 200
vasopressin 130
venlafaxine
  comorbid depression treatment 16
  OCD treatment 56–7
  pharmacokinetics 87
  side effects 97–8
  trichotillomania treatment 199
  withdrawal symptoms 114
Von Economo's encephalitis 121–2

Whiteley Index 168, 293–4
withdrawal symptoms, serotonin reuptake inhibitors
  113–14
World Wide Web resources 269–74

Yale Global Tic Severity Scale (YGTSS) 140, 290–2
Yale–Brown Obsessive–Compulsive Scale (Y–BOCS)
  37–9, 48–9, 52, 280–9
  interview questions 286–7
  shopping version (YBOCS-SV) 215–16
  symptom checklist 281–5
  to assess body dysmorphic disorder (BDD–YBOCS)
    155, 161

ziprasidone
  side effects 145–6
  Tourette's disorder treatment 145–6